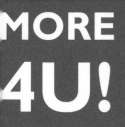

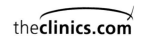

NEUROLOGIC CLINICS

Sleep Disorders

GUEST EDITOR
Robert W. Fayle, MD

November 2005 • Volume 23 • Number 4

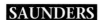

An Imprint of Elsevier, Inc.
PHILADELPHIA   LONDON   TORONTO   MONTREAL   SYDNEY   TOKYO

W.B. SAUNDERS COMPANY
A Division of Elsevier Inc.

1600 John F. Kennedy Blvd., Suite 1800, Philadelphia, PA 19103-2899

http://www.theclinics.com

NEUROLOGIC CLINICS
November 2005
Editor: Donald Mumford

Volume 23, Number 4
ISSN 0733-8619
ISBN 1-4160-2832-3

The ideas and opinions expressed in *Neurologic Clinics* do not necessarily reflect those of the Publisher. The Publisher does not assume any responsibility for any injury and/or damage to persons or property arising out of or related to any use of the material contained in this periodical. The reader is advised to check the appropriate medical literature and the product information currently provided by the manufacturer of each drug to be administered to verify the dosage, the method and duration of administration, or contraindications. It is the responsibility of the treating physician or other health care professional, relying on independent experience and knowledge of the patient, to determine drug dosages and the best treatment for the patient. Mention of any product in this issue should not be construed as endorsement by the contributors, editors, or the Publisher of the product or manufacturers' claims.

Neurologic Clinics (ISSN 0733-8619) is published quarterly by Elsevier. Corporate and editorial offices: 1600 John F. Kennedy Blvd., Suite 1800, Philadelphia, PA 19103-2899. Accounting and circulation offices: 6277 Sea Harbor Drive, Orlando, FL 32887-4800. Periodicals postage paid at Orlando, FL 32862, and additional mailing offices. Subscription prices are $175.00 per year for US individuals, $275.00 per year for US institutions, $88.00 per year for US students, $214.00 per year for Canadian individuals, $325.00 per year for Canadian institutions, and $113.00 per year for Canadian students. To receive student/resident rate, orders must be accompanied by name of affiliated institution, date of term, and the *signature* of program/ residency coordinator on institution letterhead. Orders will be billed at individual rate until proof of status is received. Foreign air speed delivery is included in all *Clinics* subscription prices. All prices are subject to change without notice. POSTMASTER: Send address changes to *Neurologic Clinics*, W.B. Saunders Company, Periodicals Fulfillment, Orlando, FL 32887-4800. **Customer Service: 1-800-654-2452 (US). From outside of the US, call 1-407-345-4000.**

Neurologic Clinics is also published in Spanish by Nueva Editorial Interamericana S.A., Mexico City, Mexico.

Neurologic Clinics is covered in *Current Contents/Clinical Medicine, Index Medicus, EMBASE/*Excerpta Medica, and *PsycINFO,* and *ISI/BIOMED.*

Printed in the United States of America.

GUEST EDITOR

ROBERT W. FAYLE, MD, Medical Director, Sleep Disorders Center at Park Plaza Hospital; Clinical Assistant Professor of Neurology, The University of Texas Medical School at Houston, Houston, Texas

CONTRIBUTORS

CHARLES H. ADLER, MD, PhD, Parkinson's Disease and Movement Disorders Center, Mayo Clinic Scottsdale, Scottsdale, Arizona

PHILIP M. BECKER, MD, President, Sleep Medicine Associates of Texas; Medical Director, Sleep Medicine Institute, Presbyterian Hospital of Dallas; and Clinical Professor, Department of Psychiatry, UT Southwestern Medical Center at Dallas, Dallas, Texas

JED E. BLACK, MD, Director, Stanford Sleep Disorders Center; Assistant Professor, Sleep Medicine Division, Department of Psychiatry and Behavioral Sciences, Stanford University, Stanford, California

STEPHEN N. BROOKS, MD, Assistant Clinical Professor, Sleep Medicine Division, Department of Psychiatry and Behavioral Sciences, Stanford University, Stanford, California

CHIEN LIN CHEN, MD, Tzu Chi University Hospital and Medical School, Huclien, Taiwan

ANTONIO CULEBRAS, MD, Professor, Department of Neurology, Upstate Medical University; and Consultant, The Sleep Center, Community General Hospital, Syracuse, New York

WILLIAM C. DEMENT, MD, PhD, Professor of Psychiatry and Behavioral Sciences, Stanford Sleep Disorders and Research Center, Palo Alto, California

MAX HIRSHKOWITZ, PhD, DABSM, Associate Professor, Department of Psychiatry and Department of Medicine, Baylor College of Medicine; Clinical Director, Houston VAMC Sleep Center; and Clinical Director, Methodist Hospital Sleep Diagnostic Laboratory, Houston, Texas

CONRAD IBER, MD, Professor of Medicine, University of Minnesota; Director, Pulmonary and Critical Care, Hennepin County Medical Center, Minneapolis, Minnesota

LENA LAVIE, PhD, Associate Professor and Head, The Lloyd Rigler Sleep Apnea Research Laboratory, Unit of Anatomy and Cell Biology, The Ruth and Bruce Rappaport Faculty of Medicine, Technion-Israel Institute of Technology, Haifa, Israel

MARK W. MAHOWALD, MD, Minnesota Regional Sleep Disorders Center; Professor, Department of Neurology, Hennepin County Medical Center; and University of Minnesota Medical School, Minneapolis, Minnesota

BETH A. MALOW, MD, MS, Associate Professor of Neurology, Department of Neurology, Vanderbilt University School of Medicine; Medical Director, Vanderbilt Sleep Disorders Center, Nashville, Tennessee

SEIJI NISHINO, MD, PhD, Associate Professor, Sleep Medicine Division, Department of Psychiatry and Behavioral Sciences, Stanford University, Stanford, California

WILLIAM G. ONDO, MD, Associate Professor of Neurology, Baylor College of Medicine, Houston, Texas

WILLIAM C. ORR, PhD, Lynn Health Science Institute, Oklahoma University Health Sciences Center, Oklahoma City, Oklahoma

CARLOS H. SCHENCK, MD, Minnesota Regional Sleep Disorders Center; Associate Professor, Department of Psychiatry, Hennepin County Medical Center; and University of Minnesota Medical School, Minneapolis, Minnesota

AMIR SHARAFKHANEH, MD, DABSM, Assistant Professor, Department of Medicine, Baylor College of Medicine; Medical Director, Houston VAMC Sleep Center; and Medical Director, Methodist Hospital Sleep Diagnostic Laboratory, Houston, Texas

TODD J. SWICK, MD, Assistant Clinical Professor of Neurology, School of Medicine, University of Texas-Houston; and Medical Director, The Houston Sleep Center, Houston, Texas

MICHAEL J. THORPY, MD, Director, Sleep-Wake Disorders Center, Montefiore Medical Center; Associate Professor of Neurology, Albert Einstein College of Medicine, Bronx, New York

CONTENTS

presented. Actuarial data for a first laboratory night are provided. Finally, the mechanisms governing sleep and wakefulness are reviewed and a model of normal sleep mechanisms going awry is outlined as an aid for understanding abnormal sleep associated with sleep disorders.

Sleep and the Gastrointestinal Tract 1007
William C. Orr and Chien Lin Chen

Advances in sleep research have elucidated marked alterations in respiratory functioning during sleep, hormonal functioning during sleep, and health consequences attributable to sleep restriction or deprivation. These discoveries have led to a broadening of the focus and importance of the applications of basic sleep physiology to clinical medicine. Lagging behind these developments is the description of gastrointestinal (GI) functioning during sleep and applications of these changes to clinical medicine, perhaps because of the inaccessibility of the GI tract for study during sleep. As a result of advances in measurement techniques, studies have increased describing alterations in GI functioning during sleep and the applications of these changes to gastroenterology.

Conditions of Primary Excessive Daytime Sleepiness 1025
Jed E. Black, Stephen N. Brooks, and Seiji Nishino

Excessive daytime sleepiness (EDS) or somnolence is common in our patients and in society. The most common cause of EDS is simply insufficient sleep in otherwise healthy individuals. Other common causes include sleep-fragmenting disorders such as the obstructive sleep apnea syndrome. Somewhat less familiar to the clinician are EDS conditions arising from central nervous system dysfunction. Of these primary disorders of somnolence, narcolepsy is the most well known and extensively studied, yet is often misunderstood and misdiagnosed. Idiopathic hypersomnia, the recurrent hypersomnias, and EDS associated with nervous system disorders also must be well understood by clinicians who wish to provide appropriate evaluation and management of patients with EDS. This review summarizes the distinguishing features of the clinical syndromes of primary EDS, provides a brief overview of the pharmacologic management of primary EDS, and highlights the tremendous advances that have occurred in the past few years in our understanding of the pathophysiology of narcolepsy.

Sleep-Related Breathing Disorders 1045
Conrad Iber

Sleep-related breathing disorders are a heterogeneous group of conditions that may be associated with alterations in the structure of sleep, in sleep quality, and in gas exchange during sleep. Obstructive sleep apnea represents the most frequent cause of sleep-related breathing disorders, which encompass a diversity of conditions that either complicate coexisting disease or present as primary disorders. Many of these disorders have consequences during both sleep and wakefulness and may produce substantial burden of symptoms and disease in untreated individuals.

disturbances associated with the primary disorder but also they are made worse by underlying sleep problems associated with aging. Recognition and management of sleep issues require in-depth assessment because of the myriad of possible sleep disorders; assessing and treating them can improve overall health, quality of life, and psychologic well-being.

Nocturnal sleep-related ventilatory alterations may occur in disproportion to the severity of the neuromuscular disorder. Diaphragm paralysis occurring with a neuromuscular disorder is an overlooked complication. Failure to thrive, daytime tiredness, and incapacitating fatigue may be the result of a correctable sleep-related abnormality, not the result of relentless progression of a neuromuscular condition. Polysomnographic evaluation is recommended for patients who have neuromuscular disorder who develop symptoms and signs of sleep-wake abnormality or nocturnal respiratory failure. Application of noninvasive positive airway ventilation and, in some cases, administration of supplemental oxygen may improve quality of life and prolong survival of patients who have neuromuscular disorder.

FORTHCOMING ISSUES

RECENT ISSUES

NEUROLOGIC
CLINICS

Neurol Clin 23 (2005) xi–xii

Preface

Sleep Disorders

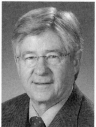

Robert W. Fayle, MD
Guest Editor

Following the excellent two-issue review of sleep disorders edited by Michael Aldrich in the *Neurologic Clinics* in 1996 [1,2], sleep disorder medicine has continued to advance. This issue is aimed at the clinical practice of sleep medicine with the neurologist in mind. Certainly, the neurophysiologic foundations of sleep make clinical sleep medicine a natural step for the neurologist, but sleep and its disorders benefit from the contributions of pulmonary medicine, psychiatry, and clinical psychology as well. Sleep medicine is truly a collaboration of multiple specialties and disciplines, and this collaboration has enriched the study and treatment of a wide variety of clinical problems. This issue of the *Neurologic Clinics* has called on clinicians from a broad background. Several of the authors will be recognized from the original two-issue review of sleep medicine, and there are new contributors with new data and ideas.

Recognition of the frequency [3] of sleep disorders in general, specifically of those discussed herein, suggests that clinicians will see patients with sleep-related complaints and sleep disorders almost daily. Additionally, the impact of the sleep disorders upon public health and modern society is being recognized with increasing clarity [4]. Physicians will be asked to contribute to the solution of these problems and will need to be educated about sleep and sleep disorders. Medical school curricula should be responsive to these needs.

The articles featured in this issue serve as an update, because a broader coverage of sleep medicine was beyond the scope of the issue. However, there are important reviews of particular importance to the neurological

doi:10.1016/j.ncl.2005.08.005

clinician. The neurophysiology of sleep, including new insights in the control of wakefulness and sleep, is clearly discussed. In addition to the article on sleep apnea, there is an article discussing probable endothelial mechanisms by which sleep apnea may account for the increased risk of ischemic cerebrovascular and cardiovascular disease. Primary parasomnias will be of interest, as will the discussions of the interactions of sleep and neurological disorders such as epilepsy, Parkinson's disease, and neuromuscular diseases. Restless legs and periodic limb movements are covered. Neurologists often have difficulty treating the insomnia patient, and a very practical discussion of both pharmacologic and nonpharmacologic treatment of the insomnias is included. The technical aspects of obtaining sleep data and the normative data with which to compare it are also covered. In addition, there is an important review of sleep and gastroenterological disorders often seen by neurologists. Finally, there is an interesting discussion of how we came to be where we are in sleep by one who was integral in getting us to this point. It is hoped that this issue will aid in recognizing and evaluating the patient with sleep disorders as well as guiding treatment or appropriate consultation.

This collection of reviews will be of use to the clinical neurologist who already has an interest in sleep disorders, and hopefully, a stimulus for those who will include it in their practice. Sleep and its disorders are fundamental to the patient; recognition of the importance of sleep and sleep medicine is growing among neurologists and the public. There is increasing need for qualified sleep medicine specialists, many of whom will need to come from the discipline of neurology.

It has been my great pleasure to work with the authors of this issue. They have uniformly contributed their expertise with enthusiasm and patience despite their own busy schedules. Likewise, the editorial staff at Elsevier has done an outstanding job in putting this issue together.

Robert W. Fayle, MD
1213 Hermann Drive, Suite 715
Houston, TX 77004, USA

E-mail address: rwfayle@robertfayle.com

References

[1] Aldrich MS, editor. Sleep disorders I. Neurol Clin 1996;14(3).
[2] Aldrich MS, editor. Sleep disorders II. Neurol Clin 1996;14(4).
[3] Partinen M, Hublin C. Epidemiology of sleep disorders. In: Kryger MH, Dement W, Roth T, editors. The principles and practice of sleep medicine. Philadelphia: WB Saunders; 2005. p. 626–47.
[4] Walsh JK, Dement WC, Dinges DF. Sleep medicine, public policy and public health. In: Kryger MH, Dement W, Roth T, editors. The principles and practice of sleep medicine. Philadelphia: WB Saunders; 2005. p. 648–56.

ELSEVIER
SAUNDERS

NEUROLOGIC
CLINICS

Neurol Clin 23 (2005) 945–965

History of Sleep Medicine

William C. Dement, MD, PhD

Stanford Sleep Disorders and Research Center, 701 Welch Road, Suite 2226,
Palo Alto, CA 94304, USA

Sleeping and dreaming always have been a fundamental part of human existence. Most early writing on these subjects almost entirely was speculation. During the twentieth century, however, scientific observation and experimentation abounded. This article emphasizes the evolution of the key concepts and research findings that characterize sleep research and sleep medicine, crucial discoveries and developments in the formative years of the field, and those principles and practices that have stood the test of time. Early writings are reviewed by others [1].

Sleep as a passive state

Sleep is the intermediate state between wakefulness and death; wakefulness is regarded as the active state of all the animal and intellectual functions and death as that of their total suspension [2].

The foregoing thought is how Robert MacNish, a member of the faculty of physicians and surgeons of Glasgow starts his book, *The Philosophy of Sleep,* published in 1834. This sentence highlights the major watershed in the history of sleep research and sleep medicine—early notions of sleep as a passive process gave way to notions of sleep as an active process. Until the discovery of rapid eye movements (REMs), sleep was regarded universally as an inactive state of the brain, which occurred as the inevitable result of reduced sensory input. Waking up and being awake were considered a reversal of this process, occurring mainly as a result of bombardment of the brain by stimulation from the environment. No clear distinction was seen between sleep and other inactive states, such as coma, stupor, intoxication, hypnosis, anesthesia, and hibernation.

In addition to the reduction of stimulation, a host of less popular assumptions was proposed to account for the onset of sleep, including vascular theories and various versions of a "hypnotoxin" theory, in which

E-mail address: grissom@stanford.edu

neurologic.theclinics.com

fatigue products, toxins, and so forth were accumulated during the day, finally causing sleep, during which they were eliminated gradually [3]. It has been observed since biblical times that alcohol and other compounds, such as opium, induce a sleep-like state and that coffee and caffeine have the power to prevent sleep.

In the 1920s, the University of Chicago physiologist, Nathaniel Kleitman, embarked on his lifelong career as a sleep researcher. He performed a series of sleep deprivation studies and made the simple but brilliant observation that individuals who stayed up all night generally were less impaired and sleepy the next morning than in the middle of their sleepless night. Kleitman argued that this observation was incompatible with the notion of a continual buildup of a hypnotoxin in the brain or blood. In addition, he believed that human beings were approximately as impaired as they could get, that is, very impaired, after approximately 60 hours of wakefulness and that longer periods of sleep deprivation produced little additional change. In the 1939 (first) edition of his landmark monograph, *Sleep and Wakefulness*, Kleitman [4] wrote,

> It is perhaps not sleep that needs to be explained, but wakefulness, and indeed, there may be different kinds of wakefulness at different stages of phylogenetic and ontogenetic development. In spite of opinions that sleep is an actively initiated process, by excitation or inhibition or cortical or subcortical structures, there is not a single fact about sleep that cannot be equally well interpreted as a let down of the waking activity.

The electrical activity of the brain

In 1875, the Scottish physiologis Richard Caton demonstrated electrical rhythms in the brains of animals. It was not until German psychiatrist Hans Berger [5] recorded electrical activity of the human brain, however, beginning in 1928, and demonstrated clear differences in these rhythms when subjects were awake or asleep that a real scientific interest commenced. Berger inferred correctly that the signals he recorded, which he called electroencephalograms, were of brain origin. For the first time, the presence of sleep could be established conclusively without disturbing the sleeper, and, equally important, sleep could be measured continuously and quantitatively without disturbing the sleeper.

Davis and Harvey and their coworkers [6–8] at Harvard University described all the major elements of sleeping brain wave patterns in an important series of articles published in 1937, 1938, and 1939. Blake and colleagues [9,10] at the University of Chicago extended those observations. In the human electroencephalogram (EEG), sleep is characterized by high-amplitude slow waves and spindles, whereas wakefulness is characterized by low-amplitude waves and alpha rhythm. The image of the sleeping brain as completely turned off gave way to the image of the sleeping brain as engaged in slow, synchronized, idling neuronal activity.

The 1930s also saw one series of investigations that seemed to establish conclusively that sleep occurred passively in response to reduction of stimulation and activity. These investigations were performed by Frederic Bremer and reported in 1935 and 1936 [11,12]. Bremer studied brain wave patterns in two cat preparations. One, which Bremer called encéphale isolé, was made by a transection in the lower part of the medulla oblongata. The other, cerveau isolé, was made by transecting the midbrain just behind the origin of the oculomotor nerves. The first preparation permitted the study of cortical electrical rhythms under the influence of olfactory, visual, auditory, vestibular, and musculocutaneous impulses; in the second preparation, the sensory input was narrowed almost entirely to the influence of olfactory and visual impulses.

In the encéphale isolé preparation, the brain continued to present manifestations of wakeful activity alternating with phases of sleep as indicated by the EEG. In the cerveau isolé preparation, however, the EEG assumed a definite deep sleep character and remained in this condition. In addition, the eyeballs immediately turned downward and the pupils became miotic. Bremer concluded that sleep is associated with a functional (reversible) deafferentiation of the cerebral cortex. The cerveau insolé preparation results in a suppression of the incessant influx of nerve impulses, particularly cutaneous and proprioceptive, which are essential for the maintenance of the waking state of the telencephalon. Bremer concluded that olfactory and visual impulses are insufficient to keep the cortex awake.

The ascending reticular system

After World War II, insulated, implantable electrodes were developed, and sleep research in animals began in earnest. In 1949, one of the most important and influential studies dealing with sleep and wakefulness was published. This was Moruzzi and Magoun's classic article, "Brain Stem Reticular Formation and Activation of the EEG." These investigators [13] concluded that

> ... transitions from sleep to wakefulness or from the less extreme states of relaxation and drowsiness to alertness and attention are all characterized by an apparent breaking up of the synchronization of discharge of the elements of the cerebral cortex, and alternation marked in the EEG by the replacements of high voltage, slow waves with low voltage fast activity.

High-frequency electrical stimulation through electrodes implanted in the brainstem reticular formation produces EEG activation and behavioral arousal. Thus, EEG activation, wakefulness, and consciousness are at one end of the continuum; sleep, EEG synchronization, and lack of consciousness are at the other end. This view is hardly different from the statement by MacNish quoted at the beginning of this article.

The demonstration by Starzl and colleagues [14] that sensory collaterals discharge into the reticular formation suggests that a mechanism is present by which sensory stimulation can be transduced into prolonged activation of the brain and sustained wakefulness. By attributing an amplifying and maintaining role to the brainstem core and the conceptual ascending reticular activating system, it was possible to account for the fact that wakefulness can be maintained in the absence of sensory stimulation.

Chronic lesions in the brainstem reticular formation produce immobility and persisting slow waves in the EEG. The usual animal for this research was the cat because excellent stereotaxic coordinates became available [15]. The theory of the reticular activating system was an anatomically based, passive theory of sleep or active theory of wakefulness. The published proceedings of a 1954 symposium, entitled *Brain Mechanisms and Consciousness* [16] (which probably was the first genuine neuroscience bestseller), contains the full flowering of the ascending reticular activating system theory.

Early observations of sleep pathology

Two early observations stand out with regard to sleep research and sleep medicine. The first is the description in 1880 of narcolepsy by Jean Baptiste Edouard Gélineau (1859–1906), who derived the name, narcolepsy, from the Greek words, narkosis (a benumbing) and lepsis (to overtake). He was the first to publish a clear description of the constellation of components that constitute the syndrome, although in 1916 Richard Henneberg coined the term, cataplexy, for the emotionally induced muscle weakness.

The second observation of what might be called the leading sleep disorder of the twentieth century, obstructive sleep apnea (OSA), was made in 1836, not by a clinician but by the novelist Charles Dickens. Dickens published a series, entitled the "Posthumous Papers of the Pickwick Club," in which he described Joe, a loud snorer who was obese and somnolent. The lad also was called Young Dropsy, suggesting he may have had right-sided heart failure. Kryger [17] and Lavie [18] have published scholarly accounts of many early references to snoring and conditions that were most certainly manifestations of sleep apnea syndrome.

Sigmund Freud and the interpretation of dreams

By far the most widespread, although indirect, interest in sleep by health professionals was engendered by the theories of Sigmund Freud. The interest really was in dreaming, with sleep as the necessary concomitant. Freud developed psychoanalysis and the technique of dream interpretation as part of his therapeutic approach to emotional and mental problems. As the ascending reticular activating system concept dominated behavioral neurophysiology, so the psychoanalytic theories about dreams dominated the psychologic side of the coin. Dreams were believed guardians of sleep and to occur in response to a disturbance to avoid waking up, as exemplified in the classic alarm clock dream. Freud's concept that dreaming discharged instinctual energy led directly to the notion of dreaming as a safety valve of the mind. At the time of the discovery of REMs during sleep (in approximately 1952), academic psychiatry was dominated by psychoanalysts, and medical students all over America were interpreting one another's dreams.

From the vantage point of today's world, the dream deprivation studies of the early 1960s, which were engendered and reified by the belief in psychoanalysis, may be regarded by some as a digression from the mainstream of sleep medicine. Alternatively, because the medical-psychiatric establishment had begun to take dreams seriously, it also was ready to support sleep research fairly generously under the guise of dream research.

Chronobiology

Most sleep specialists share the opinion that chronobiology, or the study of biologic rhythms, is a legitimate part of sleep research and sleep medicine. The 24-hour rhythms in the activities of plants and animals have been recognized for centuries. These biologic 24-hour rhythms were reasonably assumed to be a direct consequence of the 24-hour environmental fluctuation of light and darkness. In 1729, however, de Mairan described a heliotrope plant that opened its leaves during the day, even after de Mairan had moved the plant so that sunlight could not reach it. The plant opened its leaves during the day and folded them for the entire night, even though the environment constantly was dark. This first demonstration of circadian rhythms in the absence of environmental time cues is described in the book by Moore-Ede and colleagues, entitled *The Clocks That Time Us* [19].

Factors that appeared to foster a separate development of chronobiology and sleep research in earlier years were

1. The long-term studies commonly used in biologic rhythm research precluded continuous recording of brain wave activity, which was too difficult and not necessary. Thus, the measurement of wheel-running activity was a convenient and widely used method for demonstrating circadian rhythmicity.
2. The favorite animal of sleep research from the 1930s through the 1970s was the cat, and neither cats nor dogs demonstrate readily defined circadian activity rhythms. The separation was maintained further by the tendency for chronobiologists to know little about sleep and for sleep researchers to remain uninformed about such biologic clock mysteries as phase response curves, entrainment, and internal desynchronization.

The discovery of rapid eye movement sleep

The identification of the discrete organismic state known as REM sleep should be distinguished from the discovery that REMs occur during sleep.

The historical threads of the discovery of REMs are as follows: University of Chicago professor, Nathaniel Kleitman, had long been interested in cycles of activity and inactivity in infants and in the possibility that this cycle ensures that infants have a regular, recurring opportunity to respond to their own increasing hunger. He postulated that the times infants awakened to nurse on a self-demand schedule are integral multiples of this basic rest-activity cycle. Kleitman also was interested in eye mobility as a possible measure of "depth" of sleep. The reasoning for this was that eye movements have a much greater neocortical representation than any other observable motor activity. In addition, slow, rolling, or pendular eye movements were described at the onset of sleep and as gradually slowing and disappearing as sleep "deepened" [20]. In 1951, Kleitman assigned the task of observing eye movement to his graduate student, Eugene Aserinsky. Watching the closed eyes of sleeping infants was tedious, and Aserinsky found that it was easier to designate successive 5-minute epochs as "periods of motility" if he observed any movement (including a writhing or twitching of the eyelids) and "periods of no motility" when he observed no movement.

After describing an apparent rhythm in "eye motility," Kleitman and Aserinsky decided to look for a similar phenomenon in adults. Again, watching the eyes of infants during the day was tedious and at night even worse. Casting about, they came upon the technique of electro-oculography (EOG) and decided, correctly, that it was a good way of measuring eye motility continuously and relieving human observers of the tedium of direct observations. Sometime in the course of recording the EOG during sleep, bursts of electrical potential changes were seen that were different from the slow movements at sleep onset.

When they were observing infants, Aserinsky and Kleitman did not differentiate slow and rapid movements. With the EOG, however, the different nature of the slow eye movements at sleep onset and the newly observed bursts of EOG potentials became obvious. Initially, there was concern that these potentials might be electrical artifacts. With their presence in the EOG as signal, however, it was possible to watch subjects' eyes simultaneously, and when this was done, the distinct rapid movements of the eyes beneath the closed lids were easy to see.

The basic sleep cycle was not identified at this time, primarily because the EOG and other physiologic measures, notably the EEG, were not recorded continuously but were sampled only a few minutes of each hour or half hour. The sampling strategy was used to conserve paper (there was no research grant). Also, at the time, there was not a clear reason to record continuously, and sampling made it possible for investigators to nap between sampling episodes.

Aserinsky and Kleitman initiated a small series of awakenings for the purpose of eliciting dream recall either when REMs were present or when REMs were not present. They did not apply sophisticated methods of dream content analysis, but the descriptions of dream content from the two conditions generally were different, which made it possible too conclude that REMs were associated with dreaming. This was, indeed, a breakthrough in sleep research [21,22].

The occurrence of the eye movements was compatible with contemporary theories that dreams occurred when sleep lightened to prevent or delay awakening. In other words, dreaming still could be regarded as the "guardian" of sleep. It no longer could be assumed, however, that dreams were fleeting and evanescent.

All-night sleep recordings and the basic sleep cycle

The seminal Aserinsky and Kleitman article was published in 1953. To understand how little attention it attracted, it should be noted that no publications on the subject appeared from any other laboratory until 1959. In the early 1950s, most previous research on sleep physiology either had generalized a single short period of sleep to all sleep or had relied on intermittent sampling during the night. There was no motivation to obtain continuous records during typical nights of sleep.

To describe and quantify the occurrence of REM periods during the night better, however, Kleitman and I [23] performed continuous recording for a total of 126 nights from 33 subjects and, by means of a simplified categorization of EEG patterns, scored the paper recordings in their entirety. When they examined the data from 126 records, they found that there was a predictable sequence of patterns over the course of the night, which had been overlooked entirely in all previous EEG studies of sleep. This sequence of regular variations since has been observed tens of thousands of times in hundreds of laboratories, and the original description essentially has remained unchanged.

The usual sequence was that after the onset of sleep, the EEG progressed fairly rapidly to stage 4, which persisted for varying amounts of time, generally approximately 30 minutes, and then a lightening took place. Although the progression from wakefulness to stage 4 at the beginning of the cycle almost was invariable through a continuum of change, the lightening usually was abrupt and coincident with a body movement or series of body movements. After the termination of stage 4, there generally was a period of stage 2 or stage 3, which gave way to stage 1 and REMs. When the first eye movement period ended, the EEG progressed through a continuum of change to stage 3 or 4, which persisted for a time and then lightened, often abruptly, with body movement to stage 2, which again gave way to stage 1 and the second REM [23].

Kleitman and I found that this cyclical variation of EEG patterns occurred repeatedly throughout the night at intervals of 90 to 100 minutes from the end of one eye movement period to the next. The regular occurrence of REM periods and dreaming strongly suggested that dreams did not occur in response to chance disturbances of sleep.

At the time of these observations, sleep still was considered to be a single state. Kleitman and I characterized the EEG during the REM periods as "emergent stage 1" as opposed to "descending stage 1" at the onset of sleep. The percentage of the total sleep time occupied by REM sleep was between 20% and 25%, and the periods of REM sleep tended to be shorter in the early cycles of the night. This general picture of all-night sleep has been seen over and over in normal human beings of both genders, in widely different environments and cultures, and, for all intents and purposes, across the life span.

Rapid eye movement sleep in animals

The developing knowledge of the nature of sleep with REMs was in direct opposition to the ascending reticular activating system theory and constituted a paradigmatic crisis. The following observations were crucial:

- Arousal threshold in human beings was much higher during periods of REM with a low-amplitude, relatively fast (stage 1) EEG pattern than during similar "light sleep" at the onset of sleep.
- REMs during sleep were discovered in cats; the concomitant brain wave patterns (low-amplitude, fast) were completely indistinguishable from patterns associated with active wakefulness.
- By discarding the sampling approach and recording continuously, a basic 90-minute cycle of sleep without REMs alternating with sleep containing REMs was discovered. The all-night patterns had regular, lawful, predictable patterns of occurrence. Continuous recordings consistently revealed active EEG patterns during the entire period of sleep within which bursts of REM occurred.
- Observations of motor activity in human beings and animals during REM periods revealed the unique occurrence of an active suppression of spinal motor activity.

Thus, it was clear that sleep consists not of one state but rather of two distinct organismic states as different from one another as each is from wakefulness. It had to be conceded once and for all that sleep was not simply a time of brain inactivity and EEG slowing. By 1960, this fundamental advance in thinking about the nature of sleep was well established; it exists as a fact that has not changed in any way since that time.

The discovery of REMs during sleep in human beings plus the all-night sleep recordings that revealed the regular recurrence of lengthy periods during which REMs occurred and during which the brain wave patterns resembled light sleep prepared the way for the discovery of REM sleep in cats. This was in spite of the extremely powerful bias that an "activated" EEG could not be associated with sleep. In the first study of cats, the problems of maintaining the insulation of implanted electrodes was not yet solved, so an alternative, small pins in the scalp, was used. With this approach, the waking EEG was obscured totally by the electromyogram from the large temporal muscles of the cat. When the cat fell asleep, however, slow waves could be seen, and the transition to REM sleep was observed clearly because muscle potentials were suppressed completely. The cat's REMs and the twitching of the whiskers and paws could be observed directly.

The following note from a more personal account [24] is included to illustrate the power and the danger of scientific dogma.

> It is very difficult today (circa 1990) to understand and appreciate the exceedingly controversial nature of these findings. I wrote them up, but the paper was nearly impossible to publish because it was completely contradictory to the dominant neurophysiological theory of the time. The assertion by me that an activated EEG could be associated with un-ambiguous sleep was considered to be absurd. As it turned out, previous investigators had observed an activated EEG during sleep in cats [25,26], but simply could not believe it and ascribed it to arousing influences that interrupted the animals' sleep. A colleague who was assisting me was sufficiently skeptical that he preferred that I publish the scientific report as sole author. After four or five rejections, to my everlasting gratitude Editor-in-Chief Herbert Jasper accepted the paper without revision for publication in *Electroencephalography and Clinical Neurophysiology* [27].
>
> It is notable, however, that the significance of the absence of muscle potentials during the REM periods in the cats was not fully appreciated. It remained for Michel Jouvet, working in Lyon, France, to insist on the importance on the electromyographic suppression in his early papers [28,29]. Hodes and Dement began to study the "H-Reflex" in human subjects in 1960 and found complete suppression of reflexes during REM sleep [30]. Following this, Octavio Pompeiano and others in Pisa, Italy, worked out the basic mechanisms of REM atonia in the cat [31].

The duality of sleep

Even though the basic non-REM (NREM)-REM sleep cycle was well established, the realization that REM sleep qualitatively was different from the remainder of sleep took several years to evolve. Jouvet [32] and his colleagues performed an elegant series of investigations on the brainstem mechanisms of sleep that forced the inescapable conclusion that sleep consists of two fundamentally different organismic states. Among Jouvet's many early contributions were clarification of the role of pontine brainstem systems as the primary anatomic site for REM sleep mechanisms and the clear demonstration that electromyographic activity and muscle tonus are suppressed completely during REM periods and only during REM periods.

It is an established fact that muscle atonia is a fundamental characteristic of REM sleep and that it is mediated by an active and highly specialized neuronal system. The pioneering microelectrode studies of Evarts [33] in cats and monkeys and observations on cerebral blood flow in the cat by Reivich and Kety [34] provide convincing evidence that the brain during REM sleep is active. Certain areas of the brain appear to be even more active during REM sleep than during wakefulness. The notion of sleep as a passive process was demolished totally, although for many years there was a lingering attitude that NREM sleep essentially was a state of brain inactivity. By 1960, it was possible to define REM sleep as a completely separate organismic state characterized by cerebral activation, active motor inhibition, and, of course, in humans, an association with dreaming. The fundamental duality of sleep was an established fact.

Premonitions of sleep medicine

Sleep research, which emphasized all-night sleep recordings, burgeoned in the 1960s and was the legitimate precursor of sleep medicine and, in particular, its core clinical test, polysomnography. Much of the research at this time emphasized studies of dreaming and REM sleep and had its roots in a psychoanalytic approach to mental illness. After sufficient numbers of all-night sleep recordings of human volunteers had been performed to document the highly characteristic normal sleep architecture, investigators noted a significantly shortened REM latency in association with endogenous depression [35]. This phenomenon has been investigated intensively ever since. Other important precursors of sleep medicine were:

1. Discovery of sleep-onset REM periods (SOREMPs) in patients who had narcolepsy.
2. Interest, primarily in France, in sleep, epilepsy, and abnormal movement.
3. Introduction of benzodiazepines and the use of sleep laboratory studies in evaluating hypnotic efficacy.

Sleep-onset rapid eye movement periods and cataplexy

In 1959, a patient who had narcolepsy came to see Dr. Charles Fisher, who worked at the Mount Sinai Hospital in New York City. Fisher suggested that a sleep recording might be of interest. Within seconds after he fell asleep, the patient was showing dramatic, characteristic REMs and sawtooth waves in the EEG. The first article documenting SOREMPs in a single patient was published in 1960 by Vogel [36]. In a collaborative study between the University of Chicago and the Mount Sinai Hospital, nine patients were studied, and the consistent occurrence of SOREMPs was described in a 1963 article [37]. Subsequent research showed that sleepy patients who did not have cataplexy did not have SOREMPs, and those who had cataplexy always had SOREMPs [38]. Cataplectic attacks were the normal motor inhibitory mechanisms of REM sleep occurring abnormally.

The narcolepsy clinic: a false start

In January 1963, I was eager to continue studying the association between cataplexy and SOREMPs. Not a single narcoleptic patient could be identified, however. Finally, by placing a brief advertisement in the *San Francisco Chronicle*, more than 100 people responded. More than half of the respondents were bona fide narcoleptics who had sleepiness and cataplexy.

The surprising response to the advertisement was a noteworthy event in the development of sleep disorders medicine. With one or two exceptions, none of the narcoleptics ever had been diagnosed correctly. A responsibility for their clinical management had to be assumed as part of their use in research. The late Dr. Stephen Mitchell, who had completed his neurology training and was entering a psychiatry residency at Stanford University, joined me in 1964 to create a narcolepsy clinic. Soon, we were involved in the medical management of more than 100 patients. Mostly, this entailed seeing the patients at regular intervals and adjusting their medication. Nonetheless, the seeds of the modern sleep disorders clinic were sowed because at least one daytime polygraphic sleep recording was done in each patient to look for the presence of SOREMPs, and patients were questioned exhaustively about their sleep. If possible, an all-night sleep recording was performed. Unfortunately, most of the patients were unable to pay their bills, and insurance companies declared that the recordings of narcoleptic patients were experimental. Because it was unable to generate sufficient income, the clinic was discontinued and the patients were referred back to local physicians with instructions about treatment.

Benzodiazepines and hypnotic efficacy studies

Benzodiazepines were introduced in 1960 with the marketing of chlordiazepoxide. This compound offered a significant advance in terms of safety over the use of barbiturates for the purpose of tranquilizing and sedating. It was quickly followed by diazepam and the first benzodiazepine introduced specifically as a hypnotic, flurazepam. Although questionnaire studies had been done on the effects of drugs on sleep, the first use of the sleep laboratory to evaluate the effect of sleeping pills was the 1965 study by Oswald and Priest [39]. An important series of studies establishing the role of the sleep laboratory in the evaluation of hypnotic efficacy was performed by Kales and colleagues at the University of California, Los Angeles [40]. The group also performed studies of patients who had hypothyroidism, asthma, Parkinson's disease, and somnambulism [41–44].

The discovery of sleep apnea

Possibly the most important advance in the history of sleep disorders medicine occurred in Europe. Sleep apnea was discovered simultaneously by two independent groups, Gastaut and colleagues in France [45] and Jung and Kuhlo in Germany [46]. Both groups reported their findings in 1965. These important findings were ignored completely in the United States. What should have been an almost inevitable discovery by either the otolaryngologic surgery community or pulmonary medicine community did not occur because there was no tradition in either specialty for observing breathing carefully during sleep. The well-known and frequently cited study of Burwell and coworkers [47], although impressive in a literary sense in evoking the image of Dickens' somnolent fat boy, Joe, erred badly in evaluating their somnolent obese patients only during waking and attributing the cause of the somnolence to hypercapnea.

The popularity of this article essentially eliminated the possibility that the American pulmonary community would discover sleep apnea. To this day, there is no evidence that hypercapnea causes true hypersomnolence, although high levels of Pco_2 are associated with impaired cerebral function. Nevertheless, the term, pickwickian, became an instant success as a neologism. This popularity may have stimulated the interest in studying pickwickian patients' syndrome by the aforementioned European neurologists.

A small group of Italian neurologists who specialized in clinical neurophysiology and electroencephalography were in the vanguard of clinical sleep research. One of the collaborators in the French discovery of sleep apnea, Carlo Tassinari, joined Italian neurologist Elio Lugaresi in 1970. These clinical investigators, along with Coccagna and a host of others over the years, performed crucial series of clinical sleep investigations that provided a complete description of the sleep apnea syndrome, including the first observations of the occurrence of OSA in nonobese patients, an account of the cardiovascular correlates, and a clear identification of the importance of snoring and hypersomnolence as diagnostic indicators. These studies are recounted in Lugaresi and colleagues' book, *Hypersomnia with Periodic Apneas* [48].

Italian symposia

In 1967, Gastaut and Lugaresi organized an important meeting (proceedings published as *The Abnormalities of Sleep in Man* [49]), which encompassed issues across the full range of abnormal sleep in humans. This meeting took place in Bologna, Italy, and the presentations covered many of today's major topics in the sleep medicine field: insomnia, sleep apnea, narcolepsy, and periodic leg movements during sleep. It was an epic meeting from the point of view of the clinical investigation of sleep; the only major issues not represented were clear concepts of clinical practice models and clear visions of the high population prevalence of sleep disorders. The meeting that surely triggered a serious international interest in sleep apnea syndromes, however, was organized by Lugaresi in 1972 and took place in Rimini, a small resort on the Adriatic coast [50].

The evolution of sleep medicine clinical practice

The practice of sleep medicine evolved in many centers in the 1970s. The development often was a function of the original research interests of the center. The launching of the world's first sleep disorders clinic in 1970 at Stanford University is described in this article as a harbinger of how sleep medicine subsequently evolved throughout the world.

The use of patients complaining of insomnia in hypnotic efficacy studies brought the Stanford group closely into relation with many insomnia patients and demolished the notion that the majority of such patients were psychiatric subjects. One early question was, "How reliable are the descriptions of their sleep by these patients?" The classic all-night sleep recording could yield a great deal of information. A second factor was that throughout the second half of the 1960s, the research activities of the Stanford group continued to require managing patients who had narcolepsy. As the Stanford clinic's reputation for expertise in narcolepsy grew, it found itself receiving referrals for evaluation from physicians all over the United States. Although the identification of sleep apnea as a frequent cause of severe daytime sleepiness had not yet occurred, several patients referred who had the presumptive diagnosis of narcolepsy did not possess narcolepsy's two cardinal signs, SOREMPs and cataplexy. True pickwickians were an infrequent referral at this time.

In January 1972, Christian Guilleminault, a French neurologist and psychiatrist, joined the Stanford group. He had extensive knowledge of the European studies on sleep apnea. Until his arrival, the Stanford group had not used respiratory and cardiac sensors routinely in their all-night clinical sleep studies. Starting in 1972, these measurements became a routine part of the all-night diagnostic test. In 1974, Gerry Holland, a member of the Stanford group, named the all-night test, polysomnography. Publicity about narcolepsy and excessive sleepiness resulted in a flow of referrals of sleepy patients who had the presumptive diagnosis of narcolepsy to the Stanford sleep clinic. During the first year, the goal of the practice was to see at least five to ten new patients per week. To foster financial viability, the group did as much as possible, within ethical limits, to publicize its services. Accordingly, there also was a sprinkling of patient referrals, often self-referred, who had chronic insomnia. The diagnosis of OSA in patients who had profound excessive daytime sleepiness nearly always was completely unambiguous.

During 1972, the search for sleep abnormalities in patients who had sleep-related complaints continued; the intent was to conceptualize the pathophysiologic process as an entity and as the cause of the presenting symptom. With this approach, several phenomena seen during sleep rapidly were linked to the fundamental sleep-related presenting complaints. Toward the end of 1972, the basic concepts and procedures of sleep disorders medicine were established well enough such that it was possible to offer a daylong course through Stanford University's Division of Postgraduate

Medicine. The course was entitled, "The Diagnosis and Treatment of Sleep Disorders." The topics covered were normal sleep architecture; the diagnosis and treatment of insomnia with descriptions of drug-dependent insomnia, pseudoinsomnia, central sleep apnea, and periodic leg movements as diagnostic entities; and the diagnosis and treatment of excessive daytime sleepiness or hypersomnia, with narcolepsy, NREM narcolepsy, and OSA as diagnostic entities.

The disability and cardiovascular complications of severe sleep apnea were alarming. The treatment options at that time, however, were limited to weight loss and chronic tracheostomy. The dramatic results of chronic tracheostomy in ameliorating the symptoms and complications of OSA had been reported by Lugaresi and colleageus [51] in 1970. The notion of using chronic tracheostomy, however, was resisted strongly by the medical community. The first patient who was referred for investigation of his severe somnolence and eventually treated with tracheostomy was a 10-year-old boy. The challenges that were met to secure the proper management of this patient are worthy of a detailed account (Christian Guilleminault, personal communication, 1990).

Case history

Raymond M. was a 10½-year-old boy referred to the Pediatrics Clinic in 1971 for evaluation of unexplained hypertension, which had developed progressively over the preceding 6 months. There was a positive family history of high blood pressure, but never so early in life. Raymond was hospitalized and had determination of renin, angiotensin, and aldosterone; renal function studies, including contrast radiographs; and extensive cardiac evaluation. All results had been normal except that his blood pressure oscillated between 140-170/90-100. It was noticed that he was somnolent during the daytime and Dr. S. suggested that I see him for this "unrelated" symptom.

I reviewed Raymond's history with his mother. Raymond had been abnormally sleepy "all his life." However, during the past 2 to 3 years, his schoolteachers were complaining that he would fall asleep in class and was at times a "behavioral problem"—not paying attention, hyperactive, aggressive. His mother confirmed that he had been a very loud snorer since he was very young, at least since the age of 2 years, perhaps before.

Physical examination revealed an obese boy with a short neck and a very narrow airway. I recommended a sleep evaluation, which was accepted. An esophageal balloon and measurement of end tidal CO_2 was added to the usual array. His esophageal pressure reached 80 to 120 cm H_2O. He had values of 6% end tidal CO_2 at end of apnea, apneic events lasted between 25 and 65 seconds, and the apnea index was 55. His Sao_2 was frequently below 60%.

I called the pediatric resident and informed him that the sleep problem was serious. I also suggested that the sleep problem might be the cause of the alarming and unexplained hypertension. The resident could not make sense of my information and passed it on to the attending physician. I was finally asked to present my findings at the pediatric case conference, which was led by Dr. S. I came with the recordings, showed the results, and explained why I believed that there was a relationship between the hypertension and the sleep problem. There were a lot of questions. They simply could not believe it. I was asked what treatment I would recommend and I suggested a tracheostomy. I was asked how many patients had this treatment in the United States, and how many children had ever been treated with tracheostomy. When I had to answer "zero" to both questions, the audience was somewhat shocked. It was decided that such an approach was doubtful at best, and completely unacceptable in a child. However, they did concede that if no improvement was achieved by medical management, Raymond would be reinvestigated including sleep studies.

This was spring 1972. In the fall he was, if anything, worse in spite of vigorous medical treatment. At the end of 1972, Raymond finally had his tracheostomy. His blood pressure went down to 90/60 within 10 days, and he was no longer sleepy. During the 5 years we were able to follow Raymond he remained normotensive and alert, but I had to fight continuously to prevent outside doctors from closing his tracheostomy. I don't know what happened to him since.

In addition to medical skepticism, a major obstacle in the practice of sleep disorders medicine was the retroactive denial of payment by insurance companies. A 3-year period of educational efforts directed toward third-party carriers by the Stanford group finally culminated in the recognition of polysomnography as a reimbursable diagnostic test in 1975. Another issue was obtaining specific state licensure of an outpatient clinic that offered overnight testing to avoid the licensing requirements of a hospital. This, too, finally was accomplished in 1975.

Clinical significance of excessive daytime sleepiness

Guilleminault, in a series of studies, recognized excessive daytime sleepiness as one of the major presenting complaints and as a pathologic phenomenon unto itself [52]. It was recognized, however, that methods to quantify excessive daytime sleepiness in terms of improvement with treatment were not adequate. The 7-point Stanford Sleepiness Scale developed by Hoddes and colleagues [53] was a first attempt at quantification but did not give reliable results. The problem was not a crisis because patients who had severe apnea and overwhelming daytime sleepiness were improved dramatically by tracheostomy, and the reduction in daytime sleepiness was completely unambiguous. Nevertheless, documenting the objective improvement of sleepiness with pharmacologic treatment of narcolepsy and with tracheostomy in less severe sleep apnea patients continued to be a problem.

An early attempt to develop an objective measure of sleepiness was that of Yoss and coworkers [54]. They observed pupil diameter directly by video monitoring and described changes associated with sleep deprivation and narcolepsy. Subsequently designated pupillometry, this cumbersome technique has not been accepted widely.

Mary Carskadon deserves most of the credit for the development of the latter-day standard approach to the quantification of sleepiness, the Multiple Sleep Latency Test (MSLT). She noted that subjective ratings of sleepiness made before a sleep recording predicted sleep latency not infrequently. In spring 1976, she undertook to establish sleep latency as an objective measurement of the state of sleepiness alertness by measuring sleep tendency every 2 hours before, during, and after 2 days of total sleep deprivation [55]. The choices of a 20-minute duration of a single test and a 2-hour interval between tests essentially were arbitrary and dictated by the practical demands of that study. The protocol designed for this study has stood the test of time and remains the standard protocol for the MSLT. This new test formally was applied to the evaluation of sleepiness in patients who had narcolepsy [56] and later in patients who had OSA [57].

Carskadon and colleagues then undertook a monumental study of sleepiness by following children longitudinally across the second decade of life, which also is the decade of highest risk for the development of narcolepsy. Using the new MSLT measure, she found that 10-year-old children were completely alert in the daytime. By the time they reached sexual maturity, however, they were no longer fully alert with the same amount of sleep they had obtained when they were 10 years of age. Results of this remarkable decade of work and other studies are summarized in an important review [58].

The important conceptual advances that early MSLT research established were:

1. Daytime sleepiness and nighttime sleep are an interactive continuum, and the adequacy of nighttime sleep absolutely cannot be understood without a complementary measurement of the level of daytime sleepiness.
2. Excessive sleepiness, also known as impaired alertness, arguably is sleep medicine's most important symptom.

Recent history

As the decade of the 1970s drew to a close, the consolidation and formalization of the practice of sleep disorders medicine largely was completed. The Association of Sleep Disorders Centers (now the American Academy of Sleep Medicine) was founded and provided a home for professionals interested in sleep and particularly those who had begun to diagnose and treat sleep disorders. The Association was started in 1975 with five member centers. It was responsible for the launching of the scientific journal, *Sleep,* in 1978, and it fostered the setting of standards through center accreditation and an examination for practitioners, by which they were designated Accredited Clinical Polysomnographers.

The first international symposium on narcolepsy took place in the French Languedoc in summer 1975 immediately after the Second International Congress of the Association for the Psychophysiological Study of Sleep in Edinburgh. The former meeting, in addition to being scientifically productive, had landmark significance because it produced the first consensus definition of a specific sleep disorder, drafted, revised, and unanimously endorsed by 65 narcoleptologists of international reputation [59]. The first sleep disorders patient volunteer organization, the American Narcolepsy Association, also was formed in 1975. The *ASDC/APSS Diagnostic Classification of Sleep and Arousal Disorders* was published in fall 1979 after 3 years of extraordinary effort by a small group of dedicated individuals who composed the nosology committee, chaired by Roffwarg [60].

Before the 1980s, the only effective treatment for severe OSA was chronic tracheostomy. This highly effective but personally undesirable approach was replaced in 1981 by two new procedures—one surgical [61], the other mechanical [62]. The surgical approach was uvulopalatopharyngoplasty, which is giving way to more complex and effective approaches. The second was the now widely used and highly effective continuous positive nasal airway pressure technique, introduced by Australian pulmonologist Colin Sullivan. The combination of the high prevalence of OSA and the availability of effective treatments fueled a rapid increase in the number of centers and physicians practicing the diagnosis and treatment of sleep disorders. The decade of the 1980s was capped by the publication of the field's first textbook, *Principles and Practice of Sleep Medicine* [63].

The decade of the 1990s saw acceleration in the acceptance of sleep medicine throughout the world [64]. In the United States, the National Center on Sleep Disorders Research (NCSDR) was established by statute as part of the National Heart, Lung, and Blood Institute of the National Institutes of Health [65,66]. The mandate of NCSDR is to support research, promote educational activities, and coordinate sleep-related activities throughout various branches of the government. This initiative led to the development of large research projects dealing with various aspects of sleep disorders and the establishment of awards to develop educational materials at all levels of training.

The 1990s also saw the establishment of the National Sleep Foundation [67] (NSF) and other organizations for patients [68]. The NSF points out to society at large the dangers of sleepiness, and this effort is highlighted during the NSF's annual National Sleep Awareness Week. As the internet increases in size exponentially, so do its sleep resources for physicians, patients, and the public at large [69]. There currently are many Web sites devoted to sleep and its disorders.

The challenge of the future

The greatest challenge for the future is the cost-effective expansion of sleep medicine so that its benefits will be available readily throughout society. A major problem is the current failure of sleep research and sleep medicine to penetrate the mainstream educational system effectively at any level. As a consequence, the majority of human beings remain unaware of important facts of sleep and wakefulness, the fundamentals of biologic rhythms, and knowledge about sleep disorders, in particular the symptoms that suggest a serious pathologic process. The management of sleep deprivation and its serious consequences in the workplace, particularly in those industries that maintain sustained operations, is only beginning to be addressed comprehensively.

Finally, the education and training of health professionals to be sleep specialists has far to go to reach adequate numbers. Sleep medicine is fully established as a clinical scientific discipline, however. It has made a concern for the health of human beings a 24-hour enterprise and has energized a new effort to reveal the secrets of the healthy and unhealthy sleeping brain.

References

[1] Thorpy M. History of sleep and man. In: Thorpy M, Yager J, editors. The encyclopedia of sleep and sleep disorders. New York: Facts on File; 1991.

[2] MacNish R. The philoophy of sleep. New York: Appleton; 1834.

[3] Legendre R, Pieron H. The problem of the aspects of sleep. Results of vascular and intracerebral injections of insomniac liquids. C R Soc Biol 1910;68:1077–9.

[4] Kleitman N. Sleep and wakefulness. Chicago: University of Chicago Press; 1939.

[5] Berger H. On the electroencephalogram of man. J Psychol Neurol 1930;40:160–79.

[6] Davis H, Davis PA, Loomis AL, et al. Changes in human brain potentials during the onset of sleep. Science 1937;86:448–50.

[7] Davis H, Davis PA, Loomis AL, et al. Human brain potentials during the onset of sleep. J Neurophysiol 1938;1:24–38.

[8] Harvey EN, Loomis AL, Hobart GA. Cerebral states during sleep as studied by human brain potentials. Science 1937;85:443–4.

[9] Blake H, Gerard RW. Brain potentials during sleep. Am J Physiol 1937;119:692–703.

[10] Blake H, Gerard RW, Kleitman N. Factors influencing brain potentials during sleep. J Neurophysiol 1939;2:48–60.

[11] Bremer F. "Isolated" brain and the physiology of sleep. C R Soc Biol 1935;118:1235–41.

[12] Bremer F. Cerveau. New research on the mechanism of sleep. C R Soc Biol 1936;122:460–4.

[13] Moruzzi G, Magoun H. Brain stem reticular formation and activation of the EEG. Electroencephalogr Clin Neurophysiol 1949;1:455–73.

[14] Starzl TE, Taylor CW, Magoun HW. Collateral afferent excitation of reticular formation of brain stem. J Neurophysiol 1951;14:479.

[15] Jasper H, Ajmone-Marsan C. A stereotaxic atlas of the diencephalon of the cat. Ottawa (Ontario, Canada): National Research Council of Canada; 1954.

[16] Magoun HW. The ascending reticular system and wakefulness. In: Adrian ED, Bremer F, Jasper HH, editors. Brain mechanisms and consciousness. A symposium organized by The

Council for International Organizations of Medical Sciences. Springfield (IL): Charles C Thomas; 1954.

[17] Kryger MH. Sleep apnea: from the needles of Dionysius to continous positive airway pressure. Arch Intern Med 1983;143:2301–8.

[18] Lavie P. Nothing new under the moon. Historical accounts of sleep apnea syndrome. Arch Intern Med 1986;144:2025–8.

[19] Moore-Ede M, Sulzman F, Fuller C. The clocks that time us: physiology of the circadian timing system. Cambridge (MA): Harvard University Press; 1982.

[20] de Toni G. The pendular movement of the eyeballs in babies during physiological sleep and in any morbid state. Pediatria 1933;41:489–98.

[21] Aserinsky E, Kleitman N. Regularly occurring periods of eye motility, and concomitant phenomena, during sleep. Science 1953;118:273–4.

[22] Aserinsky E, Kleitman N. Two types of ocular motility occurring in sleep. J Appl Physiol 1955;8:11–8.

[23] Dement W, Kleitman N. Cyclic variations in EEG during sleeping. Electroencephalogr Clin Neurophysiol 1957;9:673–90.

[24] Dement W. A personal history of sleep disorders medicine. J Clin Neurophysiol 1990;1: 17–47.

[25] Derbyshire AJ, Rempel B, Forbes A, et al. The effects of anesthetics on action potentials in the cerebral cortex of the cat. Am J Physiol 1936;116:577–96.

[26] Hess R, Koella WP, Akert K. Cortical and subcortical recordings in natural and artificially induced sleep in cats. Electroencephalogr Clin Neurophysiol 1953;5:75–90.

[27] Dement W. The occurrence of low voltage, fast electroencephalogram patterns during behavioral sleep in the cat. Electroencephalogr Clin Neurophysiol 1958;10:291–6.

[28] Jouvet M, Michel F, Courjon J. Sur un stade d'activité électrique cérébrale rapide au cours du sommeil physiologie. C R Soc Biol 1959;153:1024–8.

[29] Jouvet M, Mounier D. Effects of lesions in the pontine reticular formation on the sleep of the cat. C R Soc Biol 1960;154:2301–5.

[30] Hodes R, Dement W. Depression of electrically induced reflexes ("H-reflexes") in man during low voltage EEG "sleep." Electroencephalogr Clin Neurophysiol 1964;17:617–29.

[31] Pompeiano O. Mechanisms responsible for spinal inhibition during desynchronized sleep: experimental study. In: Guilleminault C, Dement WC, Passouant P, editors. Advances in sleep research, vol. 3. Narcolepsy. New York: Spectrum; 1976. p. 411–49.

[32] Jouvet M. Research on the nervral structures and the mechanisms responsible for different phases of physiological sleep. Arch Ital Biol 1962;100:125–206.

[33] Evarts E. Effects of sleep and waking on spontaneous and evoked discharge of single units in visual cortex. Fed Proc 1960;4(Suppl):828–37.

[34] Reivich M, Kety S. Blood flow metabolism couple in brain. In: Plum F, editor. Brain dysfunction in metabolic disorders. New York: Raven Press; 1968. p. 125–40.

[35] Kupfer D, Foster F. Interval between onset of sleep and rapid eye movement sleep as an indicator of depression. Lancet 1972;2:684–6.

[36] Vogel G. Studies in psychophysiology of dreams, III: the dream of narcolepsy. Arch Gen Psychiatry 1960;3:421–8.

[37] Rechtschaffen A, Wolpert E, Dement W, et al. Nocturnal sleep of narcoleptics. Electro-encephalogr Clin Neurophysiol 1963;15:599–609.

[38] Dement W, Rechtschaffen A, Gulevich G. The nature of the narcoleptic sleep attack. Neurology 1966;16:18–33.

[39] Oswald I, Priest R. Five weeks to escape the sleeping pill habit. BMJ 1965;2:1093–5.

[40] Kales A, Malmstrom EJ, Scharf MB, et al. Psychophysiological and biochemical changes following use and withdrawal of hypnotics. In: Kales A, editor. Sleep: physiology and pathology. Philadelphia: JB Lippincott; 1969. p. 331–43.

[41] Kales A, Beall GN, Bajor GF, et al. Sleep studies in asthmatic adults: relationship of attacks to sleep stage and time of night. J Allergy 1968;41:164–73.

[42] Kales A, Heuser G, Jacobson A, et al. All night sleep studies in hypothyroid patients, before and after treatment. J Clin Endocrinol Metab 1967;27:1593–9.

[43] Kales A, Ansel RD, Marham CH, et al. Sleep in patients with Parkinson's disease and normal subjects prior to and following levodopa administration. Clin Pharmacol Ther 1971; 12:397–406.

[44] Kales A, Jacobson A, Paulson NJ, et al. Somnambulism: psycho-physiological correlates, I: all-night EEG studies. Arch Gen Psychiatry 1966;14:586–94.

[45] Gastaut H, Tassinari C, Duron B. Etude polygraphique des manifestations épisodiques (hypniques et respiratoires) du syndrome de Pickwick. Rev Neurol 1965;112:568–79.

[46] Jung R, Kuhlo W. Neurophysiological studies of abnormal night sleep and the pickwickian syndrome. Prog Brain Res 1965;18:140–59.

[47] Burwell CS, Robin ED, Whaley RD, et al. Extreme obesity associated with alveolar hypoventilation: a pickwickian syndrome. Am J Med 1956;21:811–8.

[48] Lugaresi E, Coccagna G, Mantovani M. Hypersomnia with periodic apneas. New York: Spectrum; 1978.

[49] Gastaut H, Lugaresi E, Berti-Ceroni G, et al, editors. The abnormalities of sleep in man. Bologna (Italy): Aulo Gaggi Editore; 1968.

[50] Lugaresi E. Organizer symposium: hypersomnia with periodic breathing. Rimini, Italy, May 25–27. Bull Physiopath Resp 1972;8:967–1292.

[51] Lugaresi E, Coccagna G, Mantovani M, et al. The effects of tracheotomy in hypersomnias with periodic breathing. Rev Neurol 1970;123:267–8.

[52] Guilleminault C, Dement W. 235 cases of excessive daytime sleepiness. Diagnosis and tentative classificiation. J Neurol Sci 1977;31:13–27.

[53] Hoddes E, Zarcone V, Smythe H, et al. Quantification of sleepiness: a new approach. Psychophysiology 1973;10:431–6.

[54] Yoss R, Moyer N, Hollenhorst R. Pupil size and spontaneous pupillary waves associated with alertness, drowsiness, and sleep. Neurology 1970;20:545–54.

[55] Carskadon M, Dement W. Effects of total sleep loss on sleep tendency. Percept Mot Skills 1979;48:495–506.

[56] Richardson G, Carskadon M, Flagg W, et al. Excessive daytime sleepiness in man: multiple sleep latency measurements in narcoleptic and control subjects. Electroencephalogr Clin Neurophysiol 1978;45:621–7.

[57] Dement W, Carskadon M, Richardson G. Excessive daytime sleepiness in the sleep apnea syndromes. In: Guilleminault C, Dement W, editors. Sleep apnea syndromes. New York: Alan R. Liss; 1978.

[58] Carskadon M, Dement W. Daytime sleepiness: qualification of a behavioral state. Neurosci Biobehav Rev 1987;11:307–17.

[59] Guilleminault C, Dement W, Passouant P, editors. Narcolepsy. New York: Spectrum; 1976.

[60] Sleep Disorders Classification Committee. Diagnostic classification of sleep and arousal disorders. 1979 first edition. Association of Sleep Disorders Centers and the Association for the Psychophysiological Study of Sleep. Sleep 1979;2:1–137.

[61] Fujita S, Conway W, Zorick F, et al. Surgical correction of anatomic abnormalities in obstructive sleep apnea syndrome: uvulopalatopharyngoplasty. Otolaryngol Head Neck Surg 1981;89:923–34.

[62] Sullivan CE, Issa FG, Berthon-Jones M, et al. Reversal of obstructive sleep apnea by continuous positive airway pressure applied through the nares. Lancet 1981;1:862–5.

[63] Kryger M, Roth T, Dement WC. Principles and practice of sleep medicine. Philadelphia: WB Saunders; 1989.

[64] University of California, Los Angeles. The world's sleep researchers. Available at http://bisleep.medsch.ucla.edu. Accessed March 4, 2001.

[65] Lefant C, Kiley JP. Sleep research: celebration and opportunity. Sleep 1988;21:665–9.

[66] National Heart, Lung, and Blood Institute. Sleep disorders information. Available at: http://www.nhlbi.gov/about/ncsdr/index.htm. Accessed January 18, 2000.

[67] National Sleep Foundation. Available at: http://www.sleepfoundation.org. Accessed January 18, 2005.

[68] Sleep Support Organizations. Available at: http://bisleep./medsch.ucla.edu/hydocs/support.html. Accessed January 18, 2005.

[69] Sleep Home Pages. Available at: http://bisleep.medsch.ucla.edu. Accessed January 2005.

The Neurology of Sleep

Todd J. Swick, MD[a,b,*]

[a]School of Medicine, University of Texas-Houston, Houston, TX, USA
[b]The Houston Sleep Center, Houston, TX, USA

Neurology, by virtue of its study of the brain, is the primary medical science for the elucidation of the anatomy, physiology, pathology, and, ultimately, the function of sleep.

Historical context

The Greco-Roman concepts of sleep were based on their belief that there were gods and goddesses that controlled the minor and major events of their lives. They identified the goddess of night (Nyx) who had two sons: Hypnos (the god of sleep) and his brother, Thanantos (the god of death). Hypnos sprinkled drops of poppy milk into people's eyes so that the opium would make them fall asleep and then fanned sleeping persons with his wings to enable them to sleep in comfort. As late as the beginning of the Common Era, Ovid wrote that Hypnos lived with his "thousand children," the Dreams, in a cave in the Caucasus. The river of Lethe (the river of forgetfulness) was believed to run through this cave [1].

In ancient Greece, if citizens were unable to sleep because of their problems, they visited one of the many sanitariums dedicated to Asclepios (the Greek god of medicine), where the afflicted spent 3 weeks in rest, thought, and meditation, soothed by gentle music, and then, having their balance restored, would be able to sleep again (obviously predating the concept of managed care) [2].

From the time of the Middle Ages until the Renaissance, there were discrete changes in the concept of sleep. More concrete explanations of sleep were enunciated by Lucretius, the Epicurean poet and philosopher, when he described "sleep as the absence of wakefulness" [3]. This was the prevailing view through the centuries. As medical science advanced with the discovery

---

* University of Texas-Houston, 7500 San Felipe, Suite 525, Houston, TX 77063.
E-mail address: tswick@houstonsleepcenter.com

0733-8619/05/$ - see front matter © 2005 Elsevier Inc. All rights reserved.
doi:10.1016/j.ncl.2005.05.006

of the circulatory system and as the young field of neurology was explored, there was renewed interest in the science of sleep and wakefulness.

In 1866, the Surgeon General of the United States, William A. Hammond, wrote a treatise, "On Wakefulness: With an Introductory Chapter on the Physiology of Sleep," arguing against the prevailing opinion of his day that sleep began as a consequence of "congestion of the cerebral vessels." He pointed out several observations that were quoted in contemporary textbooks of medical physiology of his time: (1) stupor never occurs in healthy individuals, whereas sleep is a necessity of life; (2) it is easy to awaken a person from sleep, whereas it often is impossible to arouse him from stupor; (3) in sleep the mind is active and in stupor it is as if it were dead; and (4) congestion of cerebral vessels causes stupor, not sleep. He quotes another nineteenth-century physician, Dr. Arthur Durham: "During sleep, the brain is in a comparatively bloodless condition and the blood in the encephalic vessels is not only diminished in quantity but moves with diminished rapidity. Whatever increases the activity of the cerebral circulation tends to preserve wakefulness and whatever decreases the activity of the cerebral circulation and, at the same time, is not inconsistent with the general health of the body tends to induce and favor sleep" [4].

Although still surrounded by myth and less than perfect science, the concept of the neural control of sleep was established. From 1916 through 1928, the world was ravaged by an epidemic of influenza with tens of thousands of deaths, the victims sustaining many neurologic signs and symptoms. During the acute phase of the illness, some patients exhibited severe insomnia and many more exhibited severe hypersomnia, whereas many survivors exhibited signs of Parkinsonism.

In 1917, von Economo published his first paper on encephalitis lethargica and on December 3, 1929, he read a paper before the College of Physicians and Surgeons of Columbia University in New York City entitled, "Sleep as a Problem of Localization." He stated that patients who had insomnia had lesions in the anterior portion of their hypothalamus and that patients who had hypersomnia had lesions in the posterior aspect of the hypothalamus. He designated this area of the "interbrain" as the "center for regulation of sleep." Thus, the prevailing concept espoused by such luminaries as Lhermitte and Dejerine that "sleep cannot be localized" was put to rest [5,6].

In 1928, Berger demonstrated that the brain produced clearly identifiable electrical activity that could be recorded using surface electrodes and that there existed a different pattern of electrical activity of the brain during consciousness compared with sleep [6,7].

In 1935, Bremer reported on the effects of transection of the brainstem of cats at the pontine-midbrain level (cerveau isolé) versus transection at the medullary-spinal cord level (encéphale isolé). He found that the cerveau isolé animals maintained a continuous sleep-like state with synchronous slow wave activity, whereas the encéphale isolé cats looked awake and their electroencephalograms (EEGs) contained synchronous and desynchronized activity resembling sleep-wake cycling. Bremer went on to hypothesize that sleep was a passive process and that wakefulness required a high level of continuous sensory input from the periphery to maintain activity within the cerebral hemispheres [8].

Bremer's work rekindled research concerning the observations of y Cajal and Papez. In 1909 y Cajal described an extensive network of neurons that ascended and descended through the brainstem. This was refined further by observations of Papez who in 1926 published a more complete description of the reticular formation and its caudal projections down into the spinal cord in cats [9,10].

In 1942, Morison and Dempsey published a series of articles that described a diffuse "nonspecific" thalamocortical recruiting system. They differentiated this "nonspecific" system from the primary sensory input (ie, "specific" system [described by Lorente de No in 1938], acting through direct thalamic relays) [11,12].

In 1949, Moruzzi and Magoun identified the ascending reticular activating system "whose direct stimulation activates or desynchronizes the EEG, replacing high-voltage slow waves with low-voltage fast activity." They went on to state, "the effect is exerted generally upon the cortex and is mediated, in part, at least, by the diffuse thalamic projection system" [13].

By the middle of the twentieth century it was established that sleep and wakefulness were different states that are controlled by the brain and that sleep was not a passive period of time devoid of activity. Jouvet and colleagues described more precise localizations of the neural loci of sleep and its constituents where results of lesion studies demonstrated that the brainstem contains the site of rapid eye movement (REM) sleep neural activity. Transections of a cat brain at a level just above the midbrain-pons junction preserved the appearance of REM-sleep activity, whereas transections in the pons abolished the appearance of REM sleep [14–16].

With the discoveries of REM and non-REM (NREM) sleep by Aserinsky and Kleitman and REM/NREM cycling by Dement and Kleitman, the door finally was opened for researchers to gain more exact insights into the study of the science of sleep and wakefulness [17–19].

Sleep and wake states

People exist in one of three behavioral states during normal functioning: (1) wakefulness; (2) NREM sleep; and (3) REM sleep (Fig. 1). These states are characterized by specific changes in EEG, eye movements, and muscle activity. Wakefulness is characterized by well-recognized patterns on surface EEG recording. Alpha activity (8–12 Hz waves of <50 μV amplitude) occurs when individuals are resting with their eyes closed. The rhythms are most evident in the parieto-occipital areas of the head. Alpha rhythm is attenuated or blocked by attention, especially visual (eye-opening) and

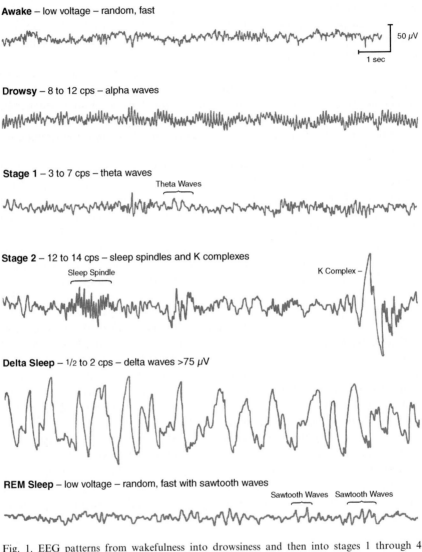

Awake – low voltage – random, fast

50 μV

1 sec

Drowsy – 8 to 12 cps – alpha waves

Stage 1 – 3 to 7 cps – theta waves

Theta Waves

Stage 2 – 12 to 14 cps – sleep spindles and K complexes

Sleep Spindle

K Complex –

Delta Sleep – 1/2 to 2 cps – delta waves >75 μV

REM Sleep – low voltage – random, fast with sawtooth waves

Sawtooth Waves   Sawtooth Waves

Fig. 1. EEG patterns from wakefulness into drowsiness and then into stages 1 through 4 NREM sleep and into REM sleep. Sleep spindles and K complexes are noted in stage 2 sleep and saw-tooth waves are seen in REM sleep. (*Adapted from* Hauri P. The sleep disorders. Curr Concepts 1982;7; with permission.)

mental effort. Eye movements are purposeful and conjugate. Muscle tone is variable but never absent.

The transition to and from sleep is not an all-or-none phenomenon but a continuum. Criteria are set (Rechtschaffen and Kales), however, that allow for the clinical and research separation of individual sleep states in a reproducible fashion [20]. Early drowsiness can be produced by boredom or fatigue and is characterized by EEG changes of gradual or rapid "alpha dropout." Theta range rhythms appear (4.5–7.5 Hz) and can be mixed with low-voltage 15- to 25-Hz activity. Deepening of drowsiness is characterized by increasing slow activity with transients of 2 to 4 Hz and 4.5 to 7 Hz. The hallmark of deep drowsiness is the appearance of vertex sharp waves that can appear as isolated events or can occur in trains of events. Accompanying the slowing of the background rhythm is the appearance of slow-rolling eye movements and moderately elevated muscle tone.

It has been stated that the first "unequivocal" stage of sleep is stage 2. This stage is characterized by the presence of sleep spindles that have a frequency of 12 to 14 Hz with progressively increasing and then progressively decreasing amplitude lasting 0.5 to 2 seconds in duration. Sleep spindles are believed to arise from generators located in the reticular nucleus of the thalamus and begin to appear as brainstem nuclei, particularly the cholinergic neurons, diminish their firing rates [21]. It is believed that sleep spindles represent the electrical signature of cerebral deafferentation that occurs when primary sensory pathways are gated.

The second hallmark of stage 2 sleep is the appearance of K complexes. These are evoked cortical responses to arousing stimuli and are characterized by a sharp negative wave followed by a slower positive wave with a minimum duration of 0.5 seconds. Slow eye movements persist generally for only a brief time after the appearance of sleep spindles and K complexes and the electromyogram shows persistence of moderate muscle tone [22].

Deep sleep, also known as slow wave sleep (SWS), comprises stage 3 and stage 4 in the Rechtschaffen and Kales criteria. Here, the background rhythm is at its slowest frequency of the sleep period (in the range of 0.5–3 Hz) with an amplitude of greater than 75 μV. Eye movements are absent and the electromyogram tone remains elevated but less than stages 1 and 2 (Fig. 2). Stage 3 is defined as delta activity comprising less than 50% of a recording epoch (30 seconds) and stage 4 represents greater than 50% in delta frequencies. The overall pattern of the EEG is one of high voltage synchronous slow wave activity seen over the entire brain. Cortical cells that are governed by cells in the dorsal thalamus and transmitted via the vast array of the thalamocortical projections generate these waves. As the dorsal and reticulothalamic nuclei become more hyperpolarized, sleep spindles diminish and slower delta waves increase. The appearance of the very low frequency slow-waves marks the virtual cessation of firing of the cholinergic neurons in the brainstem.

REM sleep, or paradoxic sleep, represents the time of cortical activation as evidenced by a rapid transition to a higher frequency rhythm of the EEG (rapid, low-voltage, irregular activity). REMs occur in phasic bursts and there is the occurrence of large burst potentials that originate in the pons and pass rapidly to the lateral geniculate body and then to the occipital lobe (Pons Geniculate Occiptal-waves) [23]. There is a marked reduction in skeletal muscle tone except for the diaphragm and the extraocular eye muscles by way of activation of the medial medulla, which inhibits motor

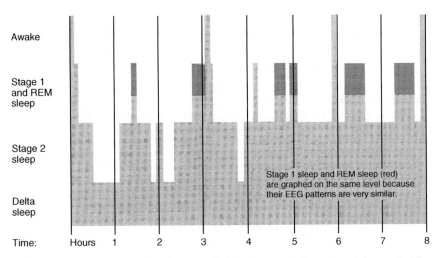

Fig. 2. Sleep hypnogram showing the course of sleep stages over the nocturnal sleep period for this young (ages 20–30) adult. Note the rapid descent into SWS (delta sleep) at the beginning of the nights and the 90-minute cycling of REM sleep. Note that most of SWS, or delta sleep, takes place in the first half of the night and REM sleep increases in period length as the night progresses, with the longest REM episode occurring just before sleep offset. (*Adapted from* Hauri P. The sleep disorders. Curr Concepts 1982;8; with permission.)

neurons by the release of glycine onto spinal and brainstem neurons producing hyperpolarization and inhibition.

Ascending reticular system

As discussed previously, Moruzzi and Magoun identified the activating system as having a significant role in the maintenance of wakefulness and its EEG correlates [13]. The neurons of the reticular activating system receive input from a range of neural networks, including visceral, somatic, and special sensory systems. The inputs travel through two pathways, a dorsal pathway to the thalamic nuclei and a ventral pathway to the hypothalamus. The neurotransmitters include acetylcholine, serotonin, noradrenalin, dopamine, histamine, and hypocretin (orexin) (Figs. 3 and 4).

Acetylcholine

Steriade and colleagues identified groups of cells in the pons-midbrain junction projecting to the thalamus that increased their firing rate approximately a minute before the first change to a desynchronized state was noted on the EEG [24]. These cell groups later were identified as the laterodorsal tegmental (LDT) and pedunculopontine tegmental (PPT) nuclei that contained acetylcholine as their neurotransmitter. These cholinergic

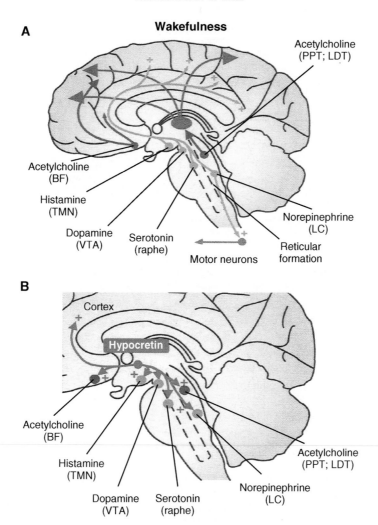

Fig. 3. (*A*) Dorsal and ventral reticular formations are shown with the dorsal cholinergic system (blue) sending fibers into the thalamus (green) and basal forebrain. The thalamus then projects out over the entire cortex by way of the thalamocortical projections. The ventral aminergic pathway is associated with wakefulness. (*B*) The hypocretin cell group in the lateral and posterior hypothalamus sends excitatory neurons to the cholinergic and monoaminergic groups of the reticular formation (all awake-promoting cell groups). (*Adapted from* España R, Scammell TE. Sleep neurobiology for the clinician. Sleep 2004;27:811–20; with permission.)

neurons send fibers via the dorsal pathway to the thalamus where they project specifically to the intralaminar nuclei, the thalamic relay nuclei, and the reticular nucleus. When active, the cholinergic projections allow flow of information through the thalamus, to and from the cerebral cortex, and promote cortical desynchronization (thalamocortical activation). The activity of the LDT-PPT neurons changes with the appearance of each of

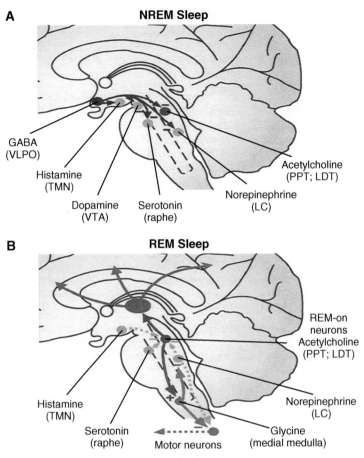

Fig. 4. (*A*) GABA-ergic VLPO neurons (blue) fire faster as sleep deepens. This causes further inhibition of arousal centers in LDT-PPT and the monoaminergic brainstem groups TMN, ventral tegmental area (VTA), the raphe, and the LC. (*B*) REM-on cells in LDT-PPT are disinhibited by GABA-ergic cells also in the LDT-PPT. This causes activation of the thalamorcortical pathways producing cortical desynchronization. There are efferents to the medial medulla from the SLD (subcoeruleus area), which they synapse on GABA-ergic and glycinergic neruons to produce inhibition of motor nuerons in the brainstem and spinal cord to produce muscle atonia. (*Adapted from* España R, Scammell TE. Sleep neurobiology for the clinician. Sleep 2004;27:811–20; with permission.)

the states of sleep and wakefulness. During wakefulness, the neurons fire rapidly. With the onset of stage 1 and 2 of NREM sleep, the LDT-PPT neurons slow their firing rate and in SWS the neurons become quiet. During REM sleep, their activity suddenly becomes active again when they are released from monoamine-mediated inhibition [25–28].

There also are cholinergic neurons in the basal forebrain (magnocellular fields in the basal nucleus of Meynert). These neurons send projections throughout the cortex, hippocampus, and amygdala. Firing rates are highest during wakefulness and REM sleep and are lowest during NREM sleep [29].

Monoaminergic systems

The second branch of the reticular activating system is the branch that innervates the hypothalamus via the ventral route. The neurons that make up these fibers are monoaminergic and include the noradrenergic locus coeruleus (LC), the serotoninergic dorsal raphe and median raphe nuclei, and dopaminergic cells in the periaqueductal gray [30,31]. These fibers are joined by fibers from the histaminergic neurons originating in the tuberomammillary nucleus (TMN) [32,33], hypocretin (orexin) input from the lateral hypothalamus, melatonin-concentrating hormone-containing neurons, and the basal forebrain cholinergic nuclei [34–36,37,38–40]. These then send fibers back to the basal forebrain, the ventral preoptic area, and, subsequently, the entire cerebral cortex.

Like the cholinergic LDT-PPT neurons, the monoaminergic neurons—noradrenergic LC, serotinergic raphe, and histaminergic (TMN)—also have a state-specific firing rate. These collectively fire fastest during wakefulness, slow down during NREM sleep, and nearly stop firing during REM sleep [28]. The specific monoamines are associated with the maintenance of wakefulness.

Norepinephrine and histamine

Norepinephrine (NE) is released during wakefulness [41], and pharmacologic manipulation with NE or NE agonist drugs uniformly produces an increase in waking behavior and exhibits inhibitory mechanisms on sleep production. Likewise, histamine is believed to be the "master" wakefulness-promoting neurotransmitter, with high activity during wakefulness and decreasing activity during NREM sleep down to its lowest levels during REM sleep. It is well known that histamine blockers promote sleep onset and increase NREM sleep [42]. Recent studies investigating H_3 receptor agonists suggest that these moieties stimulate autoinhibitory receptors on histamine and other aminergic neurons and produce augmentation of sleep onset [43].

Serotonin

The physiologic effects of serotonin on sleep and wake behavior is controversial, with conflicting reports that serotonin promotes sleep and induces wakefulness. Most recent evidence, however, shows that serotonin promotes wakefulness with an increase in sleep-onset latency and a decrease in REM sleep. Clinically, down-regulation of serotonin signaling may be the cause of hypersomnia seen when selective serotinin reuptake inhibitors first are initiated in depressed patients [44,45].

Dopamine

Dopamine (DA) and its role in sleep-wake regulation remain unclear. From a pharmacologic standpoint, the release of DA and its reuptake inhibition by powerful stimulants, such as amphetamines, shows its wakefulness-promoting properties [46–48]. Dopamine blockers (eg, chlorpromazine and haloperidol) long have been known for their sleep-inducing effects. Recent reports of the sleep of patients who have Parkinson's disease, where there is a deficiency in dopamine in the substantia nigra and the ventral tegmental area, show remarkable similarities to patients who have narcolepsy (ie, fragmented nocturnal sleep), early-onset REM periods, REM sleep behavior disorder, and multiple sleep latency test, demonstrating pathologic daytime sleepiness with an increase in sleep-onset REM periods [47]. The confound is that some patients (those who have Parkinson's disease and those who are being treated with DA receptor agonists for restless legs syndrome) on occasion experience sudden sleep attacks. One possible explanation for this incongruity is that low doses of DA receptor agonists bind to autoinhibitory receptors on DA neurons, further decreasing DA signaling and thus decreasing the wakefulness drive [49].

Hypocretin (orexin)

The recent discovery of excitatory sleep-wake neuropeptides hypocretin (HcrtR1 and HcrtR2), also known as orexin (orexin-1 and orexin-2), has added significant insight into the regulation of the sleep-wake state and offered explanations as to the cause of narcolepsy [50–53]. These neuropeptides are produced by a small cluster of neurons in the lateral, posterior, and perifornical areas of the hypothalamus that have diffuse projections throughout the central nervous system [34]. These areas of the hypothalamus receive dense input from the monoaminergic and cholinergic brainstem nuclei. The neurons of the hypocretin producing cell groups are most active during waking, particularly during periods of increased psychomotor activity, and significantly decrease in firing during NREM and REM sleep [28].

More than 90% of narcoleptics who have cataplexy have low or undetectable levels of hypocretin in their cerebrospinal fluid, and postmortem analysis of brains of patients who have narcolepsy show a marked reduction in the number of hypocretin neurons [52,53]. The hypocretin neurons are activated by glutamate that in turn increases the amount of glutamate in the surrounding cells of the hypothalamus that creates a positive feedback system to sustain the firing of the hypocretin neurons.

Recent studies suggest that the two hypocretin moieties, HcrtR1 and HcrtR2, perform distinct functions in terms of modulation of sleep and its constituent parts. Although both mediate excitatory responses, HcrtR1 binds to specific G-proteins, whereas HcrtR2 binds to specific and nonspecific proteins, signifying that there are separate functions of the two protein receptor complexes. It seems that HcrtR1 is responsible for maintenance of sleep and wake episodes and HcrtR2 is involved in the maintenance of skeletal muscle tone while awake [54]. It is believed that hypocretin deficiency leads to sleep state instability with increased numbers of transitions between sleep and wakefulness and between REM sleep phenomena and wakefulness.

The understanding of the orchestration of the timing of sleep onset and then the initiation of the ultradian rhythm of REM and NREM sleep is the Holy Grail of sleep research. Von Economo hypothesizes that within the hypothalamus there are two distinct sites, one that promotes wakefulness and a second that promotes sleep [5]. Recent findings confirm his theories and offer a better understanding of the sleep-onset and maintenance mechanisms.

By identifying modulators of the histaminergic neurons of the TMN, Sherin and coworkers show that γ-aminobutyric acid (GABA)-ergic inputs that originate in the ventrolateral preoptic (VLPO) area and the extended VLPO area of the hypothalamus inhibit the TMN [55]. There also is further inhibitory input to the TMN from fibers that have their cell bodies scattered more diffusely in the lateral hypothalamus (the extended VLPO). In addition to GABA, these neurons contain the inhibitory neuropeptide, galanin [25]. There also are inhibitory efferents to other monoaminergic nuclei, such as the raphe nuclei and the LC. Thus, by inhibiting the wake promoting action of these monoaminergic amines, the VLPO promotes the onset of sleep. Alternatively, these same monoaminergic cell groups also supply efferents back to the VLPO. There also is input from hypocretin-containing cells in the dorsolateral hypothalamus. This reciprocal innervation sets the stage for control of the sleep-wake switch. In addition, known sleep-inducing substances (somnogens), such as adenosine, increase activity in the VLPO, in turn promoting sleep, allowing more modulatory input to the sleep-wake control [56–59]. This scenario has led to the hypothesis that there is a bistable sleep-wake switch, where the VLPO and arousal systems are inhibited reciprocally [60].

The firing rates of VLPO neurons increase during sleep and get progressively faster as sleep deepens (SWS). This increased firing causes further inhibition of arousal centers that allow less interrupted and thereby deeper sleep. In the opposite scenario, wakefulness causes inhibition of the VLPO that ensures full wakefulness without letting drowsiness cause diminished cognitive abilities. Saper and coworkers describe this as a sleep-wake "flip-flop" switch, with each half of the mechanism strongly inhibiting the other. Full change of state requires overwhelming forces, such as accumulated homeostatic sleep drive, coupled with the appropriate circadian influence to drive the switch into its opposite configuration [60].

This model can explain how the behavioral states of wakefulness and sleep can transition from one to the other and maintain the state regardless of constantly changing homeostatic forces that accumulate and dissipate over the course of a day, allowing the circadian influences to ensure 24-hour rhythmicity.

Once sleep onset occurs, a second set of neuronal interactions occur that account for NREM/REM cycling. Firing of VLPO neurons increases as sleep gets deeper. A transition occurs during NREM sleep when GABA-ergic LPT neurons disinhibit REM-on neurons located in and near the cholinergic neural group of the LDT-PPT. Acetylcholine is released into the thalamus, producing cortical desynchrony [61,62]. The aminergic neurons of the TMN, raphe, and LC fall silent (most likely mediated through afferents in the area of the extended VLPO) (Fig. 5, Table 1) [28].

REM sleep can be dissociated into its different components, including muscle atonia, EEG desynchronization, PGO waves, and REMs. Each of these clinical manifestations of REM sleep is under the control of discrete cell groups within the pontine reticular formation and the midbrain reticular

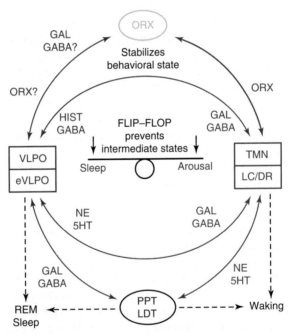

Fig. 5. The two main centers for sleep and arousal are shown. The VLPO and the extended VLPO (eVLPO) are the centers for sleep maintenance, whereas the TMN, LC, and dorsal raphe (DR) are all monoaminergic wakefulness-promoting neural groups. The inhibitory pathways are in red and the excitatory pathways are in green. Orexin/hypocretin shown at the top stabilizes the two states and prevents rapid cycling. During wakefulness there is inhibition of the VLPO and eVLPO. and during sleep there is inhibition of the monoaminergic stimulatory cell groups. (*From* Saper CB, Chou TC, Scammell TE. The sleep switch: hypothalamic control of sleep and wakefulness. Trends Neurosci 2001;24:729.)

Table 1
State-specific firing rates of brainstem and cortical neuronal groups

Site	Neurotransmitter	Wakefulness	Non–rapid eye movement sleep	Rapid eye movement sleep
Basal forebrain	Acetylcholine	++++	+	++++
Laterodorsol tegmentum/pedunculopontine tegementum	Acetylcholine	++++	+++ → 0	++++
Dorsal and median raphe	Serotonin	++++	++	0
Loceus coerulus	NE	++++	++	0
Tuberomammillary nucleus	Histamine	++++	++	0
Posterior/lateral hypothalamus	Hypocretin/orexin	++++	+	+
Ventrolateral preoptic area	GABA	+	+++	++++

formation, which includes the sublateral dorsal area (SLD), also known as the subcoeruleus area. These cell groups are called effector neurons [64]. These cell groups are silent during NREM sleep. They begin to depolarize 30 to 60 seconds before the first sign of REM sleep occurs, the PGO waves. The pontine reticular formation/midbrain reticular formation then undergoes further neuronal depolarization, leading to the development of action potentials in these cell groups. The action potentials increase as REM sleep starts and this high rate of firing is maintained throughout the REM sleep episode.

SLD neurons project to the ventrolateral medulla and the spinal cord, where they synapse on GABA-ergic and glycinergic neurons to produce hyperpolarization and inhibition of motor neurons in the brainstem and spinal cord, thus accounting for the widespread muscle atonia of REM sleep. The medial medulla inhibits motor neurons further by reducing excitatory output from the LC and red nucleus [63,66]. Lesions of the SLD cause REM without atonia [65].

Neurons in the midbrain reticular formation are important in mediating EEG desynchronization characterized by low-voltage, fast-frequency EEG.

The SLD also contains GABA-ergic efferents that feed back and can inhibit the LPT. This mutual inhibition between the LPT and SLD creates another flip-flop switch that can explain the ultradian rhythm of NREM and REM; however, this makes the REM/NREM cycling vulnerable to extrinsic perturbations. It is believed that hypocretin neurons prevent unwanted transitions by weighing in on the REM-off side during wakefulness. This can explain the intrusion of REM sleep components into wakefulness that is characteristic of narcolepsy, where lack of hypocretin signaling allows the SLD and LDT to transition independently into atonia (cataplexy) and REM forebrain phenomena (LDT causes hypnagogic hallucinations) [65].

Circadian rhythm

Suprachiasmatic nucleus

Circadian rhythms are biologic activities that recur approximately every 24 hours. In the absence of external timing cues (zeitgebers), some of these processes remain rhythmic (ie, "run free") with an approximately 24-hour period. In mammals, the suprachiasmatic nucleus (SCN) is the pacemaker for maintaining circadian sleep-wake cycles, body temperature changes, hormonal releases, and cyclic behavioral patterns. The SCN is located in the ventromedial hypothalamus immediately dorsal to the optic chiasm.

In mammals, the most important stimulus for the time-locked regulation of the circadian rhythm is light. The SCN has a direct afferent connection from the retina via the retinohypothalamic tract [67]. Activation is via a unique class of melanopsin-containing photopigment cells in the retinal ganglia providing the main input for photic entrainment. The putative neurotransmitter in the retinohypothalamic tract is the excitatory amino acid, glutamate [68].

Nonphotic entrainment remains controversial. It generally is believed that nonphotic input to the SCN is mediated by thalamic input under the influence of serotoninergic neurons [69]. There also are, however, afferents from the histaminergic TMS and cholinergic inputs from multiple forebrain and brainstem regions, in particular the pedunculopontine tegmentum [70].

There are diffuse projections from the paraventricular nucleus of the thalamus and inputs from the hypothalamus itself, via the geniculohypothalamic tract (GHT). It is believed that input from the GHT is critical in nonphotic entrainment. The GHT originates from cells in the intergeniculate leaflet (IGL), which is located between the dorsal and ventrolateral geniculate nuclei in the thalamus [71]. The IGL has inputs from the retina, the noradrenergic LC, and the serotonergic raphe [72]. Efferents project to the contralateral IGL, the SCN and the peri-SCN area, the pineal, the accessory optic system the superior colliculus, the zona incerta, and the pretectum.

Besides glutamate, other neurotransmitters associated with the SCN include GABA, vasoactive intestinal protein, neuropeptide Y (NPY), metenkephalin and orphanin-FQ [73]. NPY phase shifts circadian rhythms. Injecting antiserum to NPY into the SCN area can block its effect. Serotonin input from the median raphe nucleus goes directly into the SCN. Serotonergic input from the dorsal raphe, however, comes via projections to the IGL that then feed into the SCN via NPY [74].

Efferents from the SCN project to four main areas. One group of fibers goes dorsally to the paraventricular area of the thalamus and the posterior hypothalamus. A second group of efferents goes to nuclei located rostral to the SCN, in particular, the medial preoptic area. The third group of fibers runs caudally from the SCN to the anterior, medial, and lateral hypothalamic areas. The fourth group of fibers runs dorsal to the optic tracts into the ventrolateral geniculate nucleus. Thus, there are extensive inner-vations from the SCN back into the hypothalamus and thalamus to control a complex series of interactions involving hormonal, behavioral, and tem-perature control [75].

Clock genes

The neurons within the SCN generate the circadian rhythm by means of oscillatory protein synthesis via several clock genes. The first gene, *Period* (*Per*), which encodes a clock component protein, PER, was discovered in 1971 [76]. Since then, at least eight genes have been identified that are involved with mammalian clock regulation. There are three *Period* genes (*mPer1, mPer2,* and *mPer3*), two *Cryptochrome* genes (*mCry1* and *mCry2*), *Clock* gene, *Bmal 1* or *Mop3,* and *CkIε* [76]. Through a series of experiments that looked at mutations of these clock genes and the resultant physiologic and behavioral changes that they produced, Daan and colleagues propose a model that explains the negative feedback control that produces the 24-hour rhythms and allows for adjustment to seasonal changes in the change in the length of daylight with a morning oscillator (M) that phase advances the circadian rhythm by sensing light at dawn and an evening oscillator (E) that phase delays the rhythm keyed to decreasing light at dusk [78].

Within the nucleus of a SCN neuron, the CLOCK and BMAL1 proteins form a heterodimer that binds to the promoters of the *Per1* and *Per2* genes that activate their transcription. The PER1 and PER2 proteins, after phosphylation in the cytoplasm, interact with clock gene products, CRY1 and CRY2 proteins. These *Cry* genes have opposite effects of the *Per1* and *Per2* genes. It also is observed that *Per1* (M) and *Per2* (E) gene expression have different light responsiveness. Thus, the clock can be seen as an oscillator that is stabilized by two regulatory loops. The first is the M that is sensitive to dawn and the reappearance of sunlight. The second is an E tracking the fading of light. After the modulation by the CRY1 proteins, the PER1/CRY1 heterodime is transported back into the nucleus and turns off the transcription of CLOCK/BMAL1, thereby inhibiting *Per1* and *Cry1* transcription. Likewise, the PER2/CRY2 heterodime regulates *Per2* and *Cry2* transcription [77].

Homestatic and circadian sleep-wake interactions

Experimental studies show that in addition to the circadian timing mechanism, there is a second force that also regulates the sleep-wake cycle, known as the homeostatic sleep process. Well before the SCN was identified as the "master clock," the main theories of why humans sleep had to do with maintenance of physiologic equilibrium (homeostasis) [79].

In 1910, Legendre and Pieron found that the cerebrospinal fluid of sleep-deprived dogs induced sleep in dogs with no loss of sleep when injected into their ventricular system. The idea that there is a toxin or toxic byproduct or other sleep factor that builds up when there is sleep loss or accumulates after repeated bouts of insufficient sleep was established [80].

There is evidence that adenosine may be the sleep-inducing factor, or somnogen. Adenosine levels in the basal forebrain rise with sleep deprivation and fall rapidly during the subsequent sleep period. This may explain why caffeine, an adenosine A1 receptor blocker, is able to maintain alertness. It seems that adenosine promotes sleep by direct inhibition of wake-promoting neural groups and by disinhibiting the sleep-promoting VLPO neurons [56].

Adenosine may not be the only somnogen present. Infectious processes can induce sleep. Sleep also is induced by cytokines, such as interleukin-1β, tumor necrosis factor α, and interferon-α [81]. Cytokines also induce the production of prostaglandin D2 that promotes REM and NREM sleep.

To better understand the interaction of the two processes, several experimental paradigms were developed. One set of experiments involved sleep-deprivation studies, in which sleep was eliminated completely for extended periods of time. Even though the overall "sleep pressure" increased, there was still was a discernable 24-hour cycle, with increased sleep propensity during what ordinarily is the subject's nighttime and increased alertness during the subject's day [82]. Several studies demonstrate that there are actually two times of increased sleep propensity, one less robust period during the early afternoon and a second more powerful period at night. All studies show the greatest increase in sleepiness occurs in the early morning hours, whereas the least sleepiness occurs in the early evening [83].

A second set of experiments involved sleep displacement, where sleep-onset times were shifted. When sleep was shifted by 12 hours, there was a significant increase in wakefulness in the beginning of the sleep period accompanied by a shift of REM sleep to the first third to half of the night (REM sleep normally is maximal during the second half of the night). Thus, there was a decrease in the first REM latency and an increase in wakefulness after sleep onset [84]. This corresponds to the clinical issue of shift workers, who, after working at night, report fragmented and nonrestorative sleep when their rest cycle takes place during the day.

Some of the earliest work involved temporal isolation studies, where subjects were placed in environments where there were no discernable cues to the external environment (ie, all time cues [zeitgebers] were removed). The findings showed that the sleep-wake cycle tended to increase to somewhat less than 25 hours and the diurnal temperature curve followed suit. This was called a free-running rhythm [85].

The sleep-wake cycle is synchronized with the ambient light-dark cycle, with the peak rectal temperature occurring in the late afternoon to early evening. The nadir occurs in the second half of the sleep period. After several days in a free-running environment, however, the temperature peak advances to the first half of the activity period and the nadir changes to the first half of the sleep period. In subjects whose sleep onset occurred close to their temperature minimum, sleep offset took place on the rising limb of the temperature cycle. The total amount of sleep was reduced even when the "sleep pressure" was increasing, as measured by the total amount of prior wakefulness.

Another significant observation of these temporal isolation subjects was that many of them exhibited a spontaneous dissociation of their temperature cycles from their rest-activity cycles after several days. This is called internal desynchronization.

Zulley found that in internally desynchronized subjects, the circadian temperature curve influenced not only the duration of sleep but also the propensity of falling asleep [86]. Czeisler and coworkers show that the timing of REM sleep is dependent on the circadian phase of the temperature cycle at sleep onset and not on the amount of prior wakefulness. Further studies show that there are two "zones" of high probability for going to sleep and two "zones" of a low probability of falling asleep [87].

These findings led to what appeared to be a paradoxic conclusion (ie, it is most difficult to fall asleep shortly before what for most people is their regular bedtime). The two zones of highest sleep propensity were analyzed further using nap times in internally desynchronized subjects. Zulley and Campbell found that naps clustered at two circadian phases, one at the temperature nadir and a second at a point halfway between two successive temperature nadirs. They explained this by the existence not only of a primary sleep period but also a secondary circadian sleep period that, under normally entrained conditions, corresponds to the early afternoon [88].

Forced desynchrony

Another experimental paradigm used a forced day length close to, but not exactly, that of a 24-hour time period (eg, 22.7 or 25.3 hours). The duration of wakefulness between successive sleep periods remained constant, but sleep onset occurred at different circadian phases. The net effect was to allow the body temperature rhythm to run free and to separate the circadian dependent processes from the homeostatic processes.

Using the forced desynchrony protocol, it was established that the human circadian clock is much closer to the environmental diurnal day-night cycle (24 hours ± 10 minutes) and it is the same in all age groups. Thus, the concept that aging brings on circadian changes was challenged successfully [89].

Sleep pressure, as measured by sleep-onset latency, is maximal near the nadir of core body temperature that is close to the usual wake time in normally entrained conditions. The drive to maintain wakefulness is strongest during the evening hours near the temperature maximum that, as described previously, is close to the usual sleep-onset time [87]. Thus, the paradox: the pressure to maintain wakefulness is highest just before sleep onset and the maximal drive for sleep is just before waking. The teleologic explanation is that wakefulness is maintained right up to the point of sleep onset and sleep is maintained through the night until sleep offset.

Lavie describes a "forbidden zone" for sleep [90]. Strogatz describes this as the "wake-maintenance zone" [91,92]. This corresponds to the period of time just before sleep onset, when wakefulness is countered by an increasing circadian drive for sleep. There then occurs an abrupt transition from low sleep propensity during the evening period to the high-propensity night period. This time frame is called the "nocturnal sleep gate" and is found to be phase locked to the dark-phase hormone, melatonin. The "opening" of the sleep gate occurs approximately 2 hours after the time of the maximal nocturnal secretion of melatonin (Fig. 6) [93].

Agents of entrainment

Light

Light exposure in the early morning hours (just after the body temperature minimum) causes an advance in the sleep-wake cycle, whereas exposure to light in the early evening before the temperature minimum causes a delay in the sleep-wake cycle. Of note is that this light exposure

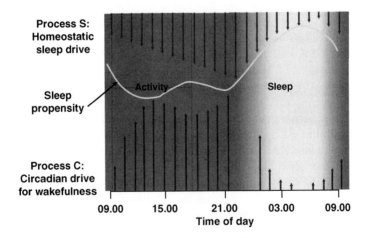

Fig. 6. The interaction of the circadian and homeostatic drives produces a sleep propensity curve that is biphasic. There is a higher sleep propensity in the midafternoon and a more robust period at night. The sleep onset occurs just after the sleep gate opens and sleep offset occurs just after the nadir of body temperature. (*Adapted from* Edgar DM, Dement W, Fuller CA. Effect of SCN lesions on sleep in squirrel monkeys: evidence for opponent processes in sleep-wake regulation. J Neurosci 1993;13:1065–79; with permission.)

does not have to be at the brightness level of sunlight and that even artificial incandescent light can cause phase shifts if exposure is present at critical times. It also is demonstrated that non–sleep-wake circadian rhythms are shifted by light exposure with changes in urine production, cortisol production, and melatonin secretion. All these rhythms exhibited a stable temporal relationship to temperature rhythms after light-induced phase shifts [94,95].

Melatonin

Melatonin is synthesized from circulating tryptophan, transformed to serotonin, and then converted into melatonin in the pineal gland. There is no pineal storage of melatonin; as it is secreted, it is distributed through the circulation. Maximum plasma concentrations occur between 3:00 and 4:00 AM and during the day, levels essentially are undetectable. Even in temporal isolation, melatonin continues to express its circadian rhythm. The rhythmicity of melatonin secretion is driven by the SCN through connections to the paraventricular nuclei and then to a multisynaptic pathway that courses through the upper part of the cervical spinal cord, synapsing on preganglionic cell bodies of the superior cervical ganglia of the cervical sympathetic chains. The superior cervical ganglia then sends noradrenergic neuronal projections directly to the pineal gland [96].

Melatonin synthesis is limited to the dark period and is inhibited by light. Exogenous melatonin exerts phase-shifting effects on the endogenous production of melatonin in humans. Melatonin administered in the morning (time of shut-down of natural melatonin production) causes phase-shift delay of the endogenous rhythm, and phase advances occur when melatonin is administered before onset of the endogenous production.

It is hypothesized that the endogenous cycle of melatonin secretion is involved in the regulation of the sleep-wake cycle, not by promoting sleep actively but by inhibiting the SCN wakefulness producing mechanism [97,98].

In this way, the evening onset of melatonin secretion, which coincides with the maximum point of the SCN-driven arousal cycle, inhibits the circadian drive for waking, enabling the sleep-onset structures to be activated, unopposed by the drive for wakefulness.

References

[1] Leadbetter R. Nyx. In: Encyclopedia mythica. Available at: Pantheon.org. 1999. Accessed April 1, 2005.
[2] Poortviliet R, Huygun W. What is sleep? In: The book of the sandman and the alphabet of sleep. New York: Harry N. Abrams; 1989.
[3] Rouse WHD, Smith MF. In: Lucretius: on the nature of things. Cambridge (MA): Harvard University Press; 1992. p. 34.

[4] Hammond WA. Physiology of sleep: on wakefulness. Philadelphia: JB Lippincott; 1866. p. 2–38.

[5] von Economo C. Sleep as a problem of localization. J Nerv Ment Dis 1930;71:249–59.

[6] Aldrich MS. Neurology of sleep. In: Sleep medicine. Contemporary neurology series, vol. 53. New York: Oxford University Press; 1999. p. 27–38.

[7] Berger H. Ueber das Elektroenkephalogramm des Menschen. J Psychol Neurol 1930;40: 160–79.

[8] Bremer F. Cerveau "isolé" et physiologie du sommeil. C R Soc Biol (Paris) 1935;118: 1235–41.

[9] y Cajal R. Histologie du systeme nerveux de L'homme et des vertebres maloine, vol. 2. Paris. Oxford University Press; 1911.

[10] Papez JW. Reticulo-spinal tracts in the cat, Marchi method. J Comp Neurol 1926;41:365–99.

[11] Morison RS, Dempsey EW. Mechanism of thalamocortical augmentation and repetition. Am J Physiol 1942;138:297–308.

[12] de No L. The cerebral cortex: architecture, intracortical connections and motor projections. In: Fulton JF, editor. Physiology of the nervous system. London: Oxford University Press; 1938. p. 291–339.

[13] Moruzzi G, Magoun HW. Communications: brain stem reticular formation and activation of the EEG. Electroencephalogr Clin Neurophysiol 1949;1:455–73.

[14] Jouvet M, Michel M. Correlations electromyographiques du sommeil chez le chat decortique et Mesencephalique chronique. C R Soc Biol (Paris) 1959;153:422–5.

[15] Jouvet M, Michel F, Courjon J. Sur un stade d'activity electrique cerebral rapide au cours du sommeil physiologique. C R Soc Biol (Paris) 1959;153:1024–8.

[16] Jouvet M, Mounier D. Effects des lesions de la formation reticulaire pontique sur le sommeil du chat. C R Soc Biol (Paris) 1960;154:2301–5.

[17] Aserinsky E, Kleitman N. Regularly occurring periods of eye movements and concomitant phenomena, during sleep. Science 1953;118:273–4.

[18] Aserinsky E, Kleitman N. Two types of ocular motility occurring in sleep. J Appl Physiol 1955;8:11–8.

[19] Dement W, Kleitman N. Cyclic variations in EEG during sleep and their relation to eye movements, body motility and dreaming. Electroencephalogr Clin Neueophysiol 1957;9: 673–90.

[20] Rechtschaffen A, Kales A. A manual of standardized terminology, techniques and scoring system for sleep stages of human subjects. Los Angeles: Brain Information Service/Brain Research Institute; 1968. p. 1–12.

[21] Steriade M, Gloor P, Llinás RR, et al. Basic mechanisms of cerebral rhythmic activities. Electroencephalogr Clin Neurophysiol 1990;76:481–508.

[22] Colrain IM. The K-complex: a 7 decade history. Sleep 2005;28:255–73.

[23] Buzsaki G, Traub RD. Physiological basis of EEG activity. In: Engel JJ, Pedley TA, editors. Epilepsy: a comprehensive textbook. New York: Raven Press; 1997. p. 819–32.

[24] Steriade M, Datta S, Paré D, et al. Neuronal activities in brain-stem cholinergic nuclei related to tonic activation processes in thalamocortical systems. J Neurosci 1990;10:2541–59.

[25] Pace-Schott EF, Hobson JA. The neurobiology of sleep: genetics, cellular physiology and subcortical networks. Nat Rev Neurosci 2002;3:591–605.

[26] Steriade M. Arousal: revisiting the reticular activating system. Science 1996;272:225–6.

[27] Armstrong DM, Saper CB, Levey AI, et al. Distribution of cholinergic neurons in rat brain: demonstrated by the immunocytochemical localization of choline acetyltransferase. J Comp Neurol 1983;216:53–68.

[28] España R, Scammell TE. Sleep neurobiology for the clinician. Sleep 2004;27:811–20.

[29] Detari L, Rasmusson DD, Semba K, et al. The role of the basal forebrain neurons in tonic and phasic activation of the cerebral cortex. Prog Neurobiol 1999;58:249.

[30] Törk I. Anatomy of the serotonergic system. Ann N Y Acad Sci 1990;600:9–34.

[31] Koella WP. Serotonin and sleep. Exp Med Surg 1969;27:157–68.

[32] Schönrock B, Büsselberg D, Haas HL. Properties of tuberomammillary histamine neurons and their response to galanin. Agents Actions 1991;33:135–7.

[33] Yang QZ, Hatton GI. Electrophysiology of excitatory and inhibitory afferents to rat histaminergic tuberomammillary nucleus neurons from hypothalamic and forebrain sites. Brain Res 1997;773:162–72.

[34] Kilduff TS, Peyron C. The hypocretin/orexin ligand-receptor system: implications for sleep and sleep disorders. Trends Neurosci 2000;23:359–65.

[35] De Lecea L, Kilduff TS, Peyron C, et al. The hypocretins: hypothalamus-specific peptides with neuroexcitatory activity. Proc Natl Acad Sci USA 1998;95:322–7.

[36] Sakurai T, Amemiya A, Ishii M, et al. Orexins and orexin receptors: a family of hypothalamic neuropeptides and G protein-coupled receptors that regulate feeding behavior. Cell 1998;92:573–85.

[37] Methippara MM, Alam N, Szymusiak R, et al. Effects of lateral preoptic area application of orexin-A on sleep-wakefulness. Sleep 2000;11:3423–6.

[38] España RA, Baldo BA, Kelley AE, et al. Wake-promoting and sleep-suppressing actions of hypocretin (orexin): basal forebrain sites of action. Neuroscience 2001;106:699–715.

[39] Li Y, Gao XB, Sakurai T, et al. Hypocretin/orexin excites hypocretin neurons via a local glutamate neuron-a potential mechanism for orchestrating the hypothalamic arousal system. Neuron 2002;36:1169–81.

[40] Torterolo P, Yamuy J, Sampogna S, et al. Hypothalamic neurons that contain hypocretin (orexin) express c-fos during active wakefulness and carbachol-induced active sleep. Available at: www.sro.org. Accessed March 15, 2005. Sleep Res Online 2001;4:25–32.

[41] Morrison JH, Foote SL. Noradrenergic and serotoninergic innervation of cortical, thalamic and tectal visual structures in Old and New World monkeys. J Comp Neurol 1986;243:117–38.

[42] Tasaka K, Chung YH, Sawada K. Excitatory effect of histamine on the arousal system and its inhibition by H1 blockers. Brain Res Bull 1989;22:271–5.

[43] Mignot E, Taheri S, Nishino S. Sleeping with the hypothalamus: emerging therapeutic targets for sleep disorders. Nat Neurosci 2002;5:1071–5.

[44] Hillarp NA, Fuxe K, Dahlström A. Demonstration and mapping of central neurons containing dopamine, noradrenalin, and 5-hydroxytryptamine and their reactions to psychopharmaca. Pharmacol Rev 1966;18:727–39.

[45] Dzoljic MR, Ukponmwan OE, Saxena PR. 5–HT1-like receptor agonists enhance wakefulness. Neuropharmacology 1992;31:623–33.

[46] Nishino S, Mao J, Sampathkumaran R, et al. Increased dopaminergic transmission mediates the wake-promoting effects of CNS stimulants. Available at: www.sro.org. Accessed March 15, 2005. Sleep Res Online 1998;1:49–61.

[47] Wisor JP, Nishino S, Sora I, et al. Dopaminergic role in stimulant-induced wakefulness. J Neurosci 2001;21:1787–94.

[48] Isaac SO, Berridge CW. Wake-promoting actions of dopamine D1 and D2 receptor stimulation. J Phamacol Exp Ther 2003;307:386–94.

[49] Rye DB. The two faces of Eve: dopamine's modulation of wakefulness and sleep. Neurology 2004;63:8(Suppl 3):S2-7.

[50] Lin L, Faraco J, Li R, et al. The sleep disorder canine narcolepsy is caused by a mutation in the hypocretin (orexin) receptor 2 gene. Cell 1999;98:365–76.

[51] Chemelli RM, Willie JT, Sinton CM, et al. Narcolepsy in orexin knockout mice: molecular genetics of sleep regulation. Cell 1999;98:437–51.

[52] Siegel JM, Moore R, Thannickal T, et al. A brief history of hypocretin/orexin and narcolepsy. Neuropyshophamacology 2001;25(S5):S14–20.

[53] Thannickal TC, Moore RY, Nienhuis R, et al. Reduced number of hypocretin neurons in human narcolepsy. Neuron 2000;27:469–74.

[54] Kisanuki YY, Chemelli RM, Sinton CM, et al. The role of orexin receptor type-1 (OX1R) in the regulation of sleep. Sleep 2000;A91.

[55] Sherin JE, Shiromani PJ, McCarley RW, et al. Activation of ventrolateral preoptic neurons during sleep. Science 1996;271:216–9.

[56] Porkka-Heiskanen T, Strecker RE, Thakkar M, et al. Adenosine: a mediator of the sleep-inducing effects of prolonged wakefulness. Science 1997;276:1265–8.

[57] Tanase D, Martin WA, Baghdoyan HA, et al. G protein activation in rat ponto-mesencephalic nuclei is enhanced by combined treatment with a mu opioid and an adenosine A1 receptor agonist. Sleep 2001;24:52–61.

[58] Chamberlin NL, Arrigoni E, Chou TC, et al. Effects of adenosine on GABAergic synaptic inputs to identified ventrolateral preoptic neurons. Neuroscience 2003;119:913–8.

[59] Ueno R, Ishikawa Y, Nakayama T, et al. Prostaglandin D2 induces sleep when microinjected into the preoptic area of conscious rats. Biochem Biophys Res Commun 1982;109:576–82.

[60] Saper CB, Chou TC, Scammell TE. The sleep switch: hypothalamic control of sleep and wakefulness. Trends Neurosci 2001;24:726–31.

[61] EL Mansari M, Saaki K, Jouvet M. Unitary characteristics of presumptive cholinergic tegmental neurons during the sleep-waking cycle in freely moving cats. Exp Brain Res 1989;76:519–29.

[62] Boissard R, Gervasoni D, Schmidt MH, et al. The rat ponto-medullary network responsible for paradoxical sleep onset and maintenance: a combined microinjection and functional neuroanatomy study. Eur J Neurosci 2002;16:1959–73.

[63] Morales FR, Engelhardt JK, Soja PJ, et al. Motoneuroneuron properties during motor inhibition produced by microinjection of carbachol into the pontine reticular formation of the decerebrate cat. J Neurophysiol 1987;57:1118–29.

[64] Sinton CM, McCarley RW. Neurophysiological mechanisms of sleep and wakefulness: a question of balance. SeminNeurol 2004;24:211–23.

[65] Saper CB. Neurobiology of sleep. In: Education program syllabus. American Academy of Neurology, 57th meeting. 2005. p. 3AC.001-1–3.

[66] Curtis DR, Hosli L, Johnston GA, et al. The hyperpolarization of spinal motorneurons by glycine and related amino acids. Exp Brain Res 1968;5:235–58.

[67] Johnson RF, Moore RY, Morin LP. Loss of entrainment and anatomical plasticity after lesions of the hamster retinohypothalamic tract. Brain Res 1988;460:297–313.

[68] Berson DM, Dunn FA, Tako M. Phototransduction by retinal ganglion cells that set the circadian clock. Science 2002;295:1070–3.

[69] Morin LP. Serotonin and the regulation of mammalian circadian rhythmicity. Ann Med 1999;31:12–33.

[70] Bina KG, Rusak B, Semba K. Localization of cholinergic neurons in the forebrain and brainstem that project to the suprachiasmatic nucleus of the hypothalamus in rat. J Comp Neurol 1993;335:295–307.

[71] Moore RY, Card JP. Intergeniculate leaflet: an anatomically and functionally distinct subdivision of the lateral genicuilate complex. J Comp Neurol 1994;344:403–30.

[72] Morin LP. The circadian visual system. Brain Res Rev 1994;67:102–27.

[73] Harrington ME, Mistlberger RE. Anatomy and physiology of the mammalian circadian system. In: Fryger MH, Roth T, Dement WC, editors. Principles and practice of sleep medicine. 2nd edition. Philadelphia: WB Saunders; 2000. p. 334–45.

[74] Biello SM, Janik D, Mrfosovsky N. Neuropeptide Y and behaviorally induced phase shifts. Neuroscience 1994;62:273–9.

[75] Watts AG, Swanson LW. Efferent projections of the suprachiasmatic nucleus, II: studies using retrograde transport of fluorescent dyes and simultaneous peptide immunochemistry in the rat. J Comp Neurol 1987;258:230–52.

[76] Konopka RJ, Benzer S. Clock mutants of Drosophila melanogaster. Proc Natl Acad Sci USA 1971;68:2112–6.

[77] Albrecht U. Functional genomics of sleep and circadian rhythm. Invited review: regulation of mammalian circadian clock genes. J Appl Physiol 2002;92:1348–55.

[78] Daan S, Beersma DG, Borbely AA. Timing of human sleep recovery process gated by a circadian pacemaker. Am J Physiology 1984;246:161–83.

[79] Borbély AA, Tobler I. Endogenous sleep-promoting substances and sleep regulation. Physiol Rev 1989;69:605–58.

[80] Legendre R, Pieron H. Le probleme des facteurs du sommeil. Resultats d'injections vasculaires et intracerebrales de liquids insomniques. C R Soc Biol (Paris) 1910;68:1077–9.

[81] Späth-Schwalbe E, Lange T, Perras B, et al. Interferon-α acutely impairs sleep in healthy humans. Cytokine 2000;12:518–21.

[82] Blake MJF. Time of day effects on performance in a range of tasks. Psychonom Sci 1967;9: 349–50.

[83] Webb WB, Agnew HW, Williams RL. Effects on sleep of a sleep period time displacement. Aerosp Med 1971;42:152–5.

[84] Aschoff J, Wever R. Spotanperiodik des menschen bei ausschluss aller zeitgeber. Naturwissenschaften 1962;49:337–42.

[85] Zulley J. Distribution of REM sleep in entrained 24 hour and free-running sleep-wake cycles. Sleep 1980;2:377–89.

[86] Zulley J, Wever R, Aschoff J. The dependence of onset and duration of sleep on the circadian rhythm of rectal temperature. Pflugers Arch 1981;391:314–8.

[87] Czeisler CA, Zimmerman JC, Ronda JM, et al. Timing of REM sleep is coupled to the circadian rhythm of body temperature in man. Sleep 1980;2:329–46.

[88] Zulley J, Campbell SS. Napping behavior during spontaneous internal desynchronization: sleep remains in synchrony with body temperature. Human Neurobiology 1985;4:123–6.

[89] Lavie P. Sleep-wake as a biological rhythm. Annu Rev Psychol 2001;52:277–303.

[90] Lavie P. Ultrashort sleep-waking schedule: III. 'Gates' and 'forbidden zones' for sleep. Electroencephal Clin Neurophysiol 1986;63:414–25.

[91] Strogatz SH. The mathematical structure of the human sleep wake cycle. New York: Springer-Verlag; 1986.

[92] Liu X, Uchiyama M, Shibui K, et al. Diurnal preference, sleep habits, circadian sleep propensity and melatonin rhytm in healthy human subjects. Neurosci Lett 2000;280: 199–202.

[93] Fröberg J. Twenty-four hour patterns in human performance, subjective and physiological variables and differences between morning and evening types. Biol Psychol 1977;5:119–34.

[94] Czeisler CA, Allan JS, Strogatz SH, et al. Bright light resets the human circadian pacemaker independent of the timing of the sleep-wake cycle. Science 1986;233:667–71.

[95] Czeisler CA, Kronauer RE, Allan JS, et al. Bright light induction of strong (type 0) resetting of the human circadian pacemaker. Science 1989;244:1328–33.

[96] Arendt J. Melatonin and the mammalian pineal gland. London: Chapman-Hall; 1995.

[97] Lewy AJ, Ahmed S, Jackson JM, Sack RL. Melatonin shifts human circadian rhythms according to a phase-response curve. Chronobiol Int 1992;9:380–92.

[98] Lavie P. Melatonin: role in gating nocturnal rise in sleep propensity. J Biol Rhythms 1997;12: 657–65.

Clinical and Technologic Approaches to Sleep Evaluation

Max Hirshkowitz, PhD, DABSM[a,b,c,d,*],
Amir Sharafkhaneh, MD, DABSM[b,c,d]

[a]*Department of Psychiatry, Baylor College of Medicine, Houston, Texas, USA*
[b]*Department of Medicine, Baylor College of Medicine, Houston, Texas, USA*
[c]*Houston VAMC Sleep Center, Houston, Texas, USA*
[d]*Methodist Hospital Sleep Diagnostic Laboratory, Houston, Texas, USA*

Background

As our planet rotates its face away from the sun and long shadows are replaced by darkness, most local inhabitants eat their evening meal and prepare for a night's sleep. Depending on the season, a locale's latitude, and individual habits, this major sleep period may last from 5 to 10 hours. During this time, sleepers' bodies cool and mostly are immobile. As with coma, arousal diminishes and individuals become less responsive. Unlike coma, this condition is rapidly reversible with associated impaired cognition fully restored. The behavioral similarity led early theorists to believe sleep, like coma, arose from a passive loss of function and metabolic depression in brainstem and cerebral cortex.

In 1909, Cajal [1] first delineated a network-intermingled collection of nerves and fibers (hence, reticular formation) extending from the spinal cord to the thalamus. Brainstem lesions high up at the midbrain (also called cerveau isole) produce continuous electroencephalogram (EEG) characteristics of sleep. Strong stimulation produces only transient arousals; however, electrical stimulation of the reticular formation produces lasting cortical excitation marked by wakefulness in cerveau isole animals [2]. In contrast, low brainstem lesions transecting at the spinal cord (or so-called "encephale isole") are associated with normal sleep-wake oscillation. Thus, process controllers necessary for wakefulness reside between the spinal cord and the

* Corresponding author. VAMC Sleep Center, 111i 2002 Holcombe Boulevard, Houston, TX 77030.

E-mail address: maxh@bcm.tmc.edu (M. Hirshkowitz).

0733-8619/05/$ - see front matter. Published by Elsevier Inc.
doi:10.1016/j.ncl.2005.08.003

midbrain [3]. But is sleep merely the absence of ascending reticular formation activation? Magoun [4] posited sleep as an active, thalamically mediated state with pacemaker roles in alpha rhythm, sleep spindles, and slow wave synchronization. As research continued, it became clear that sleep was an active brain process. Some sleep processes are so active that cortical metabolism exceeds levels normally observed during wakefulness [5,6].

Indeed, it is the brain that sleeps. Nonetheless, even though the body rests rather than sleeps, some essential body processes (eg, growth hormone release during sleep) occur only when the brain is sleeping. Furthermore, there are qualitatively different types of sleep with different characteristics and functions. Each sleep process has its own homeostatic regulatory system that responds to selective sleep-stage deprivation with sleep-stage specific rebound during recovery. As a brain process, the traditional investigative approach for studying sleep involves measuring brain activity. Thus, it is not surprising that Hans Berger [7], the father of EEG, made the first, albeit brief, sleep recordings. Berger found the predominant alpha EEG activity during wakefulness was replaced by low-voltage, mixed-frequency activity at sleep onset. Alpha cessation marks the transition from wakefulness to sleep in most individuals.

The first continuous overnight EEG sleep recordings in humans were published in 1937 [8]. The tracings on miles of paper recorded with an 8-feet long drum polygraph were summarized using a data reduction scheme called sleep staging (stages A, B, C, D, and E). Staging largely is based on the presence of particular EEG activity. EEG activity includes beta activity (>13 Hz), sleep spindles (bursts of 12–14 Hz), alpha rhythm (8–13 Hz, sometimes slower), theta rhythm (4–7 Hz), saw-tooth theta waves (4–7 Hz, with notched appearance), delta rhythm (<4 Hz), and slow waves (<2 Hz). When illustrated graphically, Loomis's sleep histograms look remarkably similar to what is used today.

The picture of human sleep was rounded out when Aserinsky and Kleitman [9] discovered episodic electro-oculographic (EOG) activity occurring every 90 to 120 minutes during stage B sleep. Initially belittled as a recording artifact, continued efforts verified that actual eye movements were occurring. These jerky eye movements eventually became known as rapid eye movements (REM). Individuals awakened during REM sleep revealed dreaming 74% of the time [9]. Although the sleep EEG correlates of dreaming were established clearly, REM sleep recording as the ultimate laboratory tool to unlock the mysteries of dreaming (by exploring "the royal road to the unconscious") [10] failed to meet researchers lofty expectations.

The final refinement to sleep state description came when Jouvet and colleagues [11] observed postural changes in cats during different sleep states. They verified muscle atonia accompanying REM sleep in normal animals electromyographically (EMG). This functional paralysis, detectable by EMG recording, was the final step toward developing what is now standard recording practice for investigating human sleep stage.

Establishing a standard for describing sleep

Sleep recording technique and sleep-stage scoring varied widely from one laboratory to the next. There were several established systems, including the Dement-Kleitman system and the Williams-Karacan system [12]. Reading the literature, it was sometimes difficult to know precisely how a polysomnogram was recorded, scored, and reduced to summary parameters. Terminology also was variable from one sleep center to the next; for example, REM sleep might be called D-sleep, paradoxic sleep, desynchronized sleep, or even unorthodox sleep. In response to this circumstance, an ad-hoc committee was formed by members of the sleep research society. This group (sometimes referred to as the R&K Committee, after the two editors Drs. Allan Rechtschaffen and Anthony Kales) included a pantheon of scientists and clinicians devoted to understanding human sleep [13]. The group included Ralph J. Berger, William C. Dement, Allan Jacobson, Laverne C. Johnson, Michel Jouvet, Anthony Kales, Lawrence J. Monroe, Ian Oswald, Allan Rechtschaffen, Howard P. Roffwarg, Bedrich Roth, and Richard D. Walter. In 1968, the United States Government Printing Office published a standardized manual. It was reprinted by the Brain Information Service (University of California, Los Angeles) [14].

The key to its success was final agreement and consensus. This is not to say that participants did not disagree heatedly; they did. In the heat of one argument, Rechtschaffen reportedly barred the doors and decreed that no one could leave until they reached consensus. And they did. Indeed, if participants had returned to his laboratory and ignored the guideline in favor of continuing to do things according to their own practice, the project would not have succeeded. The final step for defining normal human sleep was the development, publication, and widespread agreement to use *A Manual of Standardized Terminology, Techniques and Scoring System for Sleep Stages of Human Subjects* [13].

Recording

Sleep stages

Typically 4 to 5 polysomnographic channels are required to record human stages. Traditionally, EEG activity is recorded from central derivations (C3 or C4) as monopolar tracings using a mastoid reference. More recently, an occipital lead was added (O3 or O4) to improve detection of brief central nervous system (CNS) arousals. EOG activity from right and left eye (recorded from the outer canthi) and submentalis EMG also are used to define sleep stage. Each 30 seconds of recording (1 epoch) is categorized as wakefulness (W); as sleep stage 1, 2, 3, 4; or REM. Epoch length was a convention based on paper polygraph tracings. These tracings usually were recorded at a chart speed of 10 mm per second; therefore, each resulting polygraph page was 30 seconds in duration. Although paper polysomnograms mostly have gone the way of the dinosaurs, the practice of 30-second epoch sleep staging continues.

Central nervous system arousals

It is well recognized that alpha activity associated with wakefulness usually is most prominent when recorded from the occipital region. Although Williams and coworkers [12] argued as early as 1973 for including a bipolar occipital lead (O3-OZPZ) as a matter of routine, it was not adopted as standard technique until 1985 for use on the multiple sleep latency test [15] and 1992 for CNS arousal scoring on overnight polysomnograms [16]. Typically, a monopolar mastoid-referenced derivation from O1, O2, O3, or O4 is suggested.

Breathing disorders

With discovery and increasing appreciation of sleep-related breathing disorders (SRBD), polysomnographic monitoring of respiration quickly became routine. The three features of breathing measured during polysomnography are airflow, respiratory effort, and blood oxygenation. SRBD events also usually are correlated with arousals scored from the EEG. A variety of devices is available to record these breathing-related processes using the following common techniques [17].

1. Flow—A minimum of one channel of nasal/oral airflow should be recorded. Qualitative measures of flow can be obtained with thermistors, thermocouples, nasal pressure transducers, capnographs, and microphones. Semiquantitative measures of flow can be made with calibrated inductance plethysmography. Finally, flow can be measured directly using a pneumotach.
2. Effort—A minimum of one channel of respiratory effort should be recorded and can be made with piezoelectric respiratory belts, inductance plethysmography, esophageal pressure devices, or intercostals EMG electrodes.
3. Other—It is standard technique to measure blood oxygenation during polysomnography and to monitor sleeping position as supine, prone, laterally recumbent left, or laterally recumbent right.

Leg movement disorders

To detect flexion, two surface electrodes are placed on each leg on the anterior tibialis muscle 2 to 4 cm apart to detect movement of the great toe, ankle, knee, or hip. Electrode impedance should be between 10,000 to 30,000 ohms. Electrodes can be placed on the gastrocnemius muscle to assist with determining whether or not movement is artifact related; however, most sleep laboratories use only the anterior tibialis electrode placement. Left and right legs should be recorded [18].

Scoring

Sleep stages

In wakefulness (also called stage W or stage 0), the predominant EEG rhythm during eyes-closed wakefulness is alpha activity (Fig. 1). A small percentage of individuals do not have distinct alpha activity. For those recordings, alternative signs of sleep should be considered and ruled out. Differentiating between wakefulness and stage 1 can be difficult. Vertex sharp waves, high-muscle EMG, theta activity, eye movements' appearance (both rapid and slow), and blinking all should be considered when trying to differentiate wakefulness from sleep. Opening the eyes or engaging in a difficult mental task (for example, counting backward by 3's beginning with the number 982) blocks the alpha activity. Sleep-onset epoch is classified when alpha duration decreases to less than 50% of an epoch or a vertex wave, K complex, sleep spindle, or delta activity occurs for the first time in the recording. Alternatively, wakefulness is scored.

Stage 1 sleep is scored when an epoch has low-voltage, mixed-frequency EEG but there are no K complexes, spindles, or REM. Stage 1 sleep is a non-alpha state with EEG activity that has neither delta nor slow waves; however, vertex sharp waves and slow rolling eye movements may be present.

Stage 2 sleep epochs are scored when there are sleep spindles or K complexes, but high-amplitude (75 microvolts or greater) delta EEG activity totals less than 20% of the epoch duration.

Stage 3 is scored when an epoch contains 20% to 50% delta (or slow wave) activity.

Stage 4 is scored when an epoch contains 50% delta (or slow wave) activity.

REM sleep is confirmed when eye movements and muscle atonia accompany a stage 1 EEG pattern. Saw-tooth theta waves are distinctive and often accompany REM sleep. In addition to REM, a wide assortment of physiologic activities can accompany REM sleep, including middle ear muscle

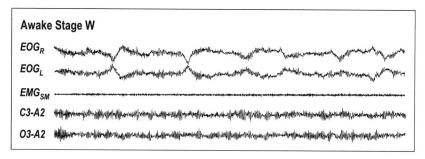

Fig. 1. Wakefulness EEG-EOG-EMG polysomnographic tracings. The figure shows a 30-second tracing of right and left EOGs (EOG$_R$ and EOG$_L$, respectively), submentalis EMG (EMG$_{SM}$), and monopolar central and occipital EEGs (C3-A2 and O3-A2, respectively).

activity, periorbital integrated potentials, and sleep-related erections. In addition to the epochs of REM in which eye movements are plentiful, some REM sleep epochs have few or no eye movements. These two faces of REM sleep are called phasic REM sleep and tonic REM sleep (Fig. 2).

Stages 1, 2, 3, and 4 sometimes are referred to collectively as non-REM (NREM) sleep.

Stages 1 and 2 sometimes are referred to as light sleep, whereas stages 3 and 4 often are combined and called slow wave sleep (SWS) or deep sleep (Figs. 3 and 4). Table 1 summarizes EEG-EOG-EMG characteristics for wakefulness and the different sleep stages.

Central nervous system arousals

Arousal scoring is specific and unambiguous [16]. Nonetheless, "variants" have emerged that rely on EMG or that consider autonomic nervous system activation. The criteria for characterizing CNS arousals from sleep are: (1) arousals are momentary events and occur intermittently; (2) arousals can be scored only in the presence of sleep; (3) arousals differ from awakenings; awakenings are occurrences of EEG alpha activity covering 50% or more of an epoch that immediately follows a recording epoch scored as stage 1, 2, 3, or 4 or REM sleep; (4) arousals can be related to specific events (eg, respiratory events or leg movements) or they may be spontaneous; (5) tonic EEG alpha intrusion into NREM sleep (eg, alpha-delta sleep) should not be scored

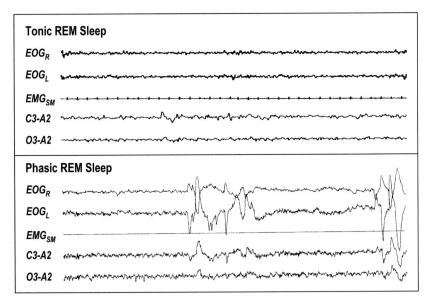

Fig. 2. Tonic and phasic REM sleep EEG-EOG-EMG polysomnographic tracings. Each panel shows a 30-second tracing of right and left EOGs (EOG$_R$ and EOG$_L$, respectively), submentalis EMG (EMG$_{SM}$), and monopolar central and occipital EEGs (C3-A2 and O3-A2, respectively).

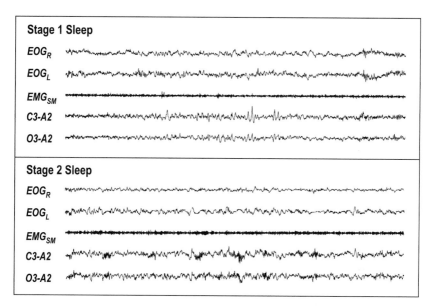

Fig. 3. Light sleep. Stages 1 and 2 EEG-EOG-EMG polysomnographic tracings. Each panel shows a 30-second tracing of right and left EOGs (EOG$_R$ and EOG$_L$, respectively), submentalis EMG (EMG$_{SM}$), and monopolar central and occipital elecroencephalograms (C3-A2 and O3-A2, respectively).

as an arousal; however, an EEG alpha burst after 10 seconds of sleep without the presence of alpha can be scored as an arousal; (6) arousals are based solely on changes in EEG except when they occur during REM sleep. In REM sleep, concomitant increased chin EMG amplitude is required because alpha and theta bursts are common occurrences in REM sleep; (7) arousals are scored in the presence of 10 seconds of uninterrupted sleep of any stage; a second arousal can be scored if there is a minimum of 10 seconds of intervening sleep; (8) scoring criteria require specific presence of a minimum 3-second shift in EEG frequency to score an arousal; (9) when artifact, K complexes, or delta waves are accompanied by a 3-second shift in EEG frequency, these occurrences also are scored as arousals; (10) K complex or delta burst alone does not constitute an arousal; (11) although chin EMG amplitude is not used to score an arousal from NREM sleep, increased chin EMG amplitude often is present; (12) in NREM sleep, a chin EMG increase without accompanying EEG change is not scored as an arousal; and (13) REM sleep arousal criteria require increased chin EMG activity.

Breathing disorders

Apnea

Apnea is a cessation of nasal/oral airflow for 10 seconds or more. Apnea episodes are classified into three categories: (1) obstructive—complete or

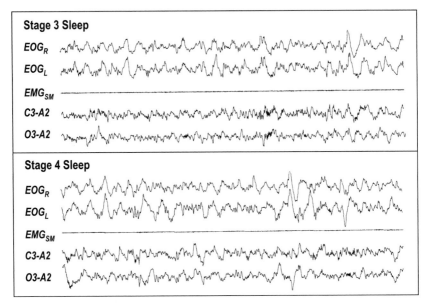

Fig. 4. Slow wave sleep. Stages 3 and 4 EEG-EOG-EMG polysomnographic tracings. Each panel shows a 30-second tracing of right and left EOGs (EOG$_R$ and EOG$_L$, respectively), sub-mentalis EMG (EMG$_{SM}$), and monopolar central and occipital EEGs (C3-A2 and O3-A2, respectively).

near complete cessation of nasal/oral airflow with continued or increased respiratory effort; (2) central—complete or near complete cessation of nasal/oral airflow and respiratory effort; and (3) mixed—a combination of central and obstructive apnea, usually beginning as a central apnea and evolving into an obstructive event.

Hypopnea

In the most general terms, a hypopnea is a shallow breath that represents a decrease in tidal volume. In sleep, hypopneas can be central or obstructive in origin; however, most of the time they are the consequence of partial airway occlusion and increased flow limitation. If a hypopnea is associated with either a disturbance of sleep (arousal, ascending stage shift, or awakening) or a significant oxyhemoglobin desaturation, it is considered pathophysiologic.

As straightforward and logical as these definitions may seem, the definition for hypopnea is controversial. The problem originates with recording technique; that is, the use of qualitative measures of flow that do not provide proportional estimates of tidal volume. Guilleminault's [19] original definition of hypopnea as a reduction in airflow without complete cessation of breathing adhered closely to the general principle but left open the question of how much decrease in airflow was minimally required to score a hypopnea. In 2001, the Clinical Practice Review Committee of the American

Table 1

Electroencephalogram–electro-oculogram–electromyogram characteristics of sleep and wakefulness

Stage	Electroencephalogram characteristics	Electro-oculogram	Electromyogram muscle activity
W	Predominant alpha activity (more than 50% of the epoch) mixed with EEG beta	Slow and rapid	High
1	Alpha activity is replaced by low voltage, mixed-frequency background activity, sometimes with vertex sharp waves	Slow	Decreased from awake
2	Sleep spindles and K complexes in a background EEG that has less than 20% delta activity	None	Decreased from awake
3	Slow wave (EEG delta activity) comprises 20–50% of the epoch; sleep spindles usually are present	None	Decreased from awake
4	More than 50% of the epoch has EEG delta activity	None	Decreased from awake
REM	Low-voltage, mixed-frequency background activity; saw-tooth theta waves may be present	Rapid	Nearly absent

Academy of Sleep Medicine published a definition for hypopnea [20] drawn largely from Sleep Heart Health epidemiologic studies [21] and that was adopted subsequently by Medicare. This definition proclaimed hypopnea as having a 30% reduction from baseline in thoracoabdominal effort or airflow that lasts at least 10 seconds accompanied by a 4% oxygen desaturation. This definition was a radical departure from previous scoring practice in its requirement of desaturation and complete disregard for sleep disturbance by arousal. To avoid confusion, this type of hypopnea can be referred to as a desaturating hypopnea.

Leg movement disorders

Periodic limb movement disorder (PLMD) events are movements in the leg caused by extension of the big toe, sometimes involving flexion of the ankle, knee, and, occasionally, the hip [22].

1. PLMD is scored in the presence of (1) a burst of EMG activity with an amplitude at least 25% or greater than the calibration movement; (2) four consecutive leg movements that are 5 to 90 seconds apart (PLM sequence); (3) leg movements that occur usually in both legs but can occur in only one leg. If movements occur in both legs, they must be separated by at least 5 seconds to be scored as a separate movement; and (4)

a duration between each burst of EMG activity that must be 0.5 seconds but less than 5 seconds; events can be terminated with arousal [17].

2. Leg movements must be distinguished from (1) sleep starts, (2) REM extremity movements, (3) phasic EMG activity, (4) fragmentary myoclonus, and (5) restless legs activity.

Interpreting results

Sleep stages

Overall pattern

Healthy young adult good sleepers spend 7 to 8 hours in bed and sleep 85% to 90% of that time. Good sleepers may have only 5% total awake time or less. Usually it takes less than 15 minutes to fall asleep and nocturnal awakenings are few and brief. Stage 2 sleep accounts for approximately 50% of the night's sleep and REM sleep accounts for another 20% to 25% [23]. Stage 1 sleep is minimal, comprising less than 5% of total sleep time, and is distributed mostly at the wakefulness-sleep transition and at light sleep transitions. SWS stages 3 and 4 make up the remainder of the sleep time. Young adult men and women do not differ much in sleep-stage percentages; however, women may have slightly more SWS. The normal sleep pattern is to transition from wakefulness to NREM sleep, usually stage 1 or 2. NREM and REM sleep then alternate with an overall cycle time of approximately 90 to 120 minutes. SWS is predominant in the first third of the night, whereas REM sleep is more plentiful in the last half of the night. REM sleep occurs episodically, usually with the early episodes short and becoming progressively longer as the night continues. Overall, there may be 4 to 6 discrete REM sleep episodes each night, with episodes generally lengthening as sleep period progresses. Stages do not occur in single long blocks; rather, there is a pattern involving repeated 90- to 120-minute–long cycles of NREM and REM sleep. With each cycle recurrence, there usually are systematic alterations in cycle properties (for example, decreasing SWS and increasing REM sleep duration). Sleep architecture refers to sleep's continuity and progression through the cycles on a given night. Fig. 5 shows a typical night with normal sleep architecture in a healthy young adult.

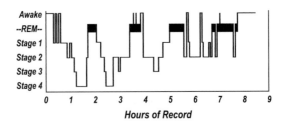

Fig. 5. Sleep architecture and composition in a normal, healthy young adult.

Sleep changes as a function of age

Overall total sleep time gradually declines. Aging, especially after middle age, is associated with increasing fragmentation in the form of arousals and awakenings. The elderly spend more time in bed but less time sleeping. SWS begins declining after adolescence and continues with advancing age, sometimes disappearing completely. REM sleep duration changes dramatically during the first few decades of life [24], decreasing from more than 50% at birth to 20% to 25% at adolescence. From adolescence until age 65, REM sleep remains stable and after 65 years, it may decline further. Sleep disturbances produced by pathophysiology (for example, arousals from sleep apnea) generally increase with age and account for poor sleep in many elders. Alternatively, some age-related sleep pattern deterioration may relate more directly to the aging process and not other factors that may affect sleep adversely.

Normal values

Data presented in this article were recorded as part of various prospective research projects. Table 2 shows first laboratory night polysomnographic results for subjects divided into five nonoverlapping age groups. All subjects were normal healthy volunteers. Informed consent was obtained from each subject. Subjects were recruited through media advertising, health fairs, posters, and referral channels.

Central nervous system arousals

Although there are no normative data concerning CNS arousals, many clinicians regard more than 10 or 15 arousals per hour of sleep as clinically significant. Often these arousals occur in conjunction with other pathophysiologic sleep events (eg, sleep apnea episodes). Sleep disturbance, in the form of arousals, adversely affect daytime function, produces sleep rebound on recovery, and increases daytime sleepiness and fatigue.

Breathing disorders

The understanding of sleep and breathing pathophysiology continues to evolve. Medicare used to consider 30 episodes of sleep apnea as the cutting score for SRBD. More recently, Medicare has recognized hypopneas (with oxygen desaturations) as clinically significant and lowered the positive airway pressure treatment criteria to 5 or more per hour of sleep when sleepiness or significant comorbidities are present and to 15 or more per hour in otherwise healthy, asymptomatic individuals. The latest criteria from the American Academy of Sleep Medicine [25] uses an index that includes apnea, hypopnea, and respiratory events provoking arousal and sets the cutting score at 5 or more events per hour of sleep in symptomatic and 15 or more in asymptomatic patients (down from 10 and 30, respectively). The increasing knowledge

Table 2
Normative sleep values for first night sleeping in the laboratory

| | Age group (number of subjects) | | | | | | | | | |
| | 20–29 years (N = 44) | | 30–39 years (N = 23) | | 40–49 years (N = 49) | | 50–59 years (N = 41) | | ≥ 60 years (N = 29) | |
	Mean	SD	Mean	SD	Mean	SD	Mean	SD	Mean	SD
General, sleep continuity, and integrity measures										
Time in bed (minutes)	404.9	44.1	393.1	58.2	404.2	49.4	393.0	51.1	395.7	42.8
Sleep latency (minutes)	11.8	13.1	13.4	10.1	14.2	14.0	8.7	11.4	15.3	14.9
Total sleep time (minutes)	347.3	62.5	340.0	70.8	329.4	54.6	331.6	63.6	298.4	61.3
Sleep efficiency index[a]	86.2	14.2	86.4	11.6	81.7	10.8	84.3	11.1	75.4	13.2
Latency to arising (minutes)	2.0	7.7	9.7	22.7	7.1	22.2	4.3	11.1	4.2	9.8
Number of awakenings	9.6	8.2	7.7	4.2	11.6	5.3	11.4	4.5	14.1	6.7
Awakenings per hour	1.5	1.2	1.3	0.8	1.8	0.8	1.8	0.7	2.2	1.0
Number of sleep stage shifts	47.1	23.6	39.9	11.8	46.7	18.8	46.3	12.7	50.8	21.9
NREM sleep-stage percentages										
Stage 1 percentage of time in bed	4.1	3.0	3.4	2.1	5.4	3.3	5.5	3.0	6.1	3.5
Stage 2 percentage of time in bed	48.7	9.2	49.7	10.1	51.8	11.7	54.2	10.2	51.0	9.1
Stage 3 percentage of time in bed	3.4	1.9	4.3	1.9	2.9	2.4	3.0	2.4	2.5	2.3
Stage 4 percentage of time in bed	12.1	5.4	10.9	5.4	5.7	6.5	4.1	5.6	2.6	3.4
REM sleep measures										
REM sleep percentage of time in bed	17.8	7.1	18.2	7.9	15.8	6.4	17.6	5.9	13.2	5.7
REM sleep episodes (number)	3.3	1.0	3.4	1.0	3.5	0.9	3.8	0.9	3.6	1.3
REMSE duration (minutes)	77.0	31.2	79.5	40.7	74.2	33.7	78.7	32.6	59.2	26.8
Mean REMSE duration (minutes)	23.1	8.4	23.6	14.1	21.1	7.1	20.3	6.3	16.3	6.5
REM Sleep Efficiency Index	91.0	18.7	93.4	8.7	88.1	11.1	89.7	10.7	90.3	12.1

Abbreviations: REM Sleep Efficiency Index, total REM sleep time percentage of total REM sleep episodes duration; REMSE, REM sleep episode.
[a] Sleep efficiency is total sleep time percentage of time in bed.

of odds ratios for cardiovascular disease continues to refine the understanding of risks posed by sleep-disordered breathing.

Leg movement disorders

Normative data and comorbidity risk ratios are not available for periodic leg movement disorder. Therefore, clinical judgment reigns. Many clinicians treat PLMD when the leg movement arousal index exceeds 10 or 15 per hour. Restless leg treatment likewise depends on clinical impression of severity and adverse affect on a patient's functioning. Systematic data are sorely needed to help establish evidence-based clinical algorithms for these disorders.

When things go awry: abnormal sleep

Three basic mechanisms coordinate sleep and wakefulness: (1) autonomic nervous system balance, (2) homeostatic sleep drive, and (3) circadian rhythms. These mechanisms maintain sleep and wakefulness in a dynamic balance and allow adaptation to sudden shifts in the timing and duration of sleep.

In general, anything that increases sympathetic outflow can disturb sleep. Additionally, sympathetic activation occurs rapidly but dissipates slowly. Finally, the autonomic process of sleep onset is amenable to classical conditioning. Conditioning sleep onset sometimes occurs inadvertently. A bed, pillow, blanket (or stuffed animal toy for children) may become a conditioned stimulus for sleep onset. Or, by contrast, a bedroom stimulus may cue an alerting response (producing psychophysiologic insomnia). Similarly, if a parent becomes a child's stimulus cue for sleep onset, parents may find themselves having to rock the baby back to sleep at any and all times of the night.

In general, the longer individuals remain awake, the sleepier they become. Homeostatic regulation of sleepiness is similar to that for thirst, hunger, and sex [26]. During extended wakefulness, however, sleepiness waxes and wanes. Sometimes, after staying up all night, persons note a surge of energy at daybreak. Although they have been awake longer, they feel less sleepy than at 5:00 AM. This violation in homeostasis reveals another factor governing sleep and wakefulness: the circadian rhythm.

Understanding what constitutes normal sleep is essential to recognizing and assessing the severity of abnormal sleep. Although better normative data are needed, sleep disturbances can be evaluated objectively and assessed quantitatively. Distinct pathophysiology leading to sleep alteration (for example, sleep-disordered, breathing-provoking awakenings) is one way disorders affect sleep adversely. Other sleep disorders arise from defective or impaired mechanisms that regulate and govern sleep. For example, a weak homeostatic drive for sleep likely produces chronic insomnia, whereas the intrusion of REM sleep phenomena into the waking state underlies narcolepsy.

In this article, normal human sleep is discussed. Discoveries leading to an understanding of human sleep, EEG definitions, and general characteristics of normal human sleep are presented. Actuarial data for a first laboratory night are presented. Finally, the mechanisms governing sleep and wakefulness are reviewed and a model of normal sleep mechanisms going awry is outlined as an aid for understanding abnormal sleep associated with sleep disorders.

References

[1] Cajal RS. Histologie du systeme nerveux de l'homme et des vertebres. Paris: Norbert Maloine; 1909.

[2] Moruzzi G, Magoun HW. Brain stem reticular formation and activation of EEG. EEG Clin Neurophysiol 1949;1:455–73.

[3] Bremmer F. Cerveau isole et physiologie du sommeil. Comp Rendus Seanes Soc Biol Filiales 1935;118:1235–41.

[4] Magoun HW. Central neural inhibition. In: Jones MR, editor. Nebraska symposium on motivation. Lincoln (NE): University of Nebraska Press; 1963. p. 161–93.

[5] Kleitman N. Sleep and wakefulness. 2nd edition. Chicago: University of Chicago; 1972.

[6] Chase MH, editor. The sleeping brain. Los Angeles: Brain Information Service/Brain Research Institute, UCLA; 1972.

[7] Berger H. Ueber das elektroenkephalogramm des menschen. J Psychol Neurol 1930;40: 160–79.

[8] Loomis AL, Harvey N, Hobart GA. Cerebral states during sleep, as studied by human brain potentials. J Exp Psychol 1937;21:127–44.

[9] Aserinsky E, Kleitman N. Regularly occurring periods of eye motility, and concomitant phenomena. Science 1953;118:273–4.

[10] Freud S. The interpretation of dreams. New York: Random House; 1950.

[11] Jouvet M, Michel F, Courjon J. Sur un stade d'activite electrique cerebrale rapide au cours du sommeil physiologique. C R Soc Biol (Paris) 1959;153:1024–8.

[12] Williams RL, Karacan I, Hursch CJ. EEG of human sleep: clinical applications. New York: Wiley; 1974.

[13] Rechtschaffen A, Kales A, editors. A manual of standardized terminology, techniques and scoring system for sleep stages of human subjects. Washington, DC: US Government Printing Office; 1968. NIH publication no. 204.

[14] Rechtschaffen A, Kales A, editors. A manual of standardized terminology, techniques and scoring system for sleep stages of human subjects. Brain Information Service, University of California, Los Angeles, 1968.

[15] Carskadon MA, Dement WC, Mitler MM, et al. Guidelines for the multiple sleep latency test (MSLT): a standard measure of sleepiness. Sleep 1986;9:519–24.

[16] Sleep Disorders Atlas Task Force. EEG arousals: scoring rules and examples—a preliminary report from the Sleep Disorders Atlas Task Force of the American Sleep Disorders Association. Sleep 1992;15:173–84.

[17] Hirshkowitz M, Kryger MH. Monitoring techniques for evaluating suspected sleep-disordered breathing in adults. In: Kryger MH, Roth T, Dement WC, editors. Principles and practice of sleep medicine. 4th edition. Philadelphia: Saunders; 2005.

[18] Sleep Disorders Atlas Task Force. Recording and scoring leg movements. Sleep 1993;16: 748–59.

[19] Guilleminault C. Sleeping and waking disorders: indications and techniques. Menlo Park (CA): Addison-Wesley; 1982.

[20] Clinical Practice Review Committee. Position paper: hypopnea sleep disorders breathing in adults. Sleep 2001;24:469–70.

[21] Iber C, Redline S, Kaplan Gilpin AM, et al. Polysomnography performed in the unattended home versus the attended laboratory setting—Sleep Heart Health Study methodology. Sleep 2004;27:536–40.

[22] Chesson AL, Wise M, Davila D, et al. Practice parameters for the treatment of restless legs syndrome and periodic limb movement disorder. Sleep 1999;22:961–8.

[23] Hirshkowitz M. Normal human sleep: an overview. Med Clin North Am 2004;88:551–65.

[24] Roffwarg HP, Muzio JN, Dement WC. Ontogenetic development of the human sleep-dream cycle. Science 1966;152:604–19.

[25] Kushida CA, Littner MR, Morgenthaler T, et al. Practice parameters for the indication for polysomnography and related procedures: an update for 2005. Sleep 2005;28:499–521.

[26] Horne J. Why we sleep. Oxford (United Kingdom): Oxford University Press; 1988.

NEUROLOGIC
CLINICS

Neurol Clin 23 (2005) 1007–1024

Sleep and the Gastrointestinal Tract

William C. Orr, PhD[a],*, Chien Lin Chen, MD[b]

[a]Lynn Health Science Institute, Oklahoma University Health Science Center,
5300 North Independence Avenue, Suite 130, Oklahoma City, OK 73112, USA
[b]Tzu Chi University Hospital and Medical School, 707, Sec 3,
Chung-Yang Road, Huclien 970, Taiwan

Recent advances in the study of sleep have elucidated marked alterations in respiratory and hormonal functioning during sleep, and major health consequences attributable to sleep restriction or deprivation. These discoveries have led to a remarkable broadening of the focus and importance of the applications of basic sleep physiology to many areas of clinical medicine. Lagging somewhat behind these developments is the description of gastrointestinal (GI) functioning during sleep and possible applications of these changes to clinical medicine. Perhaps the most obvious reason for this is the relative inaccessibility of the GI tract to easy study during sleep. As a result of advances in measurement techniques, there has been a marked increase in studies describing alterations in GI functioning during sleep and the specific applications of these changes to the practice of gastroenterology.

Upper gastrointestinal functioning during sleep

Gastroesophageal reflux

The most common and familiar problem related to the upper GI system is gastroesophageal reflux (GER) and its most common symptom, heartburn. GER is a common postprandial event and is a normal physiologic response to gastric distention, which induces a transient relaxation of the lower esophageal sphincter. Heartburn and regurgitation are the most common symptoms of esophageal mucosal contact. Because the sensation of heartburn is a waking conscious experience and many reflux events do not necessarily produce a symptom, the actual occurrence of GER during sleep

---

* Corresponding author.
E-mail address: worr@lhsi.net (W.C. Orr).

is difficult to estimate by symptoms alone. GER does occur during sleep, as documented by recent studies, but it is less common than that which occurs in the waking stage [1]. Several studies that involve the use of 24-hour esophageal pH monitoring establish that GER occurs less commonly during the sleeping interval and generally is associated with the prolongation of acid clearance [1–3]. As noted in Fig. 1, waking reflux generally is post prandial and reflux events are cleared rapidly (1–2 minutes). During sleep, however, reflux events are less frequent and generally associated with a longer period of acid contact time (Fig. 2). Subsequent studies from the authors' laboratory confirm these findings, demonstrating that the complications of reflux that result in discontinuity of the esophageal mucosa generally are associated with an increase in the percent of supine (during the sleeping interval) GER [2]. The pattern of GER is different, and the occurrence of acid mucosal contact during sleep seems to be associated with esophageal complications. What are the sleep-related physiologic alterations that facilitate this prolongation of acid mucosal contact?

Many responses are associated with acid mucosal contact in the human esophagus, including secretory, motor, and sensory responses (Fig. 3). Typically, acidification of the distal esophagus produces a marked increase in the secretion and bicarbonate concentration of saliva. This allows ample buffering potential to neutralize the acidic lining of the distal esophagus. Also, in response to an acidic distal esophagus, there is a marked increase in the rate of swallowing, which allows the delivery of the potent buffer of saliva into the distal esophagus. Swallowing and the subsequent primary peristaltic contractions of the esophagus allow the rapid removal of large volumes of refluxate from the distal esophagus. Finally, acid mucosal contact is associated with a sensation of substernal burning, which is perceived as uncomfortable or painful. These responses are determined to be present in normal waking individuals and it is immediately obvious that swallowing and the experience of heartburn generally are assumed to be

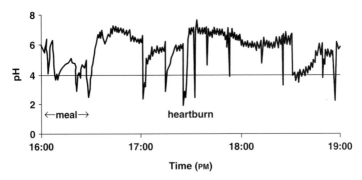

Fig. 1. Normal postprandial GER as noted by drop in the distal esophageal sensor to below 4.0. (See text for description.)

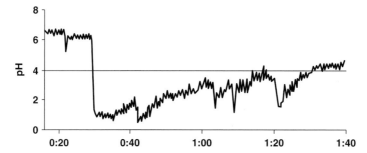

Fig. 2. Sleep-related GER in a patient who has reflux esophagitis. Note the drop in the distal esophageal pH to below 4.0 and the prolongation of the time to restore the pH to 4.0. (See text for description.)

waking conscious phenomena. The combination of these responses typically results in a rapid clearance of esophageal volume of reflux gastric contents and neutralization of the acidic mucosa. The dependence of this rapid acid clearance response on at least two waking, conscious responses logically raises the question of how these responses may be altered during sleep.

The characteristic responses to acid mucosal contact in the waking state (discussed previously) generally are absent during sleep (Fig. 4). It is these alterations in response to acid mucosal contact during sleep that result in the marked prolongation of acid clearance noted during sleep. The simple infusion of acid into the distal esophagus during polygraphically monitored sleep results in a highly significant prolongation of acid clearance time compared with infusions in the supine waking state [3]. Adding to the risks associated with reflux during sleep is the fact that the swallowing rate is diminished markedly, and salivary flow essentially is absent. Heartburn is a waking conscious phenomenon not noted absent during sleep. Thus, the combination of these alterations in acid mucosal response associated with

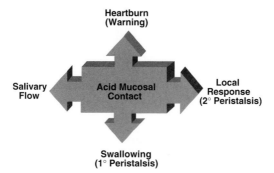

Fig. 3. Schematic diagram of normal responses to esophageal acid mucosal contact. (See text for description.)

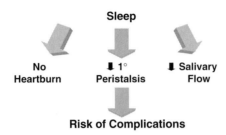

Fig. 4. Schematic diagram of changes in responses to acid mucosal contact during sleep.

sleep establishes a significant risk for the prolongation of acid mucosal contact during sleep.

The prolongation of acid mucosal contact carries significant risks. For example, the back diffusion of hydrogen ions into the esophageal mucosa is related directly to the duration of esophageal acid contact time (Fig. 5). Extrapolating from this, brief and rapidly cleared episodes of reflux seem to be relatively benign, whereas more prolonged episodes of GER are associated with a greater risk of mucosal damage. An additional risk of prolonged acid mucosal contact relates to the higher risk of the proximal migration and eventual spillover of reflux gastric contents into the tracheobronchial tree. In a study by Orr and colleagues, small (1 mL and 3 mL) volumes of acid were instilled into the esophagus during supine waking and sleep to evaluate the proximal migration of acid infused into the distal esophagus during sleep [4]. Esophageal pH sensors were located in the distal and proximal esophagus, and proximal migration was assessed by a drop in the pH in the proximal sensor subsequent to the infusion of acid. It was noted that in the awake supine position, none of the normal volunteers studied showed evidence of proximal migration of 1 mL. During sleep,

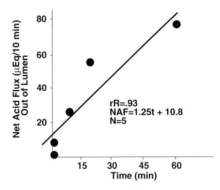

Fig. 5. Relationship of hydrogen ion back diffusion into the esophageal mucosa as a function of mucosal contact time. (*From* Johnson LF, Harmon JW. Experimental esophagitis in a rabbit model. Clinical relevance. J Clin Gastroenterol 1986;8[Suppl 1]:26–44; with permission.)

however, 40% of these same individuals showed evidence of proximal migration of acid infused into the distal esophagus during polygraphically determined non–rapid eye movement (NREM) sleep.

Thus, it can be concluded from these data that sleep itself induces considerable risk of prolonged acid mucosal contact and facilitates the occurrence of a proximal migration of refluxed gastric contents. Maintaining sleep in response to an episode of GER seems to be a maladaptive response, because an arousal from sleep is required to produce a more rapid clearance from a sleep-related reflux event. The complications of nighttime reflux are significant in that nighttime GER can lead to the development of esophagitis and other complications, such as exacerbation of bronchial asthma, chronic cough, and sleep complaints. These complications seem to be related primarily to the presence of significant nighttime reflux and the consequent prolongation of esophageal acid clearance. Of particular interest to sleep clinicians are studies done in patients who have obstructive sleep apnea. The frequent occurrence of obesity and the appreciable negative intrathoracic pressures associated with upper airway obstruction are risk factors for the occurrence of nighttime GER. Although studies do not indicate that there is a specific relationship between obstructive events and reflux events, patients tend to have an overall increase in esophageal acid contact time. Other studies show that a reduction in obstructive events, via appropriate continuous positive airway pressure treatment, results in an associated significant reduction in heartburn complaints [5,6].

Clinical manifestations of nighttime gastroesophageal reflux

Patients who have nighttime heartburn have several complaints related to disturbed sleep [7]. In addition to documenting the presence of sleep complaints, studies document the fact that in patients who have daytime and nighttime heartburn, the nighttime heartburn was significantly more bothersome. More than 50% of these individuals complained that nighttime heartburn awakened them with GER disease (GERD) symptoms, and approximately 30% were awakened by coughing and choking as a result of regurgitation. Approximately 40% of the patients who had nighttime symptoms noted that their heartburn affected their ability to function the next day and approximately 60% indicated it affected their mood. The use of sleeping pills also was increased substantially in patients who had nighttime GERD symptoms.

Nighttime GER is associated with several respiratory symptoms, such as wheezing, chronic cough, and hoarseness. Not uncommonly, patients who have GERD-related asthma or chronic cough do not have heartburn as a symptom. Thus, the presence of nighttime reflux cannot be ruled out on the basis of a negative history of nighttime heartburn. Nighttime wheezing is common in asthmatics, and approximately 41% of asthmatic patients have reflux-associated respiratory symptoms [8]. Additional support for this association is noted in an epidemiology study [9] that demonstrates that individuals who reported nighttime heartburn at least twice a week had an odds ratio of 2.0 for associated respiratory symptoms, such as coughing and wheezing. In addition, the investigators noted that nighttime heartburn is an independent risk factor for sleep complaints and daytime sleepiness.

Gastric functioning during sleep

Acid secretion

Gastric acid secretion is shown to exhibit a clear circadian rhythm, initially described by Sandweiss and colleagues [10]. It remained, however, for Moore and Englert to provide a definitive description of the circadian oscillation of gastric acid secretion in normal subjects [11]. These investigators described a peak in acid secretion occurring generally between 10 PM and 2 AM while confirming already established data that indicated that basal acid secretion in the waking state is minimal in the absence of meal stimulation. Similar results are described in patients who have duodenal ulcer (DU) disease with levels of acid secretion enhanced markedly throughout the circadian cycle [12,13]. It is clear from these results that there is an endogenous circadian rhythm of unstimulated basal acid secretion, but it is not clear that this is altered specifically in any way by sleep.

An interest in the pathogenesis of DU disease and the possible role of nocturnal gastric acid secretion in this process was stimulated further by studies by Dragstedt and Levin and coworkers [12–15]. They analyzed hourly samples of acid secretion in normal subjects and patients who had DU disease, and they identified nearly continuous acid secretion throughout the night in normal volunteers. In contrast to the normal subjects, there were increases in volume and acid concentration during sleep in patients who had DU disease. They found that the patients who had DU disease who tended to be high secreters were consistently high, and those who were low secreters were consistently low. These studies paved the way for more extensive investigations into the role of nocturnal acid secretion in the pathogenesis of DU disease. This study is at variance with the study by Sandweiss and coworkers [10], which did not find a substantial difference in nocturnal acid secretion between normal subjects and patients who had DU. These discrepant results may be the result of varying degrees of ulcer activity in the patients studied. Using hourly collections of overnight acid secretion in normal subjects and in patients who had DU disease, Dragstedt reports that the nocturnal acid secretion in patients who have DU disease is 3 to 20 times greater than that in normal subjects [14]. He reports that this greater secretion was abolished by vagotomy, which invariably produced prompt ulcer healing. These data were interpreted to be strong evidence in favor of a nervous origin for DU disease.

A subsequent study by Armstrong and colleagues reports the startling finding of a hypersecretion of acid during REM sleep in patients who have

DU disease [16]. A major problem in these early investigations was the relatively small data sample per subject, in most cases only a single night. Earlier studies document the considerable night-to-night variability in acid secretion [12–14]. Thus, studying patients or normal volunteers for a single night with a nasogastric tube undoubtedly would result in several awakenings and generally poor sleep, with correspondingly more variable acid secretion.

Stacher and coworkers [17] studied gastric acid secretion in a group of normal volunteers during polysomnographically (PSG)-monitored sleep. They report no significant differences in acid secretion during the NREM stages of sleep; however, they report that REM sleep was associated with an inhibition of acid secretion. This study used a cumbersome technique for determining acid output. It was measured by an intragastric titration from a telemetric pH capsule and involved many disruptions in the patients' sleep. Although it was natural sleep, it was by no means uninterrupted or spontaneous sleep.

The variability of these results and the various methodologic problems of previous studies prompted a study of normal subjects and patients who had DU disease. Orr and colleagues [18] studied five normal volunteers and five patients who had DU disease; each subject was studied for 5 consecutive nights in the sleep laboratory. The study involved continuous aspiration of gastric contents divided into 20-minute aliquots for gastric analysis and complete PSG monitoring for the determination of sleep stages. In addition, serum gastrin levels were assessed at 20-minute intervals throughout the study. The results did not reveal any significant correlation between the sleep stage (REM versus NREM) and acid concentration or total acid secretion. Furthermore, there was no relationship between any of these variables and serum gastrin levels. These data did show, however, that the patients who had DU failed to inhibit acid secretion during the first 2 hours of sleep, which was consistent with the previously reported studies by Levin and coworkers [12]. These studies suggested that acid secretion is poorly inhibited during sleep in patients who have DU disease.

In conclusion, the data support the presence of a clear-cut circadian rhythm in basal acid secretion, with a peak occurring in the early part of the normal sleep interval. There are no definitive data at the present time, however, that suggest a major effect of sleep stages on this process. If one conclusion can be drawn from the various studies assessing gastric acid secretion during sleep, it is that acid secretion is extremely variable from night to night and from person to person and for this reason, definitive conclusions require many replications across and within a large number of subjects and patients.

Motor function

The motor function of the stomach serves to empty solids and liquids into the duodenum at an appropriate rate and pH. The stomach is divided functionally into two sections: the fundus of the stomach functions primarily to control liquid emptying into the duodenum, whereas the antrum controls emptying of solids [19]. Because the stomach handles liquids and solids differently, the regulation of gastric emptying is correspondingly complicated, involving intrinsic regulation of motor activity and specific alterations associated with the ingestion of liquids and solids. Thus, although gastric emptying itself can be regarded as the final common pathway reflecting the motor activity of the stomach, the processes of liquid and solid emptying are regulated by different mechanisms.

There are reports of gastric motility during sleep, with contradictory results. Inhibition of gastric motility during sleep was documented in a study by Scantlebury and colleagues [20], in which they implicated the "dream mechanism" as a part of this inhibitory process. Nearly 30 years later, using somewhat more sophisticated measurement techniques, Bloom and co-workers [21] found that gastric motility was enhanced during sleep, compared with waking. Baust and Rohrwasser [22] studied gastric motility during PSG-monitored sleep, and they also described a marked enhancement in gastric motility during sleep, but their findings were restricted to REM sleep. Only a year later, a decrease in gastric motility during REM sleep was reported [23]. No consistent findings concerning alterations by sleep stage were noted in a study of unanesthetized and unrestrained cats [24].

Hall and colleagues [25] report data on gastric emptying during sleep. This study required patients to sleep with a nasogastric tube through which 750 mL of 10% glucose was administered. After 30 minutes, the gastric contents were aspirated, and the residual volume was determined. Aspiration was followed by a washout meal of 150 mL of saline. This process was done during the presleep waking interval, during NREM and REM sleep, and during postsleep waking. These data suggest a more rapid gastric emptying during REM sleep and a slower emptying during the postsleep waking state. The emptying of a hypertonic solution is controlled by vagally mediated osmoreceptors in the duodenum. These data, therefore, suggest a possible anticholinergic action during REM and a cholinergic process during the postsleep waking state. These data represent only an approximation of the alterations in gastric emptying during sleep because these measurement techniques are relatively crude, and gastric emptying is a complex process.

Dubois and coworkers [26] describe a technique that permits the simultaneous assessment of acid secretion, water secretion, and the fractional rate of emptying. These techniques have been applied to the assessment of gastric functioning during sleep; the results indicate that in normal subjects, acid secretion, water secretion, and the fractional rate of emptying showed significant decrements during sleep [27]. There did not seem to be any differences between REM and NREM sleep, but these measures demonstrate a significant difference between presleep waking and REM sleep. Data obtained by use of radionuclide emptying assessments suggest that this difference may be a circadian, rather than a sleep-dependent, effect. Studies by Goo and coworkers [28] show a marked delay in gastric emptying of solids in the evenings compared with mornings.

Gastric motor functioning is characterized by an endogenous electrical cycle generated by the gastric smooth muscle. The electrical rhythm is generated by a pacemaker located in the proximal portion of the greater curvature of the stomach [29–31]. The electrical cycle occurs at a frequency of approximately 3 per minute and represents the precursor to contractile activity of the stomach, which allows movement of gastric contents to the antrum and subsequent emptying into the duodenum. The noninvasive measurement of the gastric electrical rhythm is called electrogastrography. The progressive sophistication of the measurement and analytic techniques allows a reliable noninvasive technique to measure an important function of the GI system and is a more practical measure of determining gastric function during sleep.

It generally is believed that the gastric electrical rhythm is a product of the endogenous functioning of the gastric electrical pacemaker and that it is generally without influence from the CNS. Sleep studies from the authors' laboratory, however, challenge this traditional belief. Initially, the authors' studies showed a significant decline in the power in the 3-per-minute cycle during NREM sleep [32]. There is a significant recovery of this toward the waking state during REM sleep. Further preliminary data from the laboratory describe a profound instability in the functioning of the basic electrical cycle during NREM sleep [33]. These two studies suggest that NREM sleep is associated with a marked alteration or destabilization of the basic gastric electrical rhythm. It might be concluded from these results that higher cortical input or a degree of CNS arousal must be present to stabilize and promote normal gastric functioning and consequently normal gastric emptying.

Definitive statements concerning the alteration of gastric motor function and gastric emptying during sleep or specific sleep stages cannot be made. It would have to be concluded that gastric motor function seems to be retarded during sleep, but it is not clear if this is specifically the result of altered gastric emptying attributable to sleep or simply a natural circadian rhythm independent of sleep.

Intestinal function during sleep

Intestinal motility

The primary functions of the small and large intestine are transport and absorption. These functions are related intimately in that, for example, rapid transit through the colon results in poor absorption and loose, watery stools, whereas slow transit results in increased water absorption, slow transit of fecal material to the rectum, and the clinical consequence of infrequent defecation and complaints of constipation. Alterations in the motor function of the lower bowel are evident from clinical phenomena, such as the occurrence of nocturnal diarrhea in diabetics and nocturnal fecal incontinence, commonly noted in patients who have ileoanal anastomosis [34].

Observational techniques initially described the differences in intestinal motility during waking and sleep [35–38]. These observations report no change in intestinal motility during sleep.

Prolonged monitoring of the large and small bowel has allowed a more comprehensive description of intestinal motor activity during waking and sleep. On the basis of these studies, tonic activity in the stomach and small bowel is described as a basic electrical rhythm and as more phasic phenomena, such as the migrating motor complex (MMC), which is a wave of intestinal contraction beginning in the stomach and proceeding through the colon. The MMC consists of a dependent pattern of interdigestive motor phenomena. Subsequent to food ingestion, there is an interval of motor quiescence termed phase I. This is followed by a period of somewhat random contractions throughout the small bowel called phase II. Phase III describes a coordinated peristaltic burst of contractile activity that proceeds distally throughout the small bowel. Food ingestion establishes a pattern of vigorous contraction throughout the distal stomach and small bowel. If no food enters the stomach, the MMC cycle has a period of approximately 90 minutes [39–41].

In a study by Soffer and colleagues, the activity of the MMC subsequent to a meal was assessed during waking and during subsequent sleep [39]. They conclude that postprandial intestinal motor activity was altered substantially by sleep, primarily a reduction in the fed pattern of intestinal motility. The investigators note that responses were similar to those described after vagotomy in the waking state, suggesting that reduced levels of arousal result in diminished vagal modulation of the small bowel.

Archer and colleagues [40] describe jejunal motor activity in 20 normal subjects during sleeping and waking and find no difference in the incidence of motor complexes. Thompson and Wingate [41] find that sleep prolonged the interval between motor complexes in the small intestine. A subsequent study by the same group reveals a sleep-related diminution in the number of contractions of a specific type in the jejunum [42]. These changes also were seen in patients who had DU and vagotomies and in normal subjects, which suggests that this phenomenon is independent of vagal control and unaffected by duodenal disease.

Finch and coworkers [43] address the issue of the alteration of the MMC during sleep. Their results show a statistically significant relationship between REM sleep and the onset of MMCs originating in the duodenum [43]. Kumar and coworkers [44] describe an obvious circadian rhythm in the propagation of the MMC, with the slowest velocities occurring during sleep. This finding seems to be the effect of a circadian rhythm rather than a true modulation by sleep. These results are confirmed by Kellow and coworkers [45], who also note that the esophageal involvement in the MMC decreases during sleep, with a corresponding tendency for MMCs to originate in the jejunum at night. Kumar and colleagues [46] examined the relationship between the MMC cycle and REM sleep. They find that during sleep, there was a significant reduction in the MMC cycle length and duration of phase II of the MMC. The MMCs were distributed equally between REM and NREM sleep with no obvious alteration in the parameters of the MMC by sleep stage. These data give evidence of alteration in periodic activity in the gut during sleep, but they also are consistent with the notion that the two cycles (ie, MMCs and REM sleep) are independent. The same group of investigators examined how the presence or absence of food in the GI tract alters small bowel motility during sleep [47]. A late evening meal restored phase II activity of the MMC, normally absent during sleep. These MMC changes during the sleeping interval are confirmed substantially by subsequent ambulatory studies but without the benefit of PSG [48,49].

Sleep, intestinal motility, and symptoms of abdominal pain have been studied in patients who had irritable bowel syndrome (IBS). Kellow and coworkers [50] find striking differences between sleeping and waking small bowel motor activity. The marked increase in contractility seen in the daytime was notably absent during sleep. In a related study, Kellow and coworkers [51] note that propulsive clusters of small bowel motility were enhanced somewhat in the daytime in patients who had IBS, and this distinguished them from controls. Patients often had pain associated with these propulsive contractions, but there was no difference in small bowel activity between patients who had IBS and controls during sleep. Kumar and colleagues describe an increase in REM sleep in patients who had IBS [52]. They propose that this is evidence of a CNS abnormality in patients who have this complex, enigmatic disorder.

With the development of more sophisticated electronic measuring and recording techniques, more accurate measures of intestinal motility are possible in animals and human beings. Unfortunately, these studies have produced results that conflict with those noted earlier from direct observation. Decreases in small intestinal motility during sleep were reported in two separate studies conducted 20 years apart [53,54]. Specific duodenal recordings in human beings are conflicting, showing no change in one instance and an increase in duodenal motility during sleep in another [21,55].

A different approach to duodenal recording was employed by Spire and Tassinari, who recorded duodenal electromyographic (EMG) activity during various stages of sleep [56]. They find an inhibition of duodenal EMG activity during REM sleep and an increase in activity with changes from one sleep phase to another. In a subsequent study, a decrease in duodenal EMG activity during sleep is described by the same group [57]. They also note an activity rhythm of 80 to 120 minutes per cycle that was impervious to the changes associated with the sleep-wake cycle.

Effect of intestinal activity on sleep

Although this article concentrates on the effects of sleep on GI motility, there also are studies that address the issue of how intestinal motility may affect sleep. A practical and provocative thought concerning this issue relates to the familiar experience of postprandial somnolence. Are there changes in the intestinal motility food ingestion that could produce a hypnotic effect? Along these lines, an intriguing observation was made by Alverez [58] in 1920. He noted that distention of a jejunal balloon caused his human subject to drop off to sleep [58]. The hypnotic effects of afferent intestinal stimulation also are documented in animal studies. Perhaps the most notable work was reported by Kukorelli and Juhasz [59], who induced cortical synchronization in cats by mechanical and electrical stimulation of the small bowel. These results were interpreted as an effect of rapidly adapting phasic afferent fibers from the small intestine carried to the CNS via the splanchnic nerve. These data strongly suggest the existence of a hypnogenic effect of luminal distention.

In a subsequent study, these same investigators reported an increase in the duration of slow-wave sleep and an increase in the number of episodes of paradoxic sleep in cats subjected to low-level intestinal stimulation [60]. The investigators also acknowledged the possible hypnogenic role of intestinal hormones, such as cholecystokinin, and they cited a study by Rubenstein and Sonnenschein [61] in which administration of intestinal hormones produced a pronounced increase in paradoxic sleep episodes. The final common pathway of the afferent stimulation from the intestinal tract presumably results in an increase in sleepiness subsequent to either luminal distention or hormonal secretion postprandially. In a fascinating study concerning neuronal processing during sleep, Pigarev [62] shows that neurons in the visual cortex, which usually respond to visual stimulation in the waking state, are activated during sleep by electrical stimulation of the stomach and small bowel.

In an attempt to document the presence of postprandial sleepiness objectively, a study was undertaken by Stahl and colleagues to measure sleep onset latency with and without a prior meal [63]. Statistically, the results of this test do not support the presence of documentable postprandial sleepiness in 16 normal volunteers. It was obvious from these results, however, that there was a small group of individuals in whom there was a substantial decrease in the sleep-onset latency after ingestion of a meal. This phenomenon seems to be affected by many variables: the volume of the meal, the meal constituents, and the circadian cycle of the individual. In a follow-up study, the hypothesis that afferent stimulation from the gastric antrum enhances postprandial sleepiness was investigated [64]. This was tested by comparing an equal volume distention of the stomach with water to an equal volume and equal caloric solid meal and liquid meal. Sleep-onset latency was determined subsequent to each of these conditions. Because antral stimulation results from the digestion of a solid meal, sleep-onset latency should be shorter subsequent to the consumption of the solid meal. This was confirmed in this study in that the sleep-onset latency after the solid meal was significantly shorter than the equal volume water condition. These results are compatible with the animal studies cited earlier and lend further support to the notion that contraction of the intestinal lumen produces afferent stimulation, which induces drowsiness.

Colonic motility and irritable bowel syndrome

Studies suggest an inhibition of colonic contractile and myoelectric activity during sleep and diminished colonic tone [65]. A marked increase in colonic motor activity is noted on awakening or with brief arousals from sleep [66]. This offers a logical explanation of the common urge to defecate on awakening in the morning. Rectoanal pressures have been measured continuously during sleep, and results indicate a decrease in the minute-to-minute variation in the amplitude of spontaneous anal canal activity during sleep [67]. Another study sheds light on intrinsic anorectal functioning [68]. This study shows that intrinsic oscillation in rectal motor activity increased by 44% during sleep compared with waking activity. Of particular importance is the fact that the majority of these contractions were propagated in a retrograde direction. This activity facilitates rectal continence during periods of depressed consciousness and although anal canal pressure is decreased during sleep, it is maintained at a level somewhat higher than the intrarectal pressure, thus facilitating rectal continence during sleep [67].

These studies collectively shed important light on the mechanisms of rectal continence during sleep. There seem to be at least two mechanisms that prevent the passive escape of rectal contents during sleep. First, rectal motor activity increases substantially during sleep, but the propagation is retrograde rather than anterograde. Furthermore, these physiologic studies show that, even under the circumstances of periodic rectal contractions, the anal canal pressure consistently is above that of the rectum. Both of these mechanisms tend to protect against rectal leakage during sleep, and alterations in these mechanisms explain loss of rectal continence during sleep in individuals who have diabetes or who have undergone ileoanal anastomosis.

Several studies show a relationship between poor sleep and pain in patients who have IBS. Studies estimate the prevalence of reported sleep complaints to be as high as 25% to 30% in the population of patients who have functional bowel disorders (ie, IBS and functional dyspepsia). The high prevalence of sleep complaints in patients who have functional bowel disorders is noted in a study by Fass and colleagues in which they prospectively studied a group of patients and healthy controls using bowel symptom and sleep questionnaires [69]. In this study, patients were divided into groups that had functional dyspepsia, IBS, or a combination of dyspepsia and IBS symptoms. Patients who had IBS symptoms alone did not differ from normal controls with regard to the reported incidence of sleep complaints; however, if dyspeptic symptoms were part of the symptom complex, sleep complaints were significantly greater.

A consensus is emerging with regard to subjective and objective parameters of sleep in patients who have functional bowel disorders. Compared with normal controls, sleep architecture seems similar to normals in patients who have functional bowel disorders. In this sense, the pattern of behavior in these patients seems to resemble that of many insomniac patients, in which sleep complaints are exaggerated in terms of prolonged sleep latency and interrupted, nonrefreshing sleep. In a study by Eslenbruch and colleagues, sleep architecture was not significantly different in patients who had IBS compared with normal controls [70]. It was demonstrated that although IBS patients did have more sleep complaints, their PSG patterns were completely indistinguishable from those of age- and sex-matched controls. These results do not confirm an earlier study that describes increased REM sleep in patients who had IBS [44]. In perhaps the largest PSG study to date of patients who had IBS, it is demonstrated that there is a substantial correlation of subjective sleep complaints and depression [71]. Once again, the PSG parameters were, with the single exception of the REM onset latency, indistinguishable from normal controls.

The autonomic nervous system seems to be a mediator of visceral pain in patients who have functional bowel disorders. Studies show some disruption in autonomic functioning during the waking state in patients who have IBS, but these studies have conflicting results. Examination of autonomic functioning during sleep, however, shows an increase in sympathetic tone during REM sleep in patients who have IBS [32]. A subsequent study from the same group documents that patients who have IBS and dyspeptic symptoms did not seem to have this autonomic dysfunction; rather, it was most notable in patients who had IBS but did not have dyspeptic symptoms [72].

Collectively, these studies from sleep investigations of patients who had functional bowel disorders suggest not only that there are sleep disturbances noted in this patient population but also that the sleep disturbances may contribute to altered GI functioning. These studies confirm that there is notable autonomic dysfunction in patients who have functional bowel disorders and that these alterations perhaps are uniquely identified during sleep. Future studies of sleep and patients who have functional bowel disorders undoubtedly will provide additional understanding of the pathophysiology of the brain-gut axis in this patient population and how this may be altered during sleep.

Summary

In this review, an integration of GI functioning is attempted with regard to its relationship to sleep, how this interaction may lead to complaints of sleep disorders, and the pathogenesis of some GI disorders. Data are presented to support the notion that sleep-related GER is an important factor not only in the development of esophagitis but also in the respiratory complications of GER. Although sensory functioning is altered markedly during sleep with regard to most standard sensory functions (eg, auditory), there seems to be an enhancement of some visceral sensation during sleep that seems to protect the tracheobronchial tree from aspiration of gastric contents reflux during sleep.

Patients who have functional bowel disorders reveal an increase in sleep complaints compared with normal volunteers. The actual mechanisms of these disturbances remain somewhat obscure and studies do not demonstrate any consistent abnormalities in sleep patterns of these patients. Some studies show that autonomic functioning during sleep, particularly REM sleep, can distinguish patients who have IBS. Thus, the continued study of sleep and GI functioning promises to create a new dimension in the understanding of the pathophysiology of a variety of GI disorders.

References

[1] Freiden N, Fisher MJ, Taylor W, et al. Sleep and nocturnal acid reflux in normal subjects and patients with reflux oesophagitis. Gut 1991;32:1275–9.

[2] Orr WC, Allen ML, Robinson M. The pattern of nocturnal and diurnal esophageal acid exposure in the pathogenesis of erosive mucosal damage. Am J Gastroenterol 1994;89: 509–12.

[3] Demeester TR, Johnson LF, Joseph GJ, et al. Patterns of gastroesophageal reflux in health and disease. Ann Surg 1975;184:459–70.

[4] Orr WC, Elsenbruch S, Harnish MJ, et al. Proximal migration of esophageal acid perfusions during waking and sleep. Am J Gastroenterol 2000;95:37–42.

[5] Ing AJ, Ngu MC, Breslin AB. Obstructive sleep apnea and gastroesophageal reflux. Am J Med 2000;108(Suppl 4a):120S–5S.

[6] Green BT, Broughton WA, O'Connor JB. Marked improvement in nocturnal gastroesophageal reflux in a large cohort of patients with obstructive sleep apnea treated with continuous positive airway pressure. Arch Intern Med 2003;163:341–5.

[7] Harding SM, Sontag SJ. Asthma and gastroesophageal reflux. Amer J Gastro 2000; 95(Suppl 8):S23–32.

[8] Sontag SJ. Gastroesophageal reflux disease and asthma. J Clin Gastroenterol 2000; 39(Suppl):S9–30.

[9] Gisalson T, Janson C, Vermeire P, et al. Respiratory symptoms and nocturnal gastroesophageal reflux. Chest 2002;121:158–63.

[10] Sandweiss DJ, Friedman HF, Sugarman MH, et al. Nocturnal gastric secretion. Gastroenterology 1946;1:38–54.

[11] Moore JG, Englert E. Circadian rhythm of gastric acid secretion in man. Nature 1970;226: 1261–2.

[12] Levin E, Kirsner JB, Palmer WL, et al. A comparison of the nocturnal gastric secretion in patients with duodenal ulcer and in normal individuals. Gastroenterology 1948;10:952–64.

[13] Feldman M, Richardson CT. Total 24-hour gastric acid secretion in patients with duodenal ulcer: comparison with normal subjects and effects of cimetidine and parietal cell vagotomy. Gastroenterology 1986;90:540–4.

[14] Dragstedt LR. A concept of the etiology of gastric and duodenal ulcers. Gastroenterology 1956;30:208–20.

[15] Levin E, Kirsner JB, Palmer WL, et al. The variability and periodicity of the nocturnal gastric secretion in normal individuals. Gastroenterology 1948;10:939–51.

[16] Armstrong RH, Burnap D, Jacobson A, et al. Dreams and acid secretions in duodenal ulcer patients. New Physician 1965;33:241–3.

[17] Stacher G, Presslich B, Starker H. Gastric acid secretion and sleep stages during natural night sleep. Gastroenterology 1975;68:1449–55.

[18] Orr WC, Hall WH, Stahl ML, et al. Sleep patterns and gastric acid secretion in duodenal ulcer disease. Arch Intern Med 1976;136:655–60.

[19] Dubois A, Castell DO. Abnormal gastric emptying response to pentagastrin in duodenal ulcer disease. Dig Dis Sci 1981;26:292.

[20] Scantlebury RE, Frick HL, Patterson TL. The effect of normal and hypnotically induced dreams on the gastric hunger movements of man. J Appl Physiol 1942;26:682–91.

[21] Bloom PB, Ross DL, Stunkard AJ, et al. Gastric and duodenal motility, food intake and hunger measured in man during a 24-hour period. Dig Dis Sci 1970;15:719–25.

[22] Baust W, Rohrwasser W. Das Verhalten von pH und Motilitat des Megens in naturlichen Schlaf des Menschen. Pflugers Arch 1969;305:229–40.

[23] Yaryura-Tobias HA, Hutcheson JS, White L. Relationship between stages of sleep and gastric motility. Behav Neuropsychiatry 1970;2:22–4.

[24] Fujitani Y, Hosogai M. Circadian rhythm of electrical activity and motility of the stomach in cats and their relation to sleep-wakefulness states. Tohoku J Exp Med 1983;141:275–85.

[25] Hall WH, Orr WC, Stahl ML. Gastric function during sleep. In: Brooks FP, Evers PW, editors. Nerves and the gut. Thorofare (NJ): Slack; 1977. p. 495–502.

[26] Dubois A, Van Eerdewegh P, Gardner JD. Gastric emptying and secretion in Zollinger-Ellison syndrome. J Clin Invest 1977;59:255.

[27] Orr WC, Dubois A, Stahl ML, et al. Gastric function during sleep. Sleep Res 1978;7:72.

[28] Goo RH, Moore JG, Greenburg E, et al. Circadian variation in gastric emptying of meals in humans. Gastroenterology 1987;93:515–8.

[29] Chen JZ, McCallum RW, Familoni BO. Validity of the cutaneous electrogastrogram. In: Chen JZ, McCallum RW, editors. Electrogastrography: principles and applications. New York: Raven Press; 1994. p. 103–25.

[30] Chen JZ, McCallum RW, Smout AJPM, et al. Acquisition and analysis of electrogastrographic data. In: Chen JZ, McCallum RW, editors. Electrogastrography: principles and applications. New York: Raven Press; 1994. p. 3–30.

[31] Chen JZ, McCallum RW, Lin Z. Comparison of three running spectral analysis methods. In: Chen JZ, McCallum RW, editors. Electrogastrography: principles and applications. New York: Raven Press; 1994. p. 75–99.

[32] Orr WC, Crowell MD, Lin B, et al. Sleep and gastric function in irritable bowel syndrome: derailing the brain-gut axis. Gut 1997;41:390–3.

[33] Elsenbruch S, Harnish MJ, Orr WC, et al. Disruption of normal gastric myoelectric functioning by sleep. Sleep 1999;22:453–8.

[34] Metcalf AM, Dozois RR, Kelly KA, et al. Ileal J pouch-anal anastomosis: clinical outcome. Ann Surg 1985;202:735–9.

[35] Cannon WB. The movements of the intestine studied by means of the roentgen rays. Am J Physiol 1902;6:275–6.

[36] Barcroft J, Robinson CS. A study of some factors influencing intestinal movements. Am J Physiol 1929;67:211–20.

[37] Douglas DM, Mann FG. An experimental study of the rhythmic contractions in the small intestine of the dog. Am J Dig Dis 1977;6:318–22.

[38] Hines LE, Mead HCA. Peristalsis in a loop of small intestine. Arch Intern Med 1926;38:539.

[39] Soffer EE, Adrian TE, Launspach J, et al. Meal-induced secretion of gastrointestinal regulatory peptides is not affected by sleep. Neurogastroenterol Motil 1997;9:7–12.

[40] Archer L, Benson MJ, Green WJ, et al. Radiotelemetric measurement of normal human small bowel motor activity during prolonged fasting. J Physiol 1979;296:53.

[41] Thompson DG, Wingate DL. Characterisation of interdigestive and digestive motor activity in the normal human jejunum. Gut 1979;20:A943.

[42] Ritchie HD, Thompson DG, Wingate DL. Diurnal variation in human jejunal fasting motor activity. In: Proceedings of the American Physiological Society; March 1980. p. 54–5.

[43] Finch P, Ingram D, Henstridge J, et al. The relationship of sleep stage to the migrating gastrointestinal complex of man. In: Christensen J, editor. Gastrointestinal motility. New York: Raven Press; 1980. p. 261–5.

[44] Kumar D, Thompson PD, Wingate DL, et al. Abnormal REM sleep in the irritable bowel syndrome. Gastroenterology 1992;103:12–7.

[45] Kellow JE, Borody TJ, Phillips SF, et al. Human interdigestive motility: variations in patterns from esophagus to colon. Gastroenterology 1986;91:386–95.

[46] Kumar D, Idzikowski C, Wingate DL, et al. Relationship between enteric migrating motor complex and the sleep cycle. Am J Physiol 1990;259(6pt1):G983–90.

[47] Kumar D, Soffer EE, Wingate DL, et al. Modulation of the duration of human postprandial motor activity by sleep. Am J Physiol 1989;256(5pt1):G851–5.

[48] Wilson P, Perdikis G, Hinder RA, et al. Prolonged ambulatory antroduodenal manometry in humans. Am J Gastroenterol 1994;89:1489–95.

[49] Wilmer A, Andrioli A, Coremans G, et al. Ambulatory small Intestinal manometry. Detailed comparison of duodenal and jejunal motor activity in healthy man. Dig Dis Sci 1997;42:1618–27.

[50] Kellow JE, Gill RC, Wingate DL. Prolonged ambulant recordings of small bowel motility demonstrate abnormalities in the irritable bowel syndrome. Gastroenterology 1990;98:1208–18.

[51] Kellow JE, Phillips SF. Altered small bowel motility in irritable bowel syndrome is correlated with symptoms. Gastroenterology 1987;92:1885–93.

[52] Kumar D, Thompson PD, Wingate DL, et al. Abnormal REM sleep in the irritable bowel syndrome. Gastroenterology 1992;103:12–7.

[53] Helm JD, Kramer P, MacDonald RM, et al. Changes in motility of the human small intestine during sleep. Gastroenterology 1948;10:135–7.

[54] Sadler HH, Orten AU. The complementary relationship between the emotional state and the function of the ileum in a human subject. Am J Psychiatry 1968;124:1377–81.

[55] Bloom PB, Ross DL, Stunkard AJ, et al. Gastric and duodenal motility, food intake and hunger measured in man during a 24-hour period. Dig Dis Sci 1970;15:719–25.

[56] Spire JP, Tassinari CA. Duodenal EMG activity during sleep. Electroencephalogr Clin Neurophysiol 1971;31:179–83.

[57] Tassinari CA, Coccagna G, Mantovani M, et al. Duodenal EMG activity during sleep in man. In: Jovanovic UJ, editor. The nature of sleep. Stuttgart (Germany): Gustav Fischer Verlag; 1973.

[58] Alverez WC. Physiologic studies on the motor activities of the stomach and bowel in man. Am J Physiol 1920;88:658–60.

[59] Kukorelli T, Juhasz G. Sleep induced by intestinal stimulation in cats. Physiol Behav 1976;19:355–8.

[60] Juhasz G, Kukorelli T. Modifications of visceral evoked potentials during sleep in cats. Act Nerv Super (Praha) 1977;19:212–4.

[61] Rubenstein EH, Sonnenschein RR. Sleep cycles and feeding behavior in the cat: role of gastrointestinal hormones. Acta Cient Venez 1971;22:125–8.

[62] Pigarev IN. Neurons of visual cortex respond to visceral stimulation during slow wave sleep. Neuroscience 1994;62:1237–43.

[63] Stahl ML, Orr WC, Bollinger C. Postprandial sleepiness: objective documentation via polysomnography. Sleep 1983;6:29–35.

[64] Orr WC, Shadid G, Harnish MJ, et al. Meal composition and its effect on postprandial sleepiness. Physiol Behav 1997;62:709–12.

[65] Steadman CJ, Phillips SF, Camilleri M, et al. Variations of muscle tone in the human colon. Gastroenterology 1991;101:24.

[66] Narducci F, Bassotti G, Gaburri M, et al. Twenty-four hour manometric recording of colonic motor activity in healthy men. Gut 1987;28:17–25.

[67] Orkin BA, Hanson RB, Kelly KA, et al. Human anal motility while fasting, after feeding, and during sleep. Gastroenterology 1991;100:1016–23.

[68] Rao SS, Welcher K. Periodic rectal motor activity: the intrinsic colonic gatekeeper? Am J Gastroenterol 1996;91:890–7.

[69] Fass R, Fullerton S, Tung S, et al. Sleep disturbances in clinic patients with functional bowel disorders. Am J Gastroenterol 2000;95:1195–200.

[70] Elsenbruch S, Harnish MJ, Orr WC. Subjective and objective sleep quality in irritable bowel syndrome. Am J Gastroenterol 1999;94:2447–52.

[71] Robert JJ, Orr WC, Elsenbruch S. Modulation of sleep quality and autonomic functioning by symptoms of depression in women with irritable bowel syndrome. Dig Dis Sci 2004;49:1250–8.

[72] Thompson JJ, Elsenbruch S, Harnish MJ, et al. Autonomic functioning during REM sleep differentiates IBS symptom subgroups. Am J Gastroenterol 2002;97:3147–53.

Conditions of Primary Excessive Daytime Sleepiness

Jed E. Black, MD*, Stephen N. Brooks, MD, Seiji Nishino, MD, PhD

Stanford Sleep Disorders Center, Sleep Medicine Division, Department of Psychiatry and Behavioral Sciences, Stanford University, Stanford, CA, USA

Somnolence is a complex state, impacted by multiple determinants such as quantity and quality of prior sleep, circadian time, drugs, attention, motivation, environmental stimuli, and various medical, neurologic and psychiatric conditions. Somnolence is welcomed when sleep is desired, but it often becomes an unwanted symptom at other times. Pathologic or inappropriate somnolence is clinically termed "excessive daytime sleepiness" (EDS), which is the focus of this review, specifically, central nervous system (CNS) dysfunction yielding syndromes of EDS.

Syndromes of sleepiness

Insufficient sleep and sleep fragmentation

Critical in the evaluation of patients presenting with EDS is the determination of the presence or absence of the two most common causes of EDS: insufficient sleep in normal individuals and fragmented sleep due to extrinsic or intrinsic factors. Fragmented sleep, predominantly micro-fragmentation, resulting from conditions such as the sleep-related breathing disorders and periodic limb movement syndrome are not addressed in this review. The most common cause of daytime sleepiness is insufficient sleep, which may reflect poor sleep "hygiene" (behaviors impacting sleep) or self-imposed or work/socially-dictated sleep deprivation. Additionally, circadian rhythm disorders such as those related to shift-work or circadian phase (eg, phase delay, jet lag) contribute importantly to the common causes of EDS. In evaluating the patient with EDS, these condition(s) of insufficient sleep,

---

* Corresponding author. 401 Quarry Road #3301, Stanford, CA 94305.
E-mail address: MajorSleep@yahoo.com (J.E. Black).

0733-8619/05/$ - see front matter © 2005 Dr. J. Black. Published by Elsevier Inc. All rights reserved.
doi:10.1016/j.ncl.2005.08.002
neurologic.theclinics.com

sleep fragmentation, or circadian rhythm disturbance must be addressed even if features of a primary disorder of somnolence are apparent during the clinical assessment.

Primary disorders of somnolence

Several entities may be regarded as primary disorders of somnolence. Narcolepsy, the best known and the most completely understood disorder of this group, will be considered at greater length, whereas other clinical syndromes are reviewed more briefly.

Narcolepsy

Human narcolepsy is a syndrome of unknown etiology. Prevalence is approximately 1 in 2000 [1,2]. It is often described as a disorder of sleep-state boundary control and is characterized by the classic tetrad of EDS, cataplexy, hypnagogic/hypnopompic hallucinations, and sleep paralysis [3]. Markedly disturbed nocturnal sleep, although not included in the original literature, is reported in up to 90% of patients and is more common than cataplexy in narcolepsy. Symptoms most often begin during adolescence or young adulthood; however, narcolepsy may also occur earlier in childhood or not until the third or fourth decade of life, or even later. Quality-of-life studies suggest that the impact of narcolepsy is equal to that of Parkinson's disease [4]. No symptom or sign of narcolepsy is specific to narcolepsy; even cataplexy unrelated to narcolepsy occurs rarely either as an isolated symptom or in conjunction with other conditions. The International Classification of Sleep Disorders (ICSD-2) diagnostic criteria for narcolepsy are provided in Box 1 [3].

Narcolepsy symptoms.

Sleepiness or EDS. Patients may describe sleepiness as feeling "tired," "fatigued," "low energy," "lazy," "drowsy," "sleepy," or similar terms. EDS refers to a propensity to fall asleep, nod, or doze easily in relaxed or sedentary situations, or a need to exert extra effort to avoid sleeping in these situations. The Epworth Sleepiness Scale (ESS) provides a subjective method for measuring daytime sleepiness [5]. The ESS is not at all specific for narcolepsy, inasmuch as other more-prevalent sleep disorders can cause severe EDS, yet it manifests a fair degree of sensitivity in untreated patients. Patients with narcolepsy generally score above 12 on this scale, whereas control subjects generally score less than 10 [6]. Unwanted sleepiness may also manifest as "sleep attacks" (irresistible urges to sleep), occurring not only during monotonous situations conducive to sleep, but also in situations where the patient is actively engaged in a task. In addition to frank sleepiness, the EDS of narcolepsy or other sleep disorders can cause related symptoms, including poor memory, reduced concentration or attention, and irritability.

Box 1. International Classification of Sleep Disorders

Diagnostic Criteria (ICSD-2): Narcolepsy with Cataplexy
A. The patient has had excessive daytime sleepiness occurring almost daily for at least 3 months.
B. A definite history of cataplexy, defined as sudden and transient episodes of loss of muscle tone triggered by emotions, is present.

Note: *To be labeled as cataplexy, these episodes must be triggered by strong emotions—most reliably laughing or joking—and must be generally bilateral and brief (less than 2 minutes). Consciousness is preserved, at least at the beginning of the episode. Observed cataplexy with transient reversible loss of deep tendon reflexes is a very strong, but rare, diagnostic finding.*

C. The diagnosis of narcolepsy with cataplexy should, whenever possible, be confirmed by nocturnal polysomnography followed by an MSLT; the mean sleep latency on MSLT is less than or equal to 8 minutes and 2 or more SOREMPs are observed following sufficient nocturnal sleep (minimum 6 hours) during the night before the test. Alternatively, hypocretin-1 levels in the CSF are less than or equal to 110 pg/mL or one third of mean normal control values.

Note: *The presence of 2 or more SOREMPs during the MSLT is a very specific finding, whereas a mean sleep latency of less than 8 minutes can be found in up to 30% of the normal population. Low CSF hypocretin-1 levels (less than or equal to 110 pg/mL or one third of mean normal values) are found in over 90% of patients with narcolepsy with cataplexy and almost never in controls or in other patients with other pathologies.*

D. The hypersomnia is not better explained by another sleep disorder, medical or neurological disorder, mental disorder, medication use, or substance use disorder.

Diagnostic Criteria (ICSD-2): Narcolepsy without Cataplexy
A. The patient has a complaint of excessive daytime sleepiness occurring almost daily for at least 3 months.
B. Typical cataplexy is not present, although doubtful or atypical cataplexy-like episodes may be reported.
C. The diagnosis of narcolepsy without cataplexy must be confirmed by nocturnal polysomnography followed by an MSLT. In narcolepsy without cataplexy, the mean sleep latency on MSLT is less than or equal to 8 minutes and 2 or

more SOREMPs are observed following sufficient nocturnal
sleep (minimum 6 hours) during the night before the test.
Note: *The presence of 2 or more SOREMPs during the MSLT is
a specific finding, whereas a mean sleep latency of less than 8
minutes can be found in up to 30% of the normal population.*
D. The hypersomnia is not better explained by another sleep
disorder, medical or neurological disorder, mental disorder,
medication use, or substance use disorder.

Data from: International Classification of Sleep Disorders (ICSD). Diagnostic
and Coding Diagnostic Classification Steering Committee (Thorpy MJ, chairman).
American Sleep Disorders Association. Narcolepsy. 1990;347:38–43.

Cataplexy. Cataplexy is a sudden, partial or complete loss of voluntary
muscle tone bilaterally in response to strong emotion, most often laughter,
anger, or surprise (positive emotions are more commonly triggers for
cataplexy) [7]. It may be subtle, occurring only in a few muscle groups and
cause head drooping, slurred speech, or dropping things from the hand; or it
may be so severe that total body paralysis occurs, resulting in complete
collapse. The individual is usually alert and oriented during the spell, despite
the inability to respond. There is usually complete recollection of the events.
The retention of memory of the details of the event distinguishes complete
paralytic cataplexy attacks from syncope or seizure. Cataplexy events
usually last from a few seconds to 2 or 3 minutes, but occasionally continue
longer [8]. Startling stimuli, stress, physical fatigue, or sleepiness may also be
important triggers or factors that exacerbate cataplexy.

According to epidemiologic studies, cataplexy is found in 60% to 100%
of patients with narcolepsy. A large range in percentage affected with
cataplexy is reported because definitions of narcolepsy vary among studies.
The onset of cataplexy is most frequently simultaneous with the onset of
EDS, but in some cases, cataplexy may not develop until many years after
initial onset of EDS [8].

Nocturnal sleep disruption. An often overlooked but important feature of
narcolepsy is the experience of frequent nocturnal awakenings, often with
difficulty returning to sleep. In general, patients with narcolepsy have many
more and longer awakenings than controls. Although this sleep fragmentation may seem somewhat paradoxical, narcolepsy is a condition of
disruption of both the continuity and robustness of sleep as well as of
wakefulness.

Hypnagogic or hypnopompic hallucinations. Hypnagogic and hypnopompic hallucinations are reported to be phenomena less common in narcolepsy than is cataplexy, but when present, often occur frequently. These

hallucinations can occur in any condition of severe sleepiness, but are less common in the other sleep disorders. These sensory misperceptions occur at the transition from wakefulness to sleep (hypnagogic) or from sleep to wakefulness (hypnopompic) and are thought to result from the intrusion of dream-like brain activity into partial wakefulness. They may take many forms—visual, tactile, auditory, or multi-sensory events—and are usually brief (a minute or two) but occasionally can continue for a few minutes. Hallucinations regarding intruders in the room are common and are often coupled with sleep paralysis, resulting in an extremely disturbing experience for the patient. Hypnagogic and hypnopompic hallucinations can be distinguished from other forms of hallucinatory experiences in that the patient generally recognizes that they are not real shortly after returning to full consciousness.

Sleep paralysis. Similar to hypnagogic or hynopompic hallucinations, sleep paralysis occurs during the transition from sleep to wakefulness or vice versa. It is the inability to volitionally move any part of the body and can last from a few seconds to minutes. These episodes can be alarming to patients, particularly those who experience the sensation of being unable to breathe. Although accessory respiratory muscles may not be active during these episodes, diaphragmatic activity continues and air exchange is adequate.

Automatic behavior. Automatic behavior can be described as "absent-minded" behavior or speech that is often nonsensical and that the patient does not remember. Automatic behavior occurs more often when the patient is sleepy.

Narcolepsy evaluation.

Polysomnography (nocturnal) and multiple sleep-latency test. Although not essential in the accurate diagnosis of narcolepsy when clear-cut cataplexy is present, polysomnography (PSG) is nonetheless important in the evaluation of narcolepsy of any form. PSG is used primarily to exclude other conditions that could be the cause of sleepiness or to evaluate the coexistence of other conditions adding to the sleepiness or nocturnal sleep disruption the patient may be experiencing. Obstructive sleep apnea, periodic limb movement activity during sleep, and rapid eye movement (REM) sleep behavior disorder are all more common in narcolepsy than in the general public [9].

During PSG, episodes of REM sleep occurring at sleep-onset may be witnessed. In controls, REM sleep occurs only after 1 to 2 hours of sleep. In narcolepsy, REM sleep upon falling asleep is common.

Daytime nap studies, in the form of the multiple sleep-latency test (MSLT), usually demonstrate a substantially reduced sleep latency. Typically, the mean sleep latency during four to five daytime nap opportunities is less than 5 minutes and almost always less than 8 or 9 minutes, compared with greater than 10 to 15 minutes in controls [6]. Additionally, sleep-onset REM episodes usually occur during 50% or more of the daytime naps in patients with narcolepsy. Sleep-onset REM periods are not specific for narcolepsy (see subsequent section [CSF]), but the occurrence of two or more of these events during the MSLT, in the setting of objective sleepiness and without another explanation for their occurrence, is strongly suggestive of narcolepsy.

Cerebrospinal fluid hypocretin (orexin) assessment. As is discussed later in the section on narcolepsy pathophysiology, many, but not all, patients with narcolepsy have very low or undetectable levels of hypocretin (orexin) in the cerebrospinal fluid (CSF) [10,11]. Such low levels of CSF hypocretin are not specific for narcolepsy and occur rarely in other neurologic conditions. However, when used to assess patients for narcolepsy, low CSF hypocretin is much more specific than is the finding of two or more sleep-onset REM episodes on MSLT. Two or more sleep-onset REM episodes with MSLT occur in approximately 5% of obstructive sleep apnea patients [12] as well as in an important subset of delayed sleep phase syndrome patients. Both of these conditions are approximately 50 to 100 fold more prevalent than narcolepsy. Hence, great caution must be used to rule out at least these conditions before assuming that sleep-onset REM episodes on MSLT confirm the diagnosis of narcolepsy. In contrast, when cataplexy is absent, CSF hypocretin analysis provides a far more specific diagnostic test than MSLT when serum is positive for HLA DQB1*0602 (see HLA subsection below).

Histocompatibility human leukocyte antigen. A strong correlation exists between narcolepsy with cataplexy and the histocompatibility human leukocyte antigen (HLA) subtype DQB1*0602. This subtype, however, is very common in the general population and is not at all specific or sensitive for narcolepsy [13]. HLA testing is therefore not useful in confirming or excluding the diagnosis of narcolepsy. On the basis of estimates of DQB1*0602 prevalence in the general public of approximately 20%, coupled with the much greater prevalence of obstructive sleep apnea (OSA) and other conditions of EDS than narcolepsy, the use of HLA testing to confirm the diagnosis of narcolepsy in a patient without cataplexy will yield a false-positive diagnostic rate many times greater than the true-positive rate. The only circumstance under which HLA testing can be useful as a diagnostic tool is when cataplexy is not present and HLA testing will be followed by CSF hypocretin analysis. When HLA is negative for DQB1*0602, CSF hypocretin concentrations are normal; therefore, CSF hypocretin should only be sampled for diagnostic purposes in patients without cataplexy but who test positive for DQB1*0602.

Idiopathic hypersomnia

Idiopathic hypersomnia (also known as idiopathic CNS hypersomnia) is an incompletely defined disorder characterized by EDS. Traditionally, this diagnosis has been made for individuals with excessive somnolence but who lack the classic features of narcolepsy or another disorder known to cause

EDS (such as sleep apnea). Without doubt, many patients have been diagnosed with idiopathic hypersomnia when in fact they have suffered from other disorders, such as narcolepsy without cataplexy, delayed sleep phase syndrome, or upper airway resistance syndrome [14]. Roth [15] described monosymptomatic EDS and polysymptomatic EDS (prolonged nocturnal sleep time, marked difficulty with awakening) forms of idiopathic hypersomnia. Others have suggested that the category of idiopathic hypersomnia is heterogeneous, including individuals with EDS but with or without one or more of the other features of Roth's polysymptomatic form [16]. Idiopathic hypersomnia is thought to be less common than narcolepsy, but estimation of prevalence is difficult, because strict diagnostic criteria are lacking and no specific biologic marker has been identified. Typically, onset of symptoms occurs in adolescence or early adulthood. As denoted, the etiology of the disorder is not known, but viral illnesses, including Guillain-Barre syndrome, hepatitis, mononucleosis, and atypical viral pneumonia may herald the onset of sleepiness in a subset of patients. EDS may occur as part of the acute illness, but it persists after the other symptoms subside. Rarely, familial cases are known to occur, with increased frequency of HLA-Cw2 and HLA-DR11 [17]. Some of these patients have associated symptoms suggesting autonomic nervous system dysfunction, including orthostatic hypotension, syncope, vascular headaches, and peripheral vascular complaints. Most patients with idiopathic hypersomnia have neither a family history nor an obvious associated viral illness. Little is known about the pathophysiology of idiopathic hypersomnia. No animal model is available for study. Neurochemical studies using CSF have suggested that patients with idiopathic hypersomnia may have altered noradrenergic system function [18–20].

The clinical picture of idiopathic hypersomnia varies among individual patients. The disorder may be mistaken for narcolepsy if a careful history is not taken. The two disorders share several common features, including similar age of onset, lifelong persistence after onset (although a few patients with idiopathic hypersomnia have improved over time or attained complete remission of symptoms [21–23]), EDS as the primary symptom, and familial clustering of some cases. However, essential differences between the disorders become apparent in the history and in diagnostic studies. Patients with idiopathic CNS hypersomnia present with EDS, but without cataplexy (although some patients have episodes of sleep paralysis or hypnagogic hallucinations) or significant nocturnal sleep disruption [23]. They usually complain of daytime sleepiness that interferes with normal activities. Occupational and social functioning may be severely impacted by sleepiness. Nocturnal sleep time tends to be long, and patients are usually difficult to awaken in the morning—they may become irritable or even abusive in response to the efforts of others to rouse them. In some patients, this difficulty may be substantial and may include confusion, disorientation, and poor motor coordination, a condition called "sleep drunkenness" [24].

These patients often take naps, which may be prolonged but are usually non-refreshing. No amount of sleep relieves the EDS. "Microsleeps," with or without automatic behavior, may occur throughout the day.

Polysomnographic studies of patients with idiopathic CNS hypersomnia usually reveal shortened initial sleep latency, increased total sleep time, and normal sleep architecture (in contrast to narcoleptic patients, who exhibit significant sleep fragmentation). Using spectral analysis, Sforza et al [25] found reduced sleep pressure, as evidenced by decreased slow-wave activity during the first two non-REM (NREM) episodes of nocturnal sleep in patients with idiopathic hypersomnia. Mean sleep latency on MSLT is usually reduced, often in the 8- to 10-minute range, but sometimes dramatically shorter. Also in contrast to narcolepsy, sleep-onset REM periods (SOREMPS) are not typically seen. A study measuring evoked potentials found that subjects with idiopathic hypersomnia or severe obstructive sleep apnea had prolonged visual and auditory P300 latency compared with normals or subjects with narcolepsy, and demonstrated reduced auditory P300 amplitude compared with subjects with narcolepsy [26].

As with narcolepsy, other disorders producing EDS (such as insufficient sleep, sleep-related breathing disorders, periodic limb movement syndrome, other sleep-fragmenting disorders, psychiatric diseases, or circadian rhythm disorders) must be ruled out before the diagnosis of idiopathic hypersomnia is made.

Treatment of idiopathic CNS hypersomnia is usually less than satisfactory. Lifestyle and behavioral modifications, including good sleep hygiene, are appropriate, but treatment with stimulant or wake-promoting medication, as with narcolepsy, is usually necessary.

Recurrent hypersomnias

Kleine-Levin syndrome. This uncommon disorder, a form of recurrent hypersomnia, occurs primarily in adolescents [27]. There is a male preponderance. The disorder is characterized by the occurrence of episodes of EDS, usually, but not invariably, accompanied by hyperphagia, aggressiveness, and hypersexuality lasting days to weeks and separated by asymptomatic periods of weeks or months. During symptomatic periods, individuals sleep up to 18 hours per day and are usually drowsy (often to the degree of stupor), confused, and irritable the remainder of the time. During symptomatic episodes, polysomnographic studies show long total sleep time with high sleep efficiency and decreased slow-wave sleep. MSLT studies demonstrate short sleep latencies and SOREMPS [28]. The etiology of the syndrome remains obscure. Symptomatic cases of Kleine-Levin syndrome associated with structural brain lesions have been reported, but most cases are idiopathic. Single photon emission computed tomography (SPECT) studies have demonstrated hypoperfusion in the thalamus in one patient and in the non-dominant frontal lobe in another [29]. Treatment with stimulant medication is usually only partially effective. Effects of treatment with lithium, valproic acid, or carbamazepine have been variable but generally unsatisfactory. Fortunately, in most cases, episodes become less frequent over time and eventually subside.

Menstrual-related hypersomnia. Another form of recurrent hypersomnia is menstrual-related periodic hypersomnia, in which EDS occurs during the several days before menstruation [30,31]. The prevalence of this syndrome has not been well defined. Likewise, the etiology is not known, but presumably the symptoms are related to hormonal changes. Some cases of menstrual-related hypersomnia have responded to the blocking of ovulation with estrogen and progesterone (birth control pills) [32].

Idiopathic recurring stupor. Numerous cases have been reported in which individuals (predominately middle-aged males) are subject to stuporous episodes lasting from hours to days, in the absence of obvious toxic, metabolic, or structural cause. The individuals are normal between episodes, which occur unpredictably. Some electroencephalogram (EEG) data collected during symptomatic episodes have manifested fast background activity in the 13 to 16 Hz range. Several of these patients have been shown to have elevated plasma and CSF levels of endozepine-4, an endogenous ligand with affinity for the benzodiazepine recognition site at the $GABA_A$ receptor [33]. Administration of flumazenil, a benzodiazepine antagonist, has produced transient awakening with normalization of the EEG [34]. In some cases, the episodes resolved spontaneously after several years. Similar cases have been reported in children [35].

Nervous system disorders and EDS

EDS may be associated with various disorders of the central or peripheral nervous systems. It is a clinical feature of many toxic or metabolic encephalopathic processes. These disorders often present with other symptoms and signs, but EDS may dominate the clinical picture, particularly in chronic cases. Structural brain lesions, including strokes, tumors, cysts, abcesses, hematomas, vascular malformations, hydrocephalus, and multiple sclerosis plaques, are known to produce EDS. Somnolence may result either from direct involvement of discrete brain regions (especially the brainstem reticular formation or midline diencephalic structures) or because of effects on sleep continuity (for example, nocturnal seizure activity or secondary sleep-related breathing disorder [SRBD]).

EDS is a frequent sequela of encephalitis or head trauma. Victims of "encephalitis lethargica," described by Von Economo in the early twentieth century, were found to have lesions in the midbrain, subthalamus, and hypothalamus. Additionally, post-traumatic narcolepsy with cataplexy is well documented [36]. Epileptic patients may suffer from EDS as a consequence of medication effects or, less obviously, because of nocturnal seizure activity [37]. EDS may be associated with numerous infectious agents affecting the central nervous system, including bacteria, viruses, fungi, and parasites. Perhaps the best known is trypanosomiasis, which is called "sleeping sickness" because of the prominent hypersomnia. Sleepiness may occur with acute infectious illness, even without direct invasion of the nervous system, and may be mediated by cytokines, including interferon, interleukins, and tumor necrosis factor [38]. EDS may also persist chronically after certain viral infections [39].

Sleep disruption and EDS are common in neurodegenerative disorders, including Parkinson's disease, Alzheimer's disease, and other dementias, as well as multiple system atrophy [40–42]. Patients with neuromuscular disorders or peripheral neuropathies may also develop EDS because of associated SRBD (central or obstructive apnea), pain, or period limb movements of sleep (PLMS) [43]. Patients with myotonic dystrophy often suffer from EDS, even in the absence of sleep-disordered breathing [44].

Management of the primary disorders of somnolence

Effective treatment of narcolepsy requires both nonpharmacologic and pharmacologic strategies.

Nonpharmacologic strategies

Structured nocturnal sleep

Patients with primary EDS complain of disrupted nocturnal sleep. These patients should be instructed to maintain a structured bedtime and arising time, despite the quality or continuity of their nocturnal sleep. If the patient experiences wakeful periods during the night, he or she may arise briefly, perform a sedentary activity such as reading, then return to bed and attempt to sleep. The time scheduled for nocturnal sleep should generally be 8 hours or more.

Structured daytime naps

In addition to stimulant medications, naps may provide an important treatment for primary EDS. Naps may range from 15 or 20 minutes to longer than 1 hour. Many patients will find a short nap (<30 minutes) refreshing, but others require longer naps. Naps are often scheduled during the lunch hour and upon returning home from work. Some patients will need to schedule naps more often during the day. At least one nap, and usually two or more, can be very beneficial for most patients with narcolepsy.

Avoidance of irregular sleep–wake schedules

As already noted, patients with EDS should maintain regular sleep–wake schedules. Most will find shift work or changes in work schedule extremely difficult. Daytime work is strongly recommended.

Counseling or other assistance

Work capacity, social/family function, and quality of life may all be severely affected. In fact, a study of more than 500 narcoleptics, the largest study of its kind, revealed decrements in quality-of-life measures similar to those experienced by patients with Parkinson's disease [13]. Most patients with narcolepsy require special considerations at work or school, many benefit from marriage or family assistance/counseling, and some require full-time disability.

Driving caution for patients with EDS or cataplexy

Individuals with EDS are at a much greater risk than normal for motor vehicle accidents caused by falling asleep at the wheel or slowed reaction times. Patients should be cautioned to refrain from driving long distances and to cease driving immediately when sleepy. Some patients will not experience the sensation of sleepiness before inadvertent dosing; others will. One line of thought suggests that if a patient is able to adequately sense sleepiness, he or she may be able to drive safely if he or she will immediately pull over and take a nap when sleepy or turn over the wheel to someone else. Those who cannot predict or sense sleepiness or who are unwilling to avoid driving when sleepy should not drive. Many patients perform much better if they drive only after taking stimulant medications. Patients with cataplexy who may experience cataplectic episodes while driving must refrain from driving until the cataplexy has been adequately treated.

Pharmacologic treatment of primary disorders of somnolence

Stimulants and other alerting medications

Alerting agents provide a critical component of treatment for most patients with EDS resulting from primary disorders of somnolence. Occasionally, patients may wish to avoid medications and attempt to take extra naps during the day. This approach can be successful but usually fails to provide enough daytime alertness for adequate functioning. For most patients with narcolepsy, alerting agents will not yield a normal degree of daytime alertness, but will nonetheless produce substantial improvement [45]. Clinically, the practice of combining two alerting agents of different chemical classes has been employed when a single agent is insufficient. This technique can be useful and has been evaluated in a large international trial with modafinil and sodium oxybate in narcolepsy.

Modafinil. Modafinil is a wake-promoting therapeutic somewhat comparable to traditional stimulants in promoting alertness, but with a different mechanism of action. This mechanism is unknown, but modafinil appears to act more selectively in the brain than do the traditional stimulants [46]. The clinical duration of effect of modafinil may be longer because its serum half-life (12–15 hours) is longer than that of traditional stimulants. Modafinil has been evaluated extensively in the treatment of the EDS of narcolepsy and other sleep disorders manifesting EDS [47]. In the treatment of narcolepsy, modafinil is viewed as first-line therapy for EDS. In fact, in every condition of EDS explored, modafinil has resulted in improvement in mean ratings of sleepiness, both subjective and objective, compared with placebo.

Sodium oxybate (gamma-hydroxybutyrate). Another agent that has been found to enhance alertness in narcolepsy to a degree similar to or greater than modafinil is sodium oxybate, also known as gamma-hydroxybutyrate (GHB). These findings from a recent head-to-head trial suggest that this agent also should be viewed as first-line therapy for the EDS and cataplexy (see below) of narcolepsy. The mechanism of action of the agent has been extensively studied, but how it effects improved alertness is unknown [48]. Data from multiple studies suggest that sodium oxybate imparts a degree of alertness similar to that produced by other agents and that its effect may be additive when used in combination with other stimulants [6]. Clinical experience, but no controlled research, suggests that sodium oxybate may be useful in other conditions of primary EDS as well.

Traditional stimulants. Commonly used traditional stimulants include methylphenidate, dextro-amphetamine, and methamphetamine. Other sympathomimetic amines and sustained-release preparations are available. Patients may experience negative effects with any alerting agent. Some patients report rebound hypersomnia (exacerbation of sleepiness) as the dose wears off, or tolerance (tachyphylaxis) to the alerting effect may occur with time in some patients. In cases of tolerance, switching to a different class of medication or providing a "drug holiday" can be useful.

Medications for cataplexy (anticataplectics)

Medications useful in the treatment of cataplexy usually also improve hypnagogic/hypnopompic hallucinations and sleep paralysis.

Sodium oxybate (GHB). In addition to its effect on EDS in narcolepsy, sodium oxybate, also known as gamma-hydroxybutyrate or GHB, is remarkably effective as an anticataplectic. It has been extensively evaluated as an anticataplectic agent over many years [6]. Additionally, GHB is effective in reducing nocturnal sleep disruptions and in consolidating nocturnal sleep. Again, the mechanism of action of GHB in treating these symptoms is unknown [48].

Antidepressants. Historically, antidepressants such as the tri-cyclic anti-depressants (TCAs) and selective serotonin re-uptake inhibitors (SSRIs), especially those with CNS noradrenergic activity, have also been useful in temporizing cataplexy [49]. Tolerance to these traditional cataplexy medications can occur, requiring medication switch or drug holiday. Recently, atomoxetine, venlafaxine and other newer non–SSRI/non-TCA antidepressants, have been reported in individual cases to provide effective treatment for cataplexy, although they have not yet been rigorously studied.

Immunotherapy. Although high-dose prednisone was unsuccessful in a child with new-onset narcolepsy [50], intravenous immunoglobulin treatment early in the course of narcolepsy has been reported to be beneficial in a few case reports [51,52]. Additionally, plasmapheresis resulted in clear but very short-lived improvement in symptoms in a case of late-life onset narcolepsy. Repeated plasmapheresis treatment, however, provided only brief periods of improvement and proved impractical for chronic therapy [53]. Given the likely interplay of the immune system and the development of narcolepsy, early treatment with immunotherapy warrants further investigation.

Future directions. Work with the R-isomer of modafinil and with modafinil analogs for the treatment of EDS is in progress in humans and animals.

Of interest is that the CNS histamigergic system has long been known to function importantly in alertness; however, agents that enhance histaminergic activity have been pursued only relatively recently. Results from animal research provide evidence for wake promotion without psychomotor activation, which may enhance tolerability of such a wake-promoting agent.

Additionally, hypocretin agonists are under development. Agents that provide post-synaptic hypocretin receptor activation may be promising in the treatment of narcolepsy, particularly in the setting of hypocretin neuronal atrophy and possibly other forms of primary EDS.

Pathophysiology of narcolepsy

Narcolepsy symptoms

The similarity between cataplexy and REM sleep atonia, the presence of frequent episodes of hypnagogic hallucinations and of sleep paralysis, and the propensity for narcoleptics to transition directly from wakefulness into REM sleep led to the early perspective that narcolepsy is primarily a "disease of REM sleep" [54]. This hypothesis, however, appears too simplistic and does not explain the presence of sleepiness during the day and the short latency to both NREM and REM sleep during nocturnal and nap recordings. A more developed hypothesis is that narcolepsy results from the disruption of the control mechanisms of both sleep and wakefulness and perhaps especially of the vigilance-state boundary process [55]. According to this hypothesis, a cataplectic attack represents an intrusion of REM sleep atonia during wakefulness, while the hypnagogic hallucinations appear as dream-like imagery taking place in the waking state, especially at sleep onset in patients who frequently have SOREMPs.

Much evidence supports the view of narcolepsy as a condition of vigilance-state disturbance. Cataplexy is associated with an inhibition of the monosynaptic H-reflex and the polysynaptic deep tendon reflexes [56]. In healthy subjects, the H-reflex is completely suppressed only during REM sleep. This finding highlights the relationship between the inhibition of motor processes during REM sleep and the sudden atonia and areflexia seen during cataplexy. Studies in canine narcolepsy, however, suggest that the mechanisms for induction of cataplexy are different from those for REM sleep [57]. Furthermore, an extended human study confirmed that cataplexy correlates much more highly with hypocretin deficiency than do other REM sleep–related phenomena (see below) [58]. Cataplexy is therefore appropriately viewed as a hypocretin-deficiency pathologic phenomenon somewhat distinct from other REM-related symptoms. Patients with other sleep disorders, such as sleep apnea, and even healthy individuals can manifest SOREMPs, hypnagogic hallucinations, and sleep paralysis when their sleep/wake patterns are sufficiently disturbed. However, these subjects never develop cataplexy, further supporting the proposal that cataplexy is unrelated to other REM-associated symptoms [59–62]. Although cataplexy and REM sleep atonia have great similarity and possibly share a common executive system, it is not necessary for the regulatory mechanism of both states to be identical. The mechanism of emotional triggering of cataplexy remains undetermined.

Narcolepsy, HLA, and the immune system

A remarkably high HLA association with narcolepsy has been known since the early 1980s to exist [63]. Since the time of this initial finding, a variety of studies across multiple ethnic groups have produced findings corroborative of the existence of this strong HLA association. The most specific marker of narcolepsy in a number of different ethnic groups studied to date is DQB1*0602 [2]. This association is seen in an average of approximately 90% of those with unequivocal cataplexy [64]. Importantly, this association is substantially lower, only approximately 40%, in individuals who have received the diagnosis of narcolepsy but who do not have cataplexy.

The strong association between HLA type and narcolepsy with cataplexy would seem to suggest that narcolepsy is an autoimmune disease [65]. There is, however, no evidence of inflammatory processes or immune abnormalities associated with narcolepsy [65]. Researchers have found no classic auto-antibodies and no increase in oligoclonal CSF bands in narcoleptics [66]. Typical autoimmune pathologies (erythrocyte sedimentation rates, serum immunoglobulin levels, C-reactive protein levels, complement levels, and lymphocyte subset ratios) are apparently normal in narcoleptic patients [67]. In contrast, a variety of serological tests performed in narcoleptics, along with age- and sex-matched controls, yielded higher levels of antistreptolysine 0 and anti-Dnase antibodies in narcoleptics than in controls [68,69]. In view of these preliminary data, further exploration of possible immune-related dysfunction in narcolepsy is warranted.

Hypocretin (orexin) function deficits in canine and human narcolepsy

Narcolepsy has been observed in several domesticated animal species, including dogs, and has been produced in genetically engineered mouse models. Canine narcolepsy is a naturally occurring model, with both sporadic (17 breeds identified) and familial forms (Doberman, Labrador, and Dachshund). In Doberman pinschers and Labrador retrievers, the disease is transmitted as a recessive autosomal trait with complete penetrance [70].

In 1999, using positional cloning and gene-targeting strategies, two groups independently revealed the pathogenesis of narcolepsy in animals. The lack of the hypothalamic neuropeptide hypocretin/orexin ligand (preprohypocretin/orexin gene knockout mice [71]) or mutations in one of the two hypocretin/orexin receptor genes (hypocretin receptor 2 [*hcrtr 2*]) in autosomal recessive canine narcolepsy [72]) was observed to produce the symptom complex of narcolepsy. Extensive screening in humans, especially in familial and early-onset narcolepsy, demonstrated that mutations in hypocretin-related genes are rare; only a single case with early-onset (6 months of age) was found to be associated with a point mutation in the preprohypocretin gene [73].

Despite the lack of genetic abnormalities in the hypocretin system, the majority (85%–90%) of patients with narcolepsy-cataplexy have low or undetectable CSF hypocretin-1 ligand (Fig. 1) [10,74]. This hypocretin deficiency is tightly associated with the occurrence of cataplexy and HLA-DQB1*0602 positivity [58,75,76]. Postmortem studies in humans, although using few brains, have confirmed hypocretin ligand deficiency (both hypocretin-1 and -2) in the narcoleptic brain (Fig. 1) [73,77]. Hypocretin deficiency has also been observed in sporadic cases of canine narcolepsy

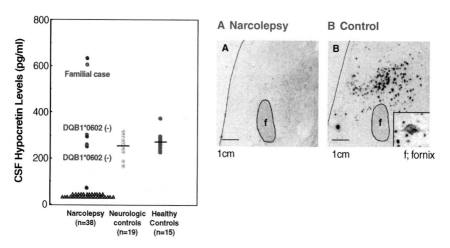

Fig. 1. Hypocretin levels in patients with narcolepsy-cataplexy.

(7 out of 7 currently studied; the results of four cases are reported), suggesting that the pathophysiology of narcolepsy in these animals mirrors that of most human cases [78].

Although positive predictive value is not 100%, low CSF hypocretin-1 levels are very specific for narcolepsy when compared with other sleep or neurologic disorders (Fig. 2) [58,75]. The establishment of CSF hypocretin measurement as a new diagnostic tool for human narcolepsy is therefore encouraging. Previously, no specific and sensitive diagnostic test for narcolepsy based on the pathophysiology of the disease was available, and the final diagnosis was often delayed for several years after disease onset [79].

Hypocretin-1 and -2 neuropeptide neurotransmitters are produced exclusively by a well-defined group of neurons localized in the lateral hypothalamus. The neurons project to the olfactory bulb, cerebral cortex, thalamus, hypothalamus, and brainstem, particularly the locus coeruleus, raphe nucleus, and cholinergic nuclei and cholinoceptive sites (such as pontine reticular formation), thought to be important for sleep regulation [80].

The hypocretin system is a major excitatory system that affects the activity of monoaminergic (dopamine, norepinephrine, serotonin, and histamine) and cholinergic systems with major effects on vigilance states

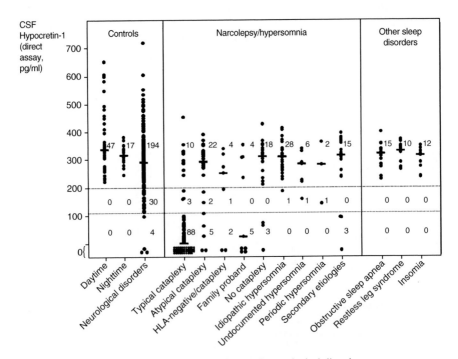

Fig. 2. Hypocretin levels in sleep and neurological disorders.

[81,82]. It is therefore likely that a deficiency in hypocretin neurotransmission induces an imbalance between these classic neurotransmitter systems, with primary effects on sleep-state organization and vigilance.

Summary

Excessive daytime somnolence is a prevalent problem in medical practice and in society. It exacts a great toll in quality of life, personal and public safety, and productivity. The causes of EDS are myriad, and careful evaluation is needed to determine the cause in each case. Although much progress has been made in discovering the pathophysiology of narcolepsy, much more remains to be understood, and far less is known about other primary conditions of EDS. Several methods have been developed to assess EDS, although each of them has limitations. Treatment is available for the great majority of cases.

References

[1] Hublin C, Kaprio J, Partinen M, et al. The prevalence of narcolepsy: an epidemiological study of the Finnish twin cohort. Ann Neurol 1994;35:709–16.

[2] Mignot E. Genetic and familial aspects of narcolepsy. Neurology 1998;50(Suppl 1):S16–22.

[3] International Classification of Sleep Disorders (ICSD). Diagnostic and Coding Diagnostic Classification Steering Committee (Thorpy MJ, chairman). American Sleep Disorders Association. Narcolepsy 1990;347:38–43.

[4] Beusterien KM, Rogers AE, Walsleben JA, et al. Health-related quality of life effects of modafinil for treatment of narcolepsy. Sleep 1999;22:757–65.

[5] Johns MW. A new method for measuring daytime sleepiness: the Epworth sleepiness scale. Sleep 1991;14:540–5.

[6] US Xyrem in Narcolepsy Multi-center Study Group. A randomized, double blind, placebo-controlled multicenter trial comparing the effects of three doses of orally administered sodium oxybate with placebo for the treatment of narcolepsy. Sleep 2002;25(1):42–9.

[7] Gelb M, Guilleminault C, Kraemer H, et al. Stability of cataplexy over several months: information for the design of therapeutic trials. Sleep 1994;17:265–73.

[8] Honda Y. Clinical features of narcolepsy: Japanese experiences. In: Honda Y, Juji T, editors. HLA in narcolepsy. Berlin: Springer-Verlag; 1988. p. 24–57.

[9] Overeem S, Mignot E, van Dijk JG, et al. Narcolepsy: clinical features, new pathophysiological insights, and future perspectives. J Clin Neurophysiol 2001;18:78–105.

[10] Nishino S, Ripley B, Overeem S, et al. Hypocretin (orexin) deficiency in human narcolepsy. Lancet 2000;355:39–40.

[11] Mignot E, Lammers GJ, Ripley B, et al. The role of cerebrospinal fluid hypocretin measurement in the diagnosis of narcolepsy and other hypersomnias. Arch Neurol 2002; 59(10):1553–62.

[12] Chervin RD, Aldrich MS. Sleep onset REM periods during multiple sleep latency tests in patients evaluated for sleep apnea. Am J Respir Crit Care Med 2000;161:426–31.

[13] Mignot E. Genetic and familial aspects of narcolepsy. Neurology 1998;50(Suppl 1):S16–22.

[14] Guilleminault C, Stoohs R, Clerk A, et al. A cause of excessive daytime sleepiness. The upper airway resistance syndrome. Chest 1993;104:781–7.

[15] Roth B. Narcolepsy and hypersomnia. Arch Neurol Psychiatr 1976;119:31–41.

[16] Aldrich MS. The clinical spectrum of narcolepsy and idiopathic hypersomnia. Neurology 1996;46:393–401.

[17] Montplaisir J, Poirier G. HLA in disorders of excessive sleepiness without cataplexy in Canada. In: Honda Y, Juji T, editors. HLA in narcolepsy. Berlin: Springer-Verlag; 1988. p. 86.

[18] Montplaisir J, De Champlain J, Young SN, et al. Narcolepsy and idiopathic hypersomnia: biogenic amines and related compounds in CSF. Neurology 1982;32:1299–302.

[19] Faull KF, Guilleminault C, Berger PA, et al. Cerebrospinal fluid monoamine metabolites in narcolepsy and hypersomnia. Ann Neurol 1983;13:258–63.

[20] Faull KF, Thiemann S, King RJ, et al. Monoamine interactions in narcolepsy and hypersomnia: a preliminary report. Sleep 1986;9:246–9.

[21] Bruck D, Parkes JD. A comparison of idiopathic hypersomnia and narcolepsy-cataplexy using self report measures and sleep diary data. J Neurol Neurosurg Psychiatr 1996;60: 576–8.

[22] Bassetti C, Aldrich MS. Idiopathic hypersomnia. A series of 42 patients. Brain 1997;120: 1423–35.

[23] Billiard M, Dauvillies Y. Idiopathic hypersomnia. Sleep Med Rev 2001;5(5):351–60.

[24] Roth B, Nevsimalova S, Rechtschaffen A. Hypersomnia with "sleep drunkenness". Arch Gen Psychiatry 1972;26:456–62.

[25] Sforza E, Gaudreau H, Petit D, et al. Homeostatic sleep regulation in patients with idiopathic hypersomnia. Clin Neurophysiol 2000;111(2):277–82.

[26] Sangal RB, Sangal JM. P300 latency: abnormal in sleep apnea with somnolence and idiopathic hypersomnia, but normal in narcolepsy. Clin Electroencephalogr 1995;26: 146–53.

[27] Critchley M. The syndrome of hypersomnia and periodical megaphagia in the adult male (Kleine-Levin): what is its natural course? Rev Neurol 1967;116(6):647–50.

[28] Rosenow F, Kotagal P, Cohen BH, et al. Multiple sleep latency test and polysomnography in diagnosing Kleine-Levin syndrome and periodic hypersomnia. J Clin Neurophysiol 2000; 17(5):519–22.

[29] Arias M, Crespo Iglesias JM, Perez J, et al. Kleine-Levin syndrome: contribution of brain SPECT in diagnosis. Rev Neurol 2003;35(6):531–3.

[30] Billiard M, Guilleminault C, Dement WC. A menstruation-linked periodic hypersomnia. Kleine-Levin syndrome or a new clinical entity? Neurology 1975;25(5):436–43.

[31] Sachs C, Persson H, Hagenfeldt K. Menstruation-associated periodic hypersomnia: a case study with successful treatment. Neurology 1982;32:1376–9.

[32] Bamford CR. Menstrual-associated sleep disorder: an unusual hypersomniac variant associated with both menstruation and amenorrhea with a possible link to prolactin and metoclopramide. Sleep 1993;16:484–6.

[33] Rothstein JD, Guidotti A, Tinuper P, et al. Endogenous benzodiazepine receptor ligands in idiopathic recurring stupor. Lancet 1992;340(8826):1002–4.

[34] Lugaresi E, Montagna P, Tinuper P, et al. Endozepine stupor. Recurring stupor linked to endozepine-4 accumulation. Brain 1998;121:127–33.

[35] Soriani S, Carrozzi M, De Carlo L, et al. Endozepine stupor in children. Cephalalgia 1997; 17(6):658–61.

[36] Francisco GE, Ivanhoe CB. Successful treatment of post-traumatic narcolepsy with methylphenidate: a case report. Am J Phys Med Rehabil 1996;75:63–5.

[37] Manni R, Tantara A. Evaluation of sleepiness in epilepsy. Clin Neurophysiol 2000; 111(Suppl 2):S111–4.

[38] Toth LA, Opp MR. Sleep and infection. In: Lee-Chiong TL, Sateia MJ, Carskadon MA, editors. Sleep medicine. Philadelphia: Hanley & Belfus; 2002. p. 77–83.

[39] Guilleminault C, Mondini S. Mononucleosis and chronic daytime sleepiness: a long-term follow-up study. Arch Intern Med 1986;146:1333–5.

[40] Askenasy JJM. Sleep in Parkinson's disease. Acta Neurol Scand 1993;87:167–70.

[41] Chokroverty S. Sleep and degenerative neurologic disorders. Neurol Clin 1996;14:807–26.

[42] Trenkwalder C. Sleep dysfunction in Parkinson's disease. Clin Neurosci 1998;5(2):107–14.

[43] George CFP. Neuromuscular disorders. In: Kryger MH, Roth T, Dement WC, editors. Principles and practice of sleep medicine. 3rd edition. Philadelphia: W.B. Saunders Co.; 2000. p. 1087–92.

[44] Gibbs JW, Ciafaloni E, Radtke RA. Excessive daytime somnolence and increased rapid eye movement pressure in myotonic dystrophy. Sleep 2002;25(6):662–5.

[45] Mitler MM, Aldrich MS, Koob GF, et al. Narcolepsy and its treatment with stimulants. ASDA standards of practice. Sleep 1994;17(4):352–71.

[46] US Modafinil in Narcolepsy Multicenter Study Group. Randomized trial of modafinil as a treatment for the excessive daytime somnolence of narcolepsy. Neurology 2000;54(5): 1166–75.

[47] US Modafinil in Narcolepsy Multicenter Study Group. Randomized trial of modafinil for the treatment of pathological somnolence in narcolepsy. Ann Neurol 1998;43(1): 88–97.

[48] Tunnicliff G, Cash CD. Gamma-hydroxybutyrate: molecular, functional and clinical aspects. New York: Taylor and Francis, Inc.; 2002.

[49] Nishino S, Mignot E. Pharmacological aspects of human and canine narcolepsy. Prog Neurobiol 1997;52:27–78.

[50] Hecht M, Lin L, Kushida CA, et al. Report of a case of immunosuppression with prednisone in an 8-year-old boy with an acute onset of hypocretin-deficiency narcolepsy. Sleep 2003; 26(7):809–10.

[51] Lecendreux M, Maret S, Bassetti C, et al. Clinical efficacy of high-dose intravenous immunoglobulins near the onset of narcolepsy in a 10-year-old boy. J Sleep Res 2003;12(4): 347–8.

[52] Dauvilliers Y, Carlander B, Rivier F, et al. Successful management of cataplexy with intravenous immunoglobulins at narcolepsy onset. Ann Neurol 2004;56(6):905–8.

[53] Chen W, Black J, Call P, et al. Late-onset narcolepsy responsive to plasmapheresis [letter]. Ann Neurol 2005;58(3):489–90.

[54] Dement W, Rechtschaffen A, Gulevich G. The nature of the narcoleptic sleep attack. Neurology 1966;16:18–33.

[55] Broughton R, Valley V, Aguirre M, et al. Excessive daytime sleepiness and pathophysiology of narcolepsy-cataplexy: a laboratory perspective. Sleep 1986;9:205–15.

[56] Guilleminault C, Wilson RA, Dement WC. A study on cataplexy. Arch Neurol 1974;31: 255–61.

[57] Nishino S, Riehl J, Hong J, et al. Is narcolepsy a REM sleep disorder? Analysis of sleep abnormalities in narcoleptic Dobermans. Neurosci Res 2000;38:437–46.

[58] Mignot E, Lammers GJ, Ripley B, et al. The role of cerebrospinal fluid hypocretin measurement in the diagnosis of narcolepsy and other hypersomnias. Arch Neurol 2002;59: 1553–62.

[59] Fukuda K, Miyasita A, Inugami M, et al. High prevalence of isolated sleep paralysis: kanashibari phenomenon in Japan. Sleep 1987;10:279–86.

[60] Bishop C, Rosenthal L, Helmus T, et al. The frequency of multiple sleep onset REM periods among subjects with no eccessive daytime sleepiness. Sleep 1996;19:727–30.

[61] Ohayon MM, Priest RG, Caulet M, et al. Hypnagogic and hypnopompic hallucinations: pathological phenomena? Br J Psychiatry 1996;169:459–67.

[62] Aldrich MS, Chervin RD, Malow BA. Value of the multiple sleep latency test (MSLT) for the diagnosis of narcolepsy. Sleep 1997;20:620–9.

[63] Juji T, Satake M, Honda Y, et al. HLA antigens in Japanese patients with narcolepsy. All the patients were DR2 positive. Tissue Antigens 1984;24:316–9.

[64] Mignot E, Hayduk R, Black J, et al. HLA Class II studies in 509 narcoleptic patients. Sleep Res 1997;26:433.

[65] Mignot E, Guilleminault C, Grumet FC, et al. Is narcolepsy an autoimmune disease? In: Smirne S, Francesci M, Ferini-Strambi L, et al, editors. Proceedings of the Third Milano International Symposium. Milan: Masson; 1992. p. 29–38.

[66] Frederickson S, Carlander B, Billiard M, et al. CSF immune variable in patients with narcolepsy. Acta Neurol Scand 1990;81:253–4.

[67] Matsuki K, Juji T, Honda Y. Immunological features of narcolepsy in Japan. In: Honda Y, Juji T, editors. HLA in narcolepsy. Berlin: Springer-Verlag; 1988. p. 150–7.

[68] Billiard M, Laaberki MF, Reygrobellet C, et al. Elevated antibodies to streptococcal antigens in narcoleptic subjects. Sleep Res 1989;18:201.

[69] Montplaisir J, Poirier G, Lapierre O, et al. Streptococcal antibodies in narcolepsy and idiopathic hypersomnia. Sleep Res 1989;18:271.

[70] Mignot E, Wang C, Rattazzi C, et al. Genetic linkage of autosomal recessive canine narcolepsy with an immunoglobulin heavy-chain switch-like segment. Proc Natl Acad Sci USA 1991;88:3475–8.

[71] Chemelli RM, Willie JT, Sinton CM, et al. Narcolepsy in orexin knockout mice: molecular genetics of sleep regulation. Cell 1999;98:437–51.

[72] Lin L, Faraco J, Li R, et al. The sleep disorder canine narcolepsy is caused by a mutation in the hypocretin (orexin) receptor 2 gene. Cell 1999;98:365–76.

[73] Peyron C, Faraco J, Rogers W, et al. A mutation in a case of early onset narcolepsy and a generalized absence of hypocretin peptides in human narcoleptic brains. Nat Med 2000;6: 991–7.

[74] Nishino S, Ripley B, Overeem S, et al. Low CSF hypocretin (orexin) and altered energy homeostasis in human narcolepsy. Ann Neurol 2001;50:381–8.

[75] Kanbayashi T, Inoue Y, Chiba S, et al. CSF hypocretin-1 (orexin-A) concentrations in narcolepsy with and without cataplexy and idiopathic hypersomnia. J Sleep Res 2002;11: 91–3.

[76] Krahn LE, Pankratz VS, Oliver L, et al. Hypocretin (orexin) levels in cerebrospinal fluid of patients with narcolepsy: relationship to cataplexy and HLA DQB1*0602 status. Sleep 2002; 25:733–6.

[77] Thannickal TC, Moore RY, Nienhuis R, et al. Reduced number of hypocretin neurons in human narcolepsy. Neuron 2000;27:469–74.

[78] Ripley B, Fujiki N, Okura M, et al. Hypocretin levels in sporadic and familial cases of canine narcolepsy. Neurobiol Dis 2001;8:525–34.

[79] Alaila SL. Life effects of narcolepsy: measures of negative impact, social support and psychological well-being. In: Goswanmi M, Pollak CP, Cohen FL, et al, editors. Loss, grief and care: psychosocial aspects of narcolepsy. New York: Haworth Press; 1992. p. 1–22.

[80] Peyron C, Tighe DK, van den Pol AN, et al. Neurons containing hypocretin (orexin) project to multiple neuronal systems. J Neurosci 1998;18:9996–10015.

[81] Willie JT, Chemelli RM, Sinton CM, et al. To eat or to sleep? Orexin in the regulation of feeding and wakefulness. Annu Rev Neurosci 2001;24:429–58.

[82] Taheri S, Zeitzer JM, Mignot E. The role of hypocretins (orexins) in sleep regulation and narcolepsy. Annu Rev Neurosci 2002;25:283–313.

ELSEVIER
SAUNDERS

Neurol Clin 23 (2005) 1045–1057

NEUROLOGIC
CLINICS

Sleep-Related Breathing Disorders

Conrad Iber, MD

University of Minnesota, Pulmonary and Critical Care, Hennepin County Medical Center,
701 Park Street South, Minneapolis, MN 55415, USA

Sleep permits a greater expression of breathing failure as compared with wakefulness and uncovers the propensity to obstruct the upper airway in susceptible individuals. This review is practical and succinct rather than comprehensive and will address the scope of prevalent sleep-related breathing disorders with emphasis on adults as well as the condition of obstructive sleep apnea. Consistent with the International Classification of Sleep Disorders (ICSD), sleep-related breathing disorders (SRBDs) span a spectrum including disorders resulting in upper airway obstruction during sleep, disorders that alter breathing patterns, and disorders that produce hypoventilation or hypoxemia (Box 1). SRBD definitions and measures have evolved since the initial consensus designed in 1999 for research purposes [1]. Readers are referred to the current ICSD for detailed descriptions of the diverse clinical categories of SRBDs [2]. In keeping with the ICSD, general reference to the diagnosis "obstructive sleep apnea" will include the clinical features associated with patients having apneas, hypopneas, and the upper airway resistance syndrome. Experimental and population studies often address more specific aspects of the condition, including snoring or the frequency of respiratory events. Because the putative consequences of obstructive sleep apnea may not require the presence of subjective sleepiness, the syndromic definition of obstructive sleep apnea with sleepiness will be de-emphasized in the discussion.

To measure the intensity of SRBD during sleep monitoring, several metrics are available. Derangements in gas exchange are typically assessed by monitoring the frequency and intensity of pulse oximetric desaturation and occasionally by indirect measures of blood carbon dioxide elevation. Interference with natural sleep is often assessed by sleep architecture or by the frequency of breathing-related events such as arousals. SRBDs may be associated with obstructive events (Fig. 1), central events (Fig. 2), or

E-mail address: iberx001@umn.edu

doi:10.1016/j.ncl.2005.08.001   *neurologic.theclinics.com*

Box 1. Current terminology for common sleep-related breathing disorders using the second edition of the International Classification of Sleep Disorders

Primary central apnea
Central sleep apnea due to
    Cheyne–Stokes breathing pattern
    high-altitude periodic breathing
    medical condition not Cheyne–Stokes
    drug or substance
Primary sleep apnea of infancy
Obstructive sleep apnea
Sleep-related nonobstructive alveolar hypoventilation, idiopathic
Congenital central alveolar hypoventilation syndrome
Sleep-related hypoventilation/hypoxemia due to
    lower airways obstruction
    neuromuscular and chest wall disorders
    pulmonary parenchymal or vascular pathology
Sleep apnea/sleep-related breathing disorder, unspecified

---

disordered breathing that is not associated with events (Fig. 3). In addition, there may be a mixture of these three components. In obstructive sleep apnea, the metric that is most commonly used to measure intensity of breathing, the apnea–hypopnea index (AHI), refers to the number of apneas and hypopneas per hour of sleep. In adults, these apnea–hypopnea events of at least 10 seconds in duration include parameters for specific changes in oxygen saturation and respiration [2]. The intensity of obstructive sleep apnea, as measured by the AHI, is exquisitely sensitive to the choice of these parameters [3]. Not all breathing disorders during sleep can be characterized by the AHI, and the choice of metric in SRBD should be tailored instead to the disorder and to the question being answered. The use of AHI, for instance, may not be an appropriate metric in disorders such as sustained hypoventilation in restrictive lung disease which is not always associated with episodic apneas or hypopneas (Fig. 3). Similarly, the AHI may not reflect the magnitude of the upper airway resistance syndrome in children [4] or adults.

Permissive effects of sleep

Sleep has several rather dramatic effects on respiration, even in normal humans. Upper airway reflex dilator responses are impaired during sleep [5], and resting lung volumes and oxygen stores are reduced. Pharyngeal muscle relaxation during sleep significantly increases in upper airway resistance [6], and sleep decreases ventilatory response to hypoxia and hypercapnia [7,8].

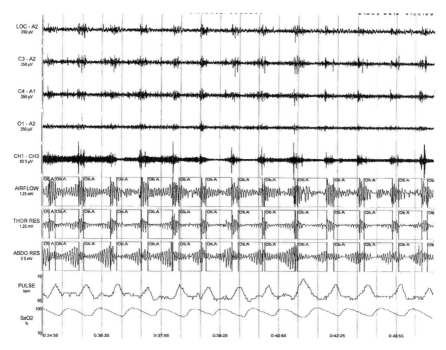

Fig. 1. Polysomnography in a patient with obstructive sleep apnea showing predominantly hypopneas.

It is likely that many of these effects contribute to the resulting 2–8 mmHg rise in carbon dioxide during sleep that occurs in the absence of disease [9]. The consequences of these effects are more severe in SRBD and may result in an exaggeration of this sleep-associated hypoventilation [9,10].

Conditions that result in hypocapnia may interrupt the regular firing of the respiratory controller. Regular breathing rhythm can become periodic during non–rapid eye movement (NREM) sleep if affected by conditions that promote continuous hypocapnia [9], such as hypoxia or the pulmonary venous congestion that may accompany heart failure. Periodic breathing may be amplified by recurrent awakenings and the intensity of ventilatory drive. In some individuals, periodicity in breathing effort may create delays in upper airway dilator activity and contribute to the development of upper airway obstruction, blurring the distinction between central and obstructive apnea. Similarly, obstructive sleep apnea may promote ventilatory overshoot and subsequent central apneas [10]. Finally, the skeletal muscle inhibition that normally accompanies rapid eye movement (REM) sleep impairs ventilation both in normal subjects and in those with respiratory disease [11].

Given the permissive effects of sleep on respiratory embarrassment, it is not surprising that SRBD may result in rather profound alterations in gas

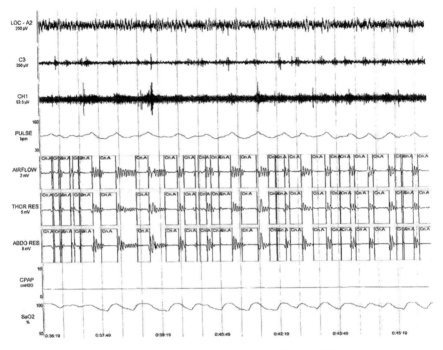

Fig. 2. Central sleep apnea in a patient with heart failure.

exchange during sleep. For instance, as compared with the typical rise in CO_2 of 2–8 mmHg with sleep in normal subjects, the CO_2 in patients with chronic obstructive pulmonary disease (COPD) may rise by 18 mmHg [12].

Specific disorders

Obstructive sleep apnea

Prevalence

It is estimated that 1% to 5% of the adult population has the syndrome of obstructive sleep apnea associated with sleepiness [13]. In a recent summary pooling three studies using AHI criteria alone for diagnosis, it was estimated that 20% of adults with a body mass index (BMI) in the range of 25–28 have sleep apnea, based on an AHI greater than 5, and 7% have sleep apnea based on an AHI greater than 15 [14]. Estimates of the prevalence of obstructive sleep apnea syndromes suggest that increasing age and male gender substantially increase the likelihood of sleep apnea in adults [15–18]. Although increasing age may increase the prevalence of sleep apnea, severity may decrease in the elderly [18]. In children, the prevalence of sleep apnea peaks between the ages of 2 and 5 years of age [19,20] and may be associated with more continuous upper airway obstruction and fewer discrete respiratory events.

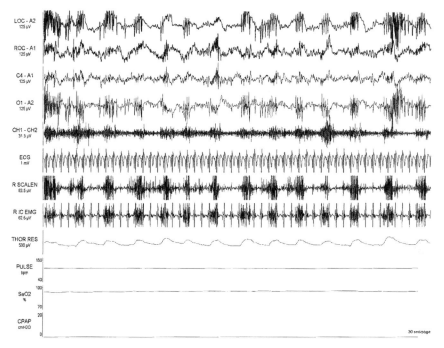

Fig. 3. Sleep-associated respiratory failure in a patient with post-polio syndrome with hypoventilation (PCO_2 76 mmHg). Note tachypnea and excessive use of accessory muscles but absence of episodic events.

Genetic predisposition

It is not entirely clear why humans have been so particularly plagued with the condition of obstructive sleep apnea. With the exception of the selectively bred English Bulldog, obstructive sleep apnea is unique to the human species. In humans, the propensity for sleep apnea may have been permitted by the evolutionary advantages of airway modification for speech and upright posture [21]. These airway skeletal and soft-tissue modifications may now interact with increasing population obesity and age to express such a high prevalence of sleep apnea. Whatever the particular susceptibility of the human, there appears to be substantial variation in the genetic risks for sleep apnea within the species. Male gender is a significant genetic risk that has been consistently associated with a twofold to threefold increased prevalence of sleep apnea [16–18,22]. Although the most obvious genetic predisposition to sleep apnea is male gender, additional genetic variation in risk has been identified. Evidence from twin studies [23] suggests that heritable factors play a substantial role in the risk of developing obstructive sleep apnea, and genome scans in population studies suggest that there are both shared and unshared genetic factors that condition the risks for obesity and sleep apnea [24,25]. Although there are limited genetic variations that are influenced by race, at least two studies have shown that BMI of younger subjects influences the risk of sleep apnea to a greater extent in whites than in African Americans or Polynesians [26,27]. Racial differences in the overall risk for sleep apnea have been more difficult to substantiate. The cross-sectional analysis performed in the Sleep Heart Health Study [28] did not substantiate an increased risk of sleep apnea in African Americans as suggested by previous population studies [27,29].

Modifiers

Obesity is associated with a smaller airway, an increase in airway collapsibility, and a propensity to develop hypoxia because of reduced lung oxygen stores and impaired efficiency of gas exchange. The frequency of apneas and hypopneas during sleep is associated in a dose-related fashion with the intensity of obesity as measured by BMI [30]. There is also more direct evidence that changes in body weight alter the severity of sleep apnea. In persons with sleep apnea, there is a positive relationship between the intensity of disordered breathing as measured by AHI and relative changes in body weight. An approximately 3% change in the AHI is expected for each 1% change in body weight, based on observational studies [31], with a similar relationship for the reduction in AHI suggested by interventional studies with weight loss [14]. Although weight loss may improve sleep apnea, successful long-term weight reduction is difficult to sustain with dietary management alone. Randomized trials suggest that low-fat diets may reduce body weight 4–5 kg over 1 year [32], although one randomized trial of dietary and behavioral intervention showing 11 kg weight loss at 1 year revealed disappointingly high failure rates after 5 years [33].

Increasing age affects the nature and severity of sleep apnea. The AHI increases modestly with age, although effects are more pronounced in habitual snorers or those with a BMI greater than 30 [14]. Increasing age in the range of 40 to 80 years, however, reduces the likelihood that reported apneas or an interval increase of BMI of greater than 5 will be associated with sleep apnea [28].

Airway structure and function have been intensively studied in obstructive sleep apnea. Both skeletal and soft-tissue structure influence the likelihood of sleep apnea. Adenotonsillar enlargement is frequently responsible for sleep apnea in children. Case reports and case series suggest that unusual skeletal abnormalities, such as retrognathia and midface hypoplasia, and soft-tissue conditions, such as macroglossia or mucopoly-saccharidoses, increase the likelihood of sleep apnea.

Many patients suffer from the coexistence of a primary pulmonary disease and sleep apnea. Although the current information on comorbidity in sleep apnea is based on referred case series, there is evidence that sleep apnea may negatively influence patient outcomes. In a case series of non-obese COPD patients, only 1 of 20 had an AHI of greater than 2 [34]. In a larger prospective study of 265 patients identified with the obstructive sleep apnea syndrome, 11% had concomitant COPD [35], and this subset was noted to have more hypoxemia, hypercapnia, and pulmonary hypertension.

Although alcohol consumption is common, its negative impact on SRBD has been somewhat inconsistently reported. Self-reporting suggests that 48.5% of Americans are regular drinkers and 15.5% consume more than four drinks on one night per month [36]. Although alcohol ingestion before bedtime causes obstructive sleep apnea in many experimental protocols [37,38], population studies have not always demonstrated an association between self-reported alcohol consumption and snoring or sleep apnea [22].

Consequences

The most immediate consequences of obstructive sleep apnea are interruptions in the normal breathing pattern, terminated by arousal. Immediate effects on respiration include relative hypoxemia and hypercapnia, and the immediate cardiovascular effects include cardiac slowing and decreased stroke volume, with a subsequent sympathetic surge that is accompanied by increases in systemic and pulmonary arterial pressures. Both ventilation and cardiac output may fluctuate below baseline levels during the obstruction and rise above baseline levels after resumption of ventilation.

Arousals accompanying obstructive sleep apnea interrupt sleep continuity, although arousals are not required for termination of all episodes of obstructive sleep apnea [39]. The immediate effects of sleep apnea produce an array of biological consequences that may result in cardiovascular stress, neurocognitive changes, and even metabolic effects.

Some outcome measures that are presumed to be related to the physiologic events have been examined in both cross-sectional and longitudinal population studies. These studies may better reflect the impact of sleep apnea on the population than do case series, which select more symptomatic individuals. For instance, although case series show a substantial impact of treatment on daytime sleepiness [40], and sleepiness may be related to the intensity of AHI [16,41], most individuals with sleep apnea in population studies may not have sleepiness that is attributable to sleep apnea [16,41]. Sleep apnea is independently associated with glucose intolerance and prevalence of cardiovascular disease, as well as cardiovascular risk factors [30,42,43]. In the Sleep Heart Health Study, these relative risks occurred within a small range for AHI (1.3 to 11.0) and were mild to moderate in magnitude (mean relative risks, 2.38 for heart failure, 1.58 for stroke, and 1.27 for coronary disease). In a dose-related fashion, sleep apnea has also been shown to increase the risk for the development of hypertension [44].

Central sleep apnea

Central sleep apnea is characterized by interruption in breathing effort that can occur as an isolated event or in a periodic pattern. Central apnea is a manifestation of instability in the regular pattern of the respiratory control system. Laryngeal stimulation and lung inflation reflexes induce non-recurring central apneas. Arousals causing deep breaths often produce brief central apneas that may be related to transient hypocapnia. Sustained patterns of central apneas and hypoponeas are typically seen in NREM rather than REM sleep and may be amplified by arousals. Hypoxemia and pulmonary edema create sustained hyperventilation and hypocapnia that results in a very regular periodic pattern of apneas or hypopneas, often associated with some degree of sleep fragmentation. In the setting of heart failure and stroke, this pattern has traditionally been called Cheyne–Stokes respiration (CSR). Factors that promote periodic breathing include frequent changes in sleep stage or state and unique individual characteristics, such as a high ventilatory response to CO_2 and a narrow margin between sleeping partial pressure of carbon dioxide (PCO_2) and the PCO_2 at which apnea occurs [9].

Heart failure and stroke

Sleep apnea is common in heart failure patients and warrants vigilance in this population and careful consideration in management strategies for heart failure. Both central sleep apnea and obstructive sleep apnea have been reported in heart failure patients. In one clinical series, sleep apnea (AHI ≥15) occurred in 61% of patients with a clinical diagnosis of heart failure (mean ejection fraction, 27%), with a nearly equal distribution of obstructive sleep apnea and CSR [45]. CSR tends to occur in heart failure patients with elevated pulmonary venous pressures and carries a particularly poor prognosis [46].

Central sleep apnea or obstructive sleep apnea frequently accompanies stroke, as shown in recent case series using unattended portable devices to identify sleep apnea (as defined as an AHI >10) in 71% to 94% of patients with acute stroke [47]. Coexisting left ventricular dysfunction and resting hypocapnia have been implicated in the risk for central sleep apnea or obstructive sleep apnea occurring in patients with stroke [48].

COPD

Although sleep apnea may coexist with COPD, sustained periods of oxygen desaturation and hypoventilation are more common than is sleep apnea in COPD. One case series demonstrated that a rise in PCO_2 of greater than 10 mmHg occurred for at least 20% of sleep time in 43% of individuals with severe COPD [12]. Two additional case series suggest that desaturation during sleep may occur in up to 80% of patients with severe COPD [49,50]. Sleep-associated desaturation typically occurs during REM sleep and may be more common in patients with daytime hypercapnia. Sustained nocturnal desaturation during REM sleep occurs as a result of decreasing tidal volume and is not necessarily associated with upper airway obstruction [51].

COPD causes subjective distress that is not necessarily associated with gas exchange abnormalities. COPD increases the frequency of symptoms such as cough, wheezing, and shortness of breath, which may contribute to changes in the structure of sleep and to sleep complaints. A large case series of patients with COPD revealed that when symptoms of wheezing and cough were present, 53% of patients reported insomnia and 23% percent complained of daytime sleepiness [52]. Patients with severe COPD have increased frequency of arousals, increased frequency of sleep stage changes, and decreased total sleep time [53,54].

Restrictive lung disease

Restriction of lung volumes because of neuromuscular disease, chest wall disease, pleural disease, and parenchymal lung disease is termed restrictive lung disease. All severe restrictive lung diseases can cause dyspnea associated with sleep disruption, and may produce sleep-associated hypoventilation and hypoxemia. Restrictive lung disease is a much more heterogeneous category than COPD, and most of our knowledge about it is based on rather small case series of patients with diverse conditions such as kyphoscoliosis, muscular dystrophies, amyotrophic lateral sclerosis, and destructive lung disease. Treatment studies employing bilevel positive airway pressure have uncovered some of the potentially treatable consequences of restrictive disease, including daytime sleepiness [55], daytime hypoventilation [56–58], altered sleep architecture [59], and even chronic respiratory muscle weakness [57,58].

Congenital central hypoventilation syndrome

Congenital central hypoventilation syndrome (CCHS) should be considered in children who express episodic or sustained hypoventilation and hypoxemia in the first few months of life in the absence of obvious cardiopulmonary disease, structural abnormalities of the brainstem, or clinical evidence of neuromuscular disease. In CCHS, there is wide variability in the expression of hypoventilation, with pronounced hypoventilation during slow-wave sleep in most individuals and hypoventilation during wakefulness in severe cases. The disease appears to be expressed commonly in heterzygotes for the PHOX2B gene [60]. There are several lines of evidence suggesting a systemic disorder, including autonomic nervous system abnormalities with diverse manifestations that include decreased heart rate variability [61], neuro-ocular findings [62], and reduction in the size of chemoreceptors [63].

Idiopathic hypoventilation

Adults with idiopathic hypoventilation may present with severe hypoventilation with absent or modest coexisting pulmonary disease and in the absence of known causes of hypoventilation, such as myxedema, structural brainstem abnormalities, or sleep apnea. Because of the impaired ventilatory drive, patients may have little dyspnea and may present instead with signs of right-heart failure. Sleep may permit more serious hypoventilation and hypoxemia in this disorder.

Sleep-related breathing disorders are a heterogeneous group of conditions that may be associated with alterations in the structure of sleep, in sleep quality, and in gas exchange during sleep. Obstructive sleep apnea represents the most frequent cause of sleep-related breathing disorders, which encompass a diversity of conditions that either complicate coexisting disease or present as primary disorders. Many of these disorders have consequences during both sleep and wakefulness and may produce substantial burden of symptoms and disease in untreated individuals.

References

[1] Sleep-related breathing disorders in adults: recommendations for syndromic definition and measurement techniques in clinical research. The Report of an American Academy of Sleep Medicine Task Force. Sleep 1999;22:667–89.

[2] Sateia M, Hauri P. The international classification of sleep disorders. 2nd edition. Westbrook, IL: The American Academy of Sleep Medicine; 2005.

[3] Redline S, Kapur VK, Sanders MH, et al. Effects of varying approaches for identifying respiratory disturbances on sleep apnea assessment. Am J Respir Crit Care Med 2000;161: 369–74.

[4] Marcus CL. Sleep-disordered breathing in children. Curr Opin Pediatr 2000;12(3):208–12.

[5] Wheatley JR, Mezzanotte WS, Tangel DJ, et al. Influence of sleep on genioglossus muscle activation by negative pressure in normal men. Am Rev Respir Dis 1993;148(3):597–605.

[6] Hudgel DW, Martin RJ, Johnson B, et al. Mechanics of the respiratory system and breathing pattern during sleep in normal humans. J Appl Physiol 1984;56(1):133–7.

[7] Douglas NJ, White DP, Weil JV, et al. Hypercapnic ventilatory response in sleeping adults. Am Rev Respir Dis 1982;126(5):758–62.

[8] Douglas NJ, White DP, Weil JV, et al. Hypoxic ventilatory response decreases during sleep in normal men. Am Rev Respir Dis 1982;125(3):286–9.

[9] Dempsey JA, Smith CA, Przybylowski T, et al. The ventilatory responsiveness to CO_2 below eupnoea as a determinant of ventilatory stability in sleep. J Physiol 2004;560:1–11.

[10] Iber C, Davies SF, Chapman RC, et al. A possible mechanism for mixed apnea in obstructive sleep apnea. Chest 1986;89(6):800–5.

[11] White JE, Drinnan MJ, Smithson AJ, et al. Respiratory muscle activity during rapid eye movement (REM) sleep in patients with chronic obstructive pulmonary disease. Thorax 1995;50(4):376–82.

[12] O'Donoghue FJ, Catcheside PG, Ellis EE, et al. Sleep hypoventilation in hypercapnic chronic obstructive pulmonary disease: prevalence and associated factors. Eur Respir J 2003; 21(6):977–84.

[13] Davies RJ, Stradling JR. The epidemiology of sleep apnoea. Thorax 1996;51(Suppl 2): S65–70.

[14] Young T, Peppard PE, Gottlieb DJ. Epidemiology of obstructive sleep apnea: a population health perspective. Am J Respir Crit Care Med 2002;165(9):1217–39.

[15] Kripke DF, Ancoli-Israel S, Klauber MR, et al. Prevalence of sleep-disordered breathing in ages 40–64 years: a population-based survey. Sleep 1997;20(1):65–76.

[16] Young T, Palta M, Dempsey J, et al. The occurrence of sleep-disordered breathing among middle-aged adults [see comment]. N Engl J Med 1993;328(17):1230–5.

[17] Bixler EO, Vgontzas AN, Lin HM, et al. Prevalence of sleep-disordered breathing in women: effects of gender [see comment]. Am J Respir Crit Care Med 2001;163:608–13.

[18] Bixler EO, Vgontzas AN, Ten Have T, et al. Effects of age on sleep apnea in men: I. Prevalence and severity. Am J Respir Crit Care Med 1998;157(1):144–8.

[19] Rosen CL. Racial differences in the diagnosis of children with obstructive sleep apnea. Am J Respir Crit Care Med 1998;157:A535.

[20] Frank Y, Kravath RE, Pollak CP, et al. Obstructive sleep apnea and its therapy: clinical and polysomnographic manifestations. Pediatrics 1983;71:737–42.

[21] Davidson TM. The great leap forward: the anatomic basis for the acquisition of speech and obstructive sleep apnea [see comment]. Sleep Med 2003;4(3):185–94.

[22] Olson LG, King MT, Hensley MJ, et al. A community study of snoring and sleep-disordered breathing. Prevalence. Am J Respir Crit Care Med 1995;152(2):711–6.

[23] Desai AV, Cherkas LF, Spector TD, et al. Genetic influences in self-reported symptoms of obstructive sleep apnoea and restless legs: a twin study. Twin Res 2004; 7(6):589–95.

[24] Palmer LJ, Buxbaum SG, Larkin E, et al. A whole-genome scan for obstructive sleep apnea and obesity. Am J Hum Genet 2003;72(2):340–50.

[25] Palmer LJ, Buxbaum SG, Larkin EK, et al. Whole genome scan for obstructive sleep apnea and obesity in African-American families [see comment]. Am J Respir Crit Care Med 2004; 169(12):1314–21.

[26] Coltman R, Taylor DR, Whyte K, et al. Craniofacial form and obstructive sleep apnea in Polynesian and Caucasian men. Sleep 2000;23(7):943–50.

[27] Redline S, Tishler PV, Hans MG, et al. Racial differences in sleep-disordered breathing in African-Americans and Caucasians. Am J Respir Crit Care Med 1997;155(1):186–92.

[28] Young T, Shahar E, Nieto FJ, et al. Predictors of sleep-disordered breathing in community-dwelling adults: the Sleep Heart Health Study. Arch Intern Med 2002;162(8):893–900.

[29] Ancoli-Israel S, Klauber MR, Stepnowsky C, et al. Sleep-disordered breathing in African-American elderly. Am J Respir Crit Care Med 1995;152:1946–9.

[30] Newman AB, Nieto FJ, Guidry U, et al. Relation of sleep-disordered breathing to cardiovascular disease risk factors: the Sleep Heart Health Study. Am J Epidemiol 2001; 154(1):50–9.

[31] Peppard PE, Young T, Palta M, et al. Longitudinal study of moderate weight change and sleep-disordered breathing. JAMA 2000;284(23):3015–21.

[32] Avenell A, Brown TJ, McGee MA, et al. What are the long-term benefits of weight reducing diets in adults? A systematic review of randomized controlled trials. J Hum Nutr Diet 2004; 17(4):317–35.

[33] Wadden TA, Sternberg JA, Letizia KA, et al. Treatment of obesity by very low calorie diet, behavior therapy, and their combination: a five-year perspective. Int J Obes 1989;13(Suppl 2):S39–46.

[34] Catteral J, Douglas NJ, Calverley PM. Transient hypoxemia during sleep in chronic obstructive pulmonary disease is not a sleep apnea syndrome. Am Rev Respir Dis 1983;128: 24–9.

[35] Chaouat A, Weitzenblum E, Krieger JI, et al. Association of chronic obstructive pulmonary disease and sleep apnea syndrome. Am J Respir Crit Care Med 1995;151(1):82–6.

[36] Health. United States, 2004. In: National Center For Health Statistics: US Department of Health and Human Services. p. 235–6.

[37] Mitler MM, Dawson A, Henriksen SJ, et al. Bedtime ethanol increases resistance of upper airways and produces sleep apneas in asymptomatic snorers. Alcohol Clin Exp Res 1988;12: 801–5.

[38] Scanlan MF, Roebuck T, Little PJ, et al. Effect of moderate alcohol upon obstructive sleep apnoea. Eur Respir J 2000;16:909–13.

[39] Younes M. Contributions of upper airway mechanics and control mechanisms to severity of obstructive apnea. Am J Respir Crit Care Med 2003;168(6):645–58.

[40] Engleman HM, Kingshott RN, Wraith PK, et al. Randomized placebo-controlled crossover trial of continuous positive airway pressure for mild sleep apnea/hypopnea syndrome. Am J Respir Crit Care Med 1999;159(2):461–7.

[41] Gottlieb DJ, Whitney CW, Bonekat WH, et al. Relation of sleepiness to respiratory disturbance index: the Sleep Heart Health Study. Am J Respir Crit Care Med 1999;159(2):502–7.

[42] Punjabi NM, Shahar E, Redline S, et al. Sleep-disordered breathing, glucose intolerance, and insulin resistance: the Sleep Heart Health Study. Am J Epidemiol 2004;160(6):521–30.

[43] Shahar E, Whitney CW, Redline S, et al. Sleep-disordered breathing and cardiovascular disease: cross-sectional results of the Sleep Heart Health Study [see comment]. Am J Respir Crit Care Med 2001;163(1):19–25.

[44] Peppard PE, Young T, Palta M, et al. Prospective study of the association between sleep-disordered breathing and hypertension. N Engl J Med 2000;342(19):1378–84.

[45] Sin DD, Fitzgerald F, Parker JD, et al. Risk factors for central and obstructive sleep apnea in 450 men and women with congestive heart failure. Am J Respir Crit Care Med 1999;160(4):1101–6.

[46] Lanfranchi PA, Braghiroli A, Bosimini E, et al. Prognostic value of nocturnal Cheyne-Stokes respiration in chronic heart failure. Circulation 1999;99(11):1435–40.

[47] Harbison J, Ford GA, James OF, et al. Sleep-disordered breathing following acute stroke. QJM 2002;95(11):741–7.

[48] Nopmaneejumruslers C, Kaneko Y, Hajek V, et al. Cheyne-Stokes respiration in stroke: relationship to hypocapnia and occult cardiac dysfunction. Am J Respir Crit Care Med 2005;171(9):1048–52.

[49] Catterall JR, Calverley PM, Power JT, et al. Ketotifen and nocturnal asthma. Thorax 1983;38(11):845–8.

[50] Douglas NJ. Nocturnal hypoxemia in patients with chronic obstructive pulmonary disease. Clin Chest Med 1992;13(3):523–32.

[51] Becker HF, Piper AJ, Flynn WEM, et al. Breathing during sleep in patients with nocturnal desaturation. Am J Respir Crit Care Med 1999;159:112–8.

[52] Klink ME, Dodge R, Quan SE. The relation of sleep complaints to respiratory symptoms in a general population. Chest 1994;105:151–4.

[53] Calverley PM, Brezinova V, Douglas NJC, et al. The effect of oxygenation on sleep quality in chronic bronchitis and emphysema. Am Rev Respir Dis 1982;126(2):206–10.

[54] Fleetham J, West P, Mezon BC, et al. Sleep, arousals, and oxygen desaturation in chronic obstructive pulmonary disease. The effect of oxygen therapy. Am Rev Respir Dis 1982;126(3):429–33.

[55] Guilleminault C, Philip P, Robinson A. Sleep and neuromuscular disease: bilevel positive airway pressure by nasal mask as a treatment for sleep disordered breathing in patients with neuromuscular disease. J Neurol Neurosurg Psychiatry 1998;65(2):225–32.

[56] Hill NS, Eveloff SE, Carlisle CC, et al. Efficacy of nocturnal nasal ventilation in patients with restrictive thoracic disease. Am Rev Respir Dis 1992;145:365–71.

[57] Ellis E, Grunstein RR, Chan S, et al. Noninvasive ventilatory support during sleep improves respiratory failure in kyphoscoliosis. Chest 1988;94:811–5.

[58] Piper AJ, Sullivan CE. Effects of long-term nocturnal nasal ventilation on spontaneous breathing during sleep in neuromuscular and chest wall disorders. Eur Respir J 1996;9(7):1515–22.

[59] Schonhofer B, Kohler D. Effect of non-invasive mechanical ventilation on sleep and nocturnal ventilation in patients with chronic respiratory failure. Thorax 2000;55:308–13.

[60] Gaultier C, Amiel J, Dauger S, et al. Genetics and early disturbances of breathing control. Pediatr Res 2004;55(5):729–33.

[61] Woo MS, Woo MA, Gozal D, et al. Heart rate variability in congenital central hypoventilation syndrome. Pediatr Res 1992;31(3):291–6.

[62] Goldberg DS, Ludwig IH. Congenital central hypoventilation syndrome: ocular findings in 37 children. J Pediatr Ophthalmol Strabismus 1996;33(3):175–80.

[63] Cutz E, Ma TK, Perrin DG, et al. Peripheral chemoreceptors in congenital central hypoventilation syndrome. Am J Respir Crit Care Med 1997;155(1):358–63.

ELSEVIER
SAUNDERS

NEUROLOGIC
CLINICS

Neurol Clin 23 (2005) 1059–1075

Sleep-Disordered Breathing and Cerebrovascular Disease: A Mechanistic Approach

Lena Lavie, PhD

*The Lloyd Rigler Sleep Apnea Research Laboratory, Unit of Anatomy and Cell Biology,
The Ruth and Bruce Rappaport Faculty of Medicine, Technion-Israel Institute of Technology,
POB 9649, 31096, Haifa, Israel*

Sleep apnea syndrome, which is characterized by repeated apneic events and associated with hypoxemia and brief arousals during sleep, is recognized as a major public health problem [1]. Approximately one in four men and one in ten women have at least five apneas or hypopneas in each hour of sleep. In 4% of men and in 2% of women, these are associated with excessive daytime sleepiness which, when combined with the breathing events in sleep, define the obstructive sleep apnea (OSA) syndrome [2]. Loud snoring, nonrefreshing sleep and chronic fatigue also are characteristic complaints of patients who have OSA. The nightly occurrence of complete or partial cessations of breathing has a profound impact on patients' daytime behavior, quality of life, and health. Sleep fragmentation resulting from apnea-related awakenings alters sleep architecture, which results in reduced deep sleep, stages 3-4, and REM sleep and an increase in wake and light sleep after sleep onset. Consequently, patients display excessive daytime sleepiness, which affects their proneness to motor vehicle or work-related accidents. Cognitive and neuropsychologic impairments also are common [3].

The most dramatic impact of OSA is its far-reaching clinical consequences on the cardiovascular system. This association has been recognized since the first patients were investigated in a sleep laboratory [4]. Clinical observations made during the early 1980s documented higher rates of cardiovascular diseases, particularly hypertension, but also ischemic heart disease, myocardial infarction, and stroke, in patients who had OSA. Conversely, OSA was a prevalent finding in nonselected patients who had cardiovascular diseases. More recently, these associations are corroborated by large-scale

---

E-mail address: lenal@tx.technion.ac.il

epidemiologic and prospective studies and by animal models. Furthermore, there also is rapid progress in understanding the underlying mechanisms mediating this association. These include elevated nocturnal and diurnal sympathetic activation, intracranial hemodynamic changes, alteration in platelet aggregability, and occurrence of apnea-related nocturnal ischemia, intrathoracic pressure swings, and oxidative stress and inflammatory cell activation [5–7].

This article addresses the evidence that OSA is associated with cellular and molecular processes that promote atherogenesis, thereby increasing the risk of cerebrovascular diseases. As cerebrovascular diseases and OSA are prevalent phenomena, a great deal of effort has been invested in an attempt to determine if one constitutes a risk factor for the other and what the direction is of this association. These studies are the subject of recent reviews [8,9] and, therefore, are summarized only briefly. Specifically, this article focuses on atherosclerotic processes that are associated with intermittent hypoxia and, therefore, may promote stroke. Evidence that links sleep apnea to stroke with a particular emphasis on oxidative stress, inflammation, and endothelial dysfunction is presented and corroborated by in-vitro and animal studies.

Sleep apnea and strokes

The first hints that disordered breathing in sleep may be associated with increased risk of stroke came from studies that investigated the association of self-reported snoring with various health-related factors. Epidemiologic and case-control studies reported a statistical association between habitual snoring and stroke independent of other potential risk factors, such as gender, obesity, smoking, and alcohol consumption. The relative risk of stroke in individuals who had habitual snoring was between two- and tenfold higher than in nonsnorers [10,11]. Risk of stroke increased if snoring was combined with other characteristic symptoms of OSA, such as excessive daytime sleepiness [12]. The association between snoring and stroke also is found in two prospective studies. A 3-year follow-up study of 4388 men, ages 40 to 69, reveals a twofold higher risk of ischemic heart disease, stroke, or both in snorers compared with nonsnorers. This was independent of age, body mass index, history of hypertension, smoking, and alcohol [13]. Similarly, in an 8-year follow-up study in women ages 40 to 65, there was a modest but significant independent association between the incidence of cardiovascular morbidity and snoring [14]. There was no such relationship, however, in individuals older than 70 [15].

Even though snoring is a ubiquitous sign of sleep apnea, not all snorers suffer from the syndrome. Further cross-sectional and case-control studies examine the association between sleep apnea, determined objectively by polyosmnographic recordings, and stroke. These reveal that 63% to 95% of stroke patients had clinically significant disordered breathing in sleep in comparison with 10% to 20% in the matched control groups [16]. In the Sleep Heart Health Study, in which disordered breathing in sleep was examined in 6424 free-living individuals, even mild forms of disordered breathing in sleep within the normal range were associated with self-reported stroke. The association of disordered breathing in sleep with stroke was stronger than with coronary artery disease [17].

The statistical association between disordered breathing in sleep and strokes, based on cross-sectional epidemiologic or case control studies, does not lead to a firm conclusion as to its direction. Without any evidence that OSA precedes stroke, it cannot be concluded that OSA is the cause rather than the consequence of the stroke. There is, however, some indirect evidence that supports the assumption that OSA precedes stroke. Patients suffering from a transient ischemic stroke, who had either no or minor residual side effects, had the same frequency of OSA as patients who had ischemic stroke, that was significantly higher in stroke patients than the control group [18]. A weaker association between transient ischemic stroke and OSA was reported by McArdle and colleagues [19] in a case control study of 86 patients. The association of different stroke subtypes with similar frequencies of sleep apnea and a decline in the frequency of central but not obstructive apneas from the time period immediately after the stroke to several months afterwards provide support that OSA precedes cerebrovascular events [20].

The time of onset of stroke symptoms also provides clues to the direction of the relationship between disordered breathing in sleep and strokes. Accumulated data show that the time of occurrence of all types of strokes is not distributed randomly during a 24-hour period but tends to cluster during the first 2 hours after waking from sleep and in some types of strokes during sleep itself [21]. Although there is no data linking strokes during sleep or after waking from sleep with OSA except for a few case reports [22], snoring was the only predictor of strokes that occurred either during sleep or within 30 minutes after waking from sleep [23]. The morning occurrence of endothelial dysfunction that is prognostic of future cardiovascular events may make these patients particularly prone to cardiovascular events at this specific time period [24–26].

Atherogenesis, oxidadive stress, and inflammation

Recent years have witnessed progress in the understanding of the natural evolution of cardio- and cerebrovascular diseases. Atherosclerosis, the culprit behind cardiovascular and cerebrovascular events, currently is viewed as a dynamic and progressive disease arising from the subclinical condition of endothelial dysfunction [27]. Likewise, oxidative stress and inflammation are gaining widespread attention as fundamental mechanisms that participate in the initiation and progression of atherosclerosis and its major complications, such as ischemic heart disease and stroke [28–30].

Both of these underlying mechanisms—oxidative stress and inflammation—are exaggerated in patients who have OSA. It is, therefore, reasonable to assume that alterations in these fundamental mechanisms in the setting of OSA may promote cardiocerebrovascular events.

Cellular and molecular mechanisms that promote endothelial dysfunction in obstructive sleep apnea

Hypoxia/reoxygenation and oxidative stress

The hallmark of sleep apnea—intermittent hypoxia—is characterized by repetitive episodes of hypoxia/reoxygenation [7]. The ischemia/reperfusion or hypoxia/reoxygenation is accompanied by injury, that is, the damage that occurs as a result of restoration of blood circulation to a hypoxic tissue [30]. This phenomenon also is characterized by complex metabolic and molecular changes that elicit increased production of reactive oxygen species (ROS) during the reoxygenation period by various mechanisms. Apart from inflicting injury to the surrounding tissues, these oxidant molecules have an essential role: they can activate redox-sensitive signaling pathways that initiate adaptive responses to hypoxia (such as hypoxia inducible factor 1α [not discussed in this article]) (Fig. 1) [7] and or inflammatory pathways [31]. Consequently, endothelial cells, leukocytes, and platelets undergo activation [29]. These activated cells can contribute further to reperfusion injury through a further release of ROS and increased expression of adhesion molecules on leukocytes, platelets, and endothelial cells [32], thereby facilitating endothelial cell-leukocyte interactions that can further exaggerate inflammatory responses. Moreover, circulating activated leukocytes, which express adhesion molecules, also can block cerebral capillaries by attaching to endothelial cells, a phenomenon referred to as no-flow [30,33]. Taken together, all the intermittent hypoxia-related cellular processes described previously may lead to stroke and other cardiovascular morbidities [33].

Reactive oxygen species formation in sleep apnea patients

In the brain, hypoxia/reoxygenation affects several enzymatic systems responsible for increased ROS formation, including enzymes of the mitochondrial respiration chain, xanthine oxidase, and nicotinamide adenine dinucleotide phosphate (NADPH) oxidase from leukocytes and endothelial cells (see Lavie for a comprehensive description [7]). There currently is substantial evidence suggesting that the intermittent hypoxia experienced by patients who have OSA affects these enzymatic pathways in a similar manner to the experimentally induced hypoxia/reperfusion in animal models. For instance, hypoxia/reperfusion–induced mitochondrial dysfunction, which results in excessive free radical formation, is shown by measurement of changes in cytochrome oxidase redox state during OSAs [34]. By using near-infrared spectroscopy, McGown and colleagues show that the oxidation state

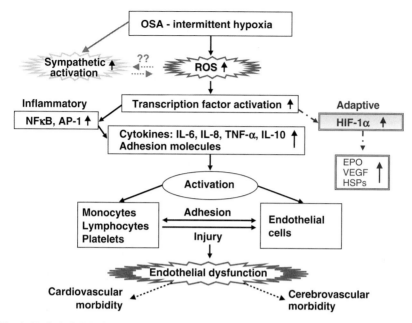

Fig. 1. Endothelial dysfunction in sleep apnea. This figure summarizes the possible course of events starting with intermittent hypoxia and oxidative stress through activation of inflammatory mechanisms that promote endothelial dysfunction and ending with cardiocerebrovascular morbidity. The sleep apnea–related intermittent hypoxia elicits the formation of ROS by several mechanisms. This induces the activation of redox-regulated transcription factors of the adaptive and of the inflammatory response. The adaptive response is characterized by increased expression of HIF-1α gene products, such as erythropoietin (EPO), vascular endothelial growth factor (VEGF), and heat shock proteins (HSPs). The inflammatory response is triggered via activation of the transcription factors NFκb and AP-1, which upregulate the expression of inflammatory cytokines, adhesion molecules, and CRP. These promote activation of endothelial cells, circulating leukocytes, and platelets and facilitate the interactions between circulating cells and endothelial cells lining the vasculature, further amplifying the inflammatory response. Increased adhesiveness between activated leukocytes platelets and endothelial cells injures endothelial cells and elicits endothelial dysfunction, which is the initial step in atherosclerosis.

Given that sleep apnea also is characterized by increased surges of sympathetic nerve activity, sympathetic activation also is shown to affect the expression of adhesion molecules and proinflammatory cytokines; this, however, is beyond the scope of this article. The link, if any, between excessive formation of ROS and sympathetic nerve activity remains to be elucidated.

of the mitochondrial cytocrome oxidase, which is responsible for the final metabolism of molecular oxygen to produce adenosine triphosphate in the respiratory chain, is altered, as are cerebral oxygenation levels, arterial saturation, and cerebral blood flow velocity [34]. Indirect evidence also implicates xanthine oxidase in the pathology of OSA. This is supported by the observations that metabolic byproducts in this pathway, such as uric acid and adenosine, are elevated, suggesting that xanthine oxidase also is a likely source of ROS in OSA [35–38].

A well-established source of increased ROS formation in patients who have OSA is activated monocytes and neutrophils, which implicates NADPH oxidase in this process. NADPH oxidase is the primary enzyme used by these inflammatory cells for generating ROS as a protective mechanism against microbial invasion [30]. Yet this enzyme is activated by a variety of additional stimuli, including hypoxia/reoxygenation. Moreover, an NADPH oxidase isoform, which is expressed by activated endothelial cells and serves signaling purposes, is implicated in the pathogenesis of hypertension that also confers a risk factor for stroke [39]. In OSA, neutrophils and monocytes are activated and release two- to threefold higher amounts of ROS [40,41]. Although endothelial cell activation is suggested as a result of increased expression of adhesion molecules [42,43], there is no direct evidence that corroborates increased endothelial NADPH oxidase expression in OSA.

Another line of evidence that attests to increased oxidative stress in patients who have OSA is the findings of increased lipid peroxidation [44]. The increased lipid peroxidation is apnea-hypopnea index (AHI) (ie, the number of apneas plus hypopneas divided by hours of sleep) severity dependent and less affected by comorbidities, such as hypertension and cardiovascular diseases, or by age and body mass index. The fact that lipid peroxidation, which is a surrogate marker of atherosclerosis and cardiovascular morbidity, is AHI severity dependent emphasizes the possible involvement of ROS in amplifying atherosclerotic processes in these patients.

Because oxidative stress results from an altered balance of oxidant-producing systems and antioxidant defense mechanisms, increased oxidative stress also can result from lower antioxidant capabilities. Antioxidant systems, which protect cells from injury inflicted by oxidative stress, also are affected in OSA. Christou and coworkers demonstrate attenuated antioxidant capacity in severe OSA [45]. Lavie and coworkers demonstrate lower activity of paraoxonase-1 (PON1) in patients who had OSA that was more pronounced in those who had cardiovascular comorbidities [44]. PON1 is a protective enzyme located exclusively on high-density lipoproteins. It also protects low- and high-density lipoprotein from oxidative modification by acting as an antioxidant [46,47]. In a clinical setting, PON1 activity is decreased in patients who have acute myocardial infarction, hypercholesterolmia, and diabetes mellitus [48].

Collectively, these data demonstrate altered balance between oxidant and antioxidant capacities in favor of the former, implicating oxidative stress as one of the fundamental mechanisms that underlie the increased prevalence of cardiocerebrovascular events in OSA.

Inflammatory responses to hypoxia/reoxygenation and stroke

The understanding of the pathophysiology of hypoxia/reoxygenation has increased in recent years largely based on experimental evidence derived from animal models and tissue culture studies. A series of elegant studies using intravital microscopy—a technique that allows visualization of events that occur within microvessels—document vascular interactions during hypoxia/reoxygenation [33,49]. By following the fate of fluorescent molecules, Granger and colleagues demonstrate the contribution of increased expression of various adhesion molecules in enhancing platelet-leukocyte and endothelial cell interactions in the microvasculature. By using mice genetically deficient in a specific adhesion molecule, they show that the adhesion molecules involved elicit a prothrombotic and a proinflammatory phenotype in the cerebral microvascular circulation that also is oxidative stress dependent [49,50].

Similarly, in OSA using monocytes and various subpopulations of cytotoxic T lymphocytes that underwent intermittent hypoxia/reperfusion epochs in vivo (in patients' circulation during sleep), Dyugovskaya and coworkers [41] document activation and altered functions of leukocytes in patients who had OSA. Hence, monocytes and lymphocytes from patients who had OSA expressed higher amounts of adhesion molecules and increased avidity to human endothelial cells in culture. Additionally, various cytotoxic T-lymphocyte subpopulations, such as CD8+, CD4+, and γδ T cells from OSA patients, exhibited higher then control killing capacities against human endothelial cells [51–53]. Such cellular interactions can promote increased adhesion of leukocytes to the vascular walls, initiating atherogenic processes [54].

Adhesion molecules and leukocytes/endothelial cells interactions in obstructive sleep apnea

Adhesion molecules represent a set of molecules that are upregulated in endothelial cells and in leukocytes in response to a variety of stimuli, including hypoxia/reoxygenation. Their expression is a highly regulated, sequential process that is manifested in endothelial cells and leukocytes, thereby facilitating the interactions between these cell types. These sequential interactions entail three independent steps: rolling, firm adhesion, and transmigration [28]. Each step involves a specific set of adhesion molecules, having specific receptors and counter receptors on leukocytes and endothelial cells. The selectins that mediate leukocyte rolling are designated according to the cell type they are expressed on. L-selectins are expressed in leukocytes, E-selectins are expressed in endothelial cells, and P-selectins, which are stored in α granules of platelets and in Weibel-Palade bodies of endothelial cells, are expressed on stimulation.

Rolling is characterized by slowing down the flow of leukocytes in the blood stream, thereby promoting the initial binding to the endothelium. The slowing down of the leukocytes allows interactions with inflammatory mediators released from endothelial cells, and if both leukocytes and endothelial cells undergo activation, they attach to each other firmly via adhesion molecules. The firm adhesion involves integrins (mainly of the

CD18/CD11) on leukocytes and the counter receptors of the immunoglobu-lin superfamily—intracellular adhesion molecules (ICAM-1) and vascular cell adhesion molecules (VCAM-1)—on endothelial cells. The firm adhesion between leukocytes and endothelial cells is followed by migration of the leukocytes from postcapillary venules to the interstitum, where they release lytic enzymes proinflammatory cytokines and free radicals [28,54]. Soluble isoforms of the various adhesion molecules detected in the circulation, such as P-selectin, E-selectin, ICAM-1, and VCAM-1, that are shed from activated enothelium are considered markers of active atherosclerotic diseases and predictors of future cardiovascular disease [55]. Their ex-pression and significance in the setting of OSA are discussed later.

Monocytes

In patients who have OSA, two adhesion molecules on monocytes are increased: the expression of the CD15 moiety on selectins (of the family of adhesion molecules that mediates rolling) and CD11c, a β subunit of the integrins (and a counter receptor for ICAM-1 on endothelial cells), which promotes firm adhesion [41]. This implicates exaggerated rolling and firm adhesion in the pathogenesis of vascular complications in OSA. The finding that monocytes in patients who have OSA adhere significantly more avidly to nonstimulated endothelial cells in culture emphasizes the functional significance of the increased expression of these molecules in OSA. Furthermore, CD15 upregulation is associated directly with the amount of hypoxia these patients experienced, as attested by the severity of the syndrome (unpublished observation). Additionally, increased CD15 expres-sion also is observed after exposing monocytes of control subjects to hypoxia in vitro [41]. Of note, nasal continuous positive airway pressure (nCPAP) treatment, which ameliorates the condition of OSA, proportion-ally reduced the percentage of monocytes expressing CD15 and CD11c, decreased basal ROS formation of CD11c expressing monocytes, and attenuated monocytes/endothelial cells interactions in culture. Also, by pretreating endothelial cells with antibodies against E-selectin/P-selectin or ICAM-1, the relative contribution of each of these adhesion molecules to the interactions that occurred between monocytes and endothelial cells was demonstrated. Jointly, these data indicate that monocytes of patients who have OSA undergo activation.

T lymphocytes

Investigations the functional and phenotypic characteristics of CD8+, CD4+, and γδ+ subpopulations of cytotoxic T lymphocytes from patients who have OSA reveal that these T cell subpopulations acquire an activated phenotype and a higher-than-control ability to kill endothelial cells in culture. Moreover, the killing abilities of CD8+ T lymphocytes also are AHI severity dependent. Yet, each subpopulation uses different killing mechanisms to damage endothelial cells. Whereas CD8+ T lymphocytes primarily express higher amounts of the CD56 natural killer receptors and perforin, CD4+ killing relies on the presence of CD4+/CD^{28null} T cells, and the killing by γδ+ T lymphocytes primarily is mediated by the presence of the proinflammatory cytokine, tumor necrosis factor α (TNF-α), that was found elevated in patients who had OSA [51–53].

The higher expression of adhesion molecules, the higher avidity and ability to strongly attach to endothelial cells in culture conditions, and the stronger cytotoxicity against endothelial cells are markers of activation of the various leukocyte subpopulations studied in patients who have OSA and can be considered indicators of the possible ongoing processes that may damage the endothelium.

Platelets

As with circulating leukocytes, platelets acquire an activated and a prothrombotic phenotype in response to hypoxia/reoxygenation. In animal models, the changes elicited in the cerebral microcirculation by hypoxia/reoxygenation are accompanied by platelets attaching firmly to the leukocytes and to the endothelium, with the adherent leukocytes preceding the recruitment of platelets [49]. In OSA, platelet activation and aggregability in vitro are increased. The percentage of platelets expressing P-selectin (CD62P) is higher [56,57], particularly in patients who have severe OSA [58] and is lowered effectively after nCPAP treatment [59]. Additionally, owing to increases in hematocrit, blood viscosity, and fibrinogen, patients who have OSA may be predisposed further to hypercoagulability [60,61]. In view of the fact that platelets play a key role in ischemic cardiovascular diseases, their altered activation state and hyperaggregability also may contribute to increased cardiocerebrovascular morbidity in OSA.

Endothelial cells and adhesion molecules in the circulation

Although endothelial cells from the vasculature of patients who have OSA are unobtainable, one way of following their responses is through activation markers in the circulation. Adhesion molecules in the circulation that originate from endothelial cells also increase in OSA [42,43]. Moreover, elevated ICAM-1, VCAM-1, L-selectin, and E-selectin levels [43] are attenuated by nCPAP treatment [42]. Jointly, these observations suggest that the endothelium and leukocytes of these patients are activated and that treatment with nCPAP could ameliorate this condition. Also, expression of soluble adhesion molecules (ICAM-1, VCAM-1, L-selectin, and E-selectin) was determined in patients who had coronary artery disease with and without OSA to eliminate the possible contribution of comorbidities. All but L-selectin increased in patients who had coronary artery disease and OSA. The investigators conclude that in the setting of cardiovascular disease, OSA modulates proinflammatory mediators [62]. Furthermore, the authors recently found that levels of E-selectin were elevated in patients who have OSA in a severity-dependent manner compared with control values and increased further in OSA who also suffer from hypertension and cardiovascular morbidity (unpublished observations). These data further support the notion that the endothelium of patients who have OSA is activated.

C-reactive protein

Another potential molecule linking OSA to inflammation and athero-sclerosis is the acute phase reactant C-reactive protein (CRP), a marker of inflammation and a strong predictor of future cardiovascular events [55]. It also is an independent predictor of congestive heart failure in patients who have stroke [63] and of stroke patients who have a poor outcome [64]. Moreover, CRP levels affect endothelial cells, induce expression of adhesion molecules (such as E-selectin, ICAM-1, and VCAM-1) in vitro by endo-thelial cells [65], and sensitize endothelial cells to killing by T cells [66]. These data suggest that CRP is not merely an inflammatory marker but has modulatory functions that may contribute to the development of inflam-matory/atherosclerotic processes [65].

In OSA, the question of whether or not CRP levels are elevated is controversial. Earlier, CRP was reported to be elevated in a severity-dependent manner [67] and to decrease with nCPAP [68]. More recently, however, obesity, rather than OSA, was suggested as a risk factor for elevated CRP [69]. Yet, the fact that CRP levels also are affected by sleep duration [70] makes it difficult to separate the independent contribution of each of the factors affecting CRP in OSA. Most likely, all contribute to varying degrees and there is a need for large-scale studies to resolve this issue. Yet, a patient who has OSA and also high CRP levels should be considered at high risk for cardiocerebrovascular complications.

Cytokines, atherogenesis, and sleep apnea

Given that cytokines participate and amplify inflammatory responses, their role in OSA also was investigated. Cytokines are secreted by activated T cells and control macrophage activation, scavenger receptor expression, and metalloproteinase secretion; modulate smooth muscle cell proliferation, nitric oxide (NO) production, and apoptosis; and induce endothelial cell activation. The classical proinflammatory cytokines, TNF-α, interleukin (IL) 6, and IL-8, are regulated by oxygen tension and free radicals via activation of transcription factors of the inflammatory response, such as nuclear factor κB (NFκB) and activator protein 1 (AP-1) [71]. The anti-inflammatory and antioxidant, IL-10, which is an important pleiotropic cytokine and a regulator of immune and inflammatory responses [72], also is regulated by oxygen tension and free radicals and controls proinflammatory cytokine production [73]. Therefore, it could be expected that regulation and synthesis of cytokines also are affected by sleep apnea. For instance, TNF-α, which acts as a proatherogenic agent because of its ability to cause cell necrosis and also is implicated in atheroma formation and in cytotoxicity and thrombogenicity against endothelial cells [74], is elevated in patients who have OSA [75,76]. Increases in TNF-α and IL-8 (the chemotactic peptide for neutrophils) content in γδ T cells [51] and IL-6 and IL-8 in the circulation [68,76,77] also support this paradigm. Moreover, an imbalance is noted between the levels of TNF-α and IL-10 in OSA CD4+ and CD8+ T cells. When TNF-α is elevated, IL-10 also is elevated, perhaps as a compensatory mechanism to protect from the deleterious effects of TNF-α. As the severity of OSA increases (in an AHI-dependent manner), however, IL-10 does not increase proportionally, resulting in an imbalance between TNF-α and IL-10 in favor of the former [53]. Also, elevated levels of TNF-α and IL-10 are suggested as involved in the pathogenesis of stroke after cardiac surgery with cardiopulmonary bypass [78].

Endothelial dysfunction in sleep apnea

Under normal physiologic conditions, the endothelium regulates vascular tone and interactions between the vessel wall and circulating substances and blood cells. It thus maintains homeostasis by keeping the balance between vasoconstrictors and vasodilators. On disruption of this balance, the endothelium is activated and can acquire a proatherogenic and proinflammatory phenotype [28,79], which, as described previously, is characterized by overexpression of adhesion molecules and initiation of inflammatory pathways.

Endothelial dysfunction represents a state where NO bioavailability is compromised, resulting in vasoconstriction [27]. In addition to its strong vasodilatory properties, NO mediates many of the protective functions of the endothelium. It limits leukocyte recruitment and expression of leukocyte adhesion molecules. Vascular smooth muscle cell proliferation and platelet aggregation and adhesion also are inhibited. Likewise, it inhibits tissue factor production and thereby limits atherosclerotic plaque disruption and intravascular thrombosis [27,28]. Diminished NO bioavailability, measured as nitrite/nitrate concentrations, is detected in patients who have OSA [80,81] and treatment with nCPAP restores NO levels [81]. Concomitantly, vasoconstrictors levels also are elevated [82,83].

Exposure to oxidative stress, characteristic of sleep apnea, to inflammatory mediators, such as TNF-α and IL-6, or the presence of cardiovascular risk factors, such as hypercholesterolemia or hyperhomocysteinemia, promotes endothelial cell activation and endothelial dysfunction [84]. Thus, impaired endothelial function correlates with well-established inflammatory biomarkers of vascular disease, such as CRP and TNF-α, that are increased in patients who have OSA. Moreover, inflammatory biomarkers, such as

CRP, and soluble adhesion molecules, such as ICAM-1, currently are viewed as surrogate markers of endothelial dysfunction and, like endothelial dysfunction itself, are predictive of future cardiovascular events [55].

Impaired endothelial-dependent vasodilatation is reported predominantly in male patients who have OSA and are free of any overt cardiovascular morbidity. Carlson and colleagues [24] report that endothelial function in forearm resistance vessels is impaired in patients who have OSA in comparison with healthy subjects. Kato and colleagues [25] report that patients who have OSA have a blunted vasodilatation response to acetylcholine in the forearm in comparison with carefully matched nonapneic obese subjects. Kraiczi and coworkers [85] report a significant association between sleep apnea severity and reduced endothelium-dependent dilatory capacity. More recently, Ip and colleagues [86] demonstrate that sleep apnea–associated endothelial dysfunction is AHI severity dependent and can be reversed by nCPAP treatment. Furthermore, by omitting nCPAP in otherwise treated patients, they also show that endothelial dysfunction is re-established [86]. A recent study from the authors' laboratory, using a novel technique of measuring the peripheral arterial tone response to reactive hyperemia, also confirms the existence of endothelial dysfunction in a severity-dependent manner [26]. Furthermore, in a group of patients who had OSA and also cardiovascular morbidity, the association between the severity of OSA and endothelial dysfunction was stronger than in patients who had OSA alone [26]. In patients who have stroke, evidence suggests that endothelial dysfunction can play a major role in the pathogenesis of ischemic stroke, endothelial dysfunction was long recognized for elevated blood pressure [87].

Collectively, patients who have OSA and are free of any overt cardiovascular disease display impaired endothelial function as determined by various methods and protocols. This measure, if standardized, has an important prognostic value that may provide useful clinical information. As the underlying mechanisms of endothelial dysfunction, atherosclerosis and its clinical manifestations are being delineated; this measure can be used as a noninvasive surrogate marker to evaluate patients at risk and, alternatively, to monitor the reversal of endothelial dysfunction by nCPAP or other treatment modalities.

Summary

The observations described in this article point to the existence of increased oxidative stress and systemic inflammation in sleep apnea and have paved the way for establishing sleep apnea as an independent risk factor for cardio- and cerebrovascular morbidities. The proposed course of events is summarized in Fig. 1. It is suggested that hypoxia/reoxygenation, characteristic of sleep apnea, promotes the formation of ROS, particularly during the reoxygenation period, and can be deleterious to cells and tissues. ROS, however, regulate the activation of critical transcription factors that are redox sensitive, resulting in increased expression of sets of genes that encode proteins essential to adaptation to hypoxia (via hypoxia inducible factor 1 [hypoxia inducible factor-1α]). Yet, redox-sensitive transcription factors (NFκB and AP-1) that elicit inflammatory pathways also are activated, thereby affecting inflammatory and immune responses by promoting activation of endothelial cells, leukocytes, and platelets. These activated cells express adhesion molecules and proinflammatory cytokines that may lead to endothelial injury and dysfunction and consequently to the development of cardio- and cerebrovascular morbidities. These may be exaggerated in patients who have sleep apnea in response to the intermittent hypoxia.

Acknowledgments

The author would like to thank Professor P. Lavie for the helpful suggestions and critical reading of the manuscript, the staff of The Lloyd Rigler Sleep Apnea Research Laboratory, and the staff of the Sleep Medicine Center, RAMBAM Hospital, Haifa, Isreal, for their invaluable help.

References

[1] Phillipson EA. Sleep apnea—a major public health problem. N Engl J Med 1993;328:1271–3.
[2] Young T, Palta M, Dempsey J, et al. The occurrence of sleep-disordered breathing among middle-aged adults. N Engl J Med 1993;328:1230–5.
[3] Malhotra A, White DP. Obstructive sleep apnoea. Lancet 2002;360:237–45.
[4] Shamsuzzaman AS, Gersh BJ, Somers VK. Obstructive sleep apnea: implications for cardiac and vascular disease. JAMA 2003;290:1906–14.
[5] Narkiewicz K, Somers VK. Sympathetic nerve activity in obstructive sleep apnoea. Acta Physiol Scand 2003;177:385–90.
[6] Marrone O, Bonsignore MR. Pulmonary haemodynamics in obstructive sleep apnoea. Sleep Med Rev 2002;6:175–93.
[7] Lavie L. Obstructive sleep apnoea syndrome–an oxidative stress disorder. Sleep Med Rev 2003;7:35–51.
[8] Yaggi H, Mohsenin V. Obstructive sleep apnoea and stroke. Lancet Neurol 2004;3:333–42.
[9] Hermann DM, Bassetti CL. Sleep-disordered breathing and stroke. Curr Opin Neurol 2003; 16:87–90.
[10] Smirne S, Palazzi S, Zucconi M, et al. Habitual snoring as a risk factor for acute vascular disease. Eur Respir J 1993;6:1357–61.
[11] Neau JP, Meurice JC, Paquereau J, et al. Habitual snoring as a risk factor for brain infarction. Acta Neurol Scand 1995;92:63–8.
[12] Palomaki H. Snoring and the risk of ischemic brain infarction. Stroke 1991;22:1021–5.
[13] Koskenvuo M, Kaprio J, Telakivi T, et al. Snoring as a risk factor for ischaemic heart disease and stroke in men. Br Med J (Clin Res Ed) 1987;294:16–9.
[14] Hu FB, Willett WC, Manson JE, et al. Snoring and risk of cardiovascular disease in women. J Am Coll Cardiol 2000;35:308–13.
[15] Jennum P, Schultz-Larsen K, Davidsen M, et al. Snoring and risk of stroke and ischaemic heart disease in a 70 year old population. A 6-year follow-up study. Int J Epidemiol 1994;23: 1159–64.

[16] Wessendorf TE, Teschler H, Wang YM, et al. Sleep-disordered breathing among patients with first-ever stroke. J Neurol 2000;247:41–7.

[17] Shahar E, Whitney CW, Redline S, et al. Sleep-disordered breathing and cardiovascular disease: cross-sectional results of the Sleep Heart Health Study. Am J Respir Crit Care Med 2001;163:19–25.

[18] Bassetti C, Aldrich MS. Sleep apnea in acute cerebrovascular diseases: final report on 128 patients. Sleep 1999;15:217–23.

[19] McArdle N, Riha RL, Vennelle M, et al. Sleep-disordered breathing as a risk factor for cerebrovascular disease: a case-control study in patients with transient ischemic attacks. Stroke 2003;34:2916–21.

[20] Parra O, Arboix A, Bechich S, et al. Time course of sleep-related breathing disorders in first-ever stroke or transient ischemic attack. Am J Respir Crit Care Med 2000;161(2 Pt 1): 375–80.

[21] Muller JE. Circadian variation in cardiovascular events. Am J Hypertens 1999;12(2 Pt 2): 35S–42S.

[22] Kario K, Morinari M, Murata M, et al. Nocturnal onset ischemic stroke provoked by sleep-disordered breathing advanced with congestive heart failure. Am J Hypertens 2004;17: 636–7.

[23] Palomaki H, Partinen M, Juvela S, et al. Snoring as a risk factor for sleep-related brain infarction. Stroke 1989;20:1311–5.

[24] Carlson JT, Rangemark C, Hedner JA. Attenuated endothelium-dependent vascular relaxation in patients with sleep apnoea. J Hypertens 1996;14:577–84.

[25] Kato M, Roberts-Thomson P, Phillips BG, et al. Impairment of endothelium-dependent vasodilation of resistance vessels in patients with obstructive sleep apnea. Circulation 2000; 102:2607–10.

[26] Itzhaki S, Lavie L, Pillar G, et al. Endothelial dysfunction in obstructive sleep apnea measured by peripheral arterial tone response in the finger to reactive hyperemia. Sleep 2005; 28:594–600.

[27] Davignon J, Ganz P. Role of endothelial dysfunction in atherosclerosis. Circulation 2004; 109(23 Suppl 1):III27–32.

[28] Libby P. Inflammation in atherosclerosis. Nature 2002;420:868–74.

[29] Lefer DJ, Granger DN. Oxidative stress and cardiac disease. Am J Med 2000;109:315–23.

[30] Babior BM. Phagocytes and oxidative stress. Am J Med 2000;109:33–44.

[31] McCord JM. The evolution of free radicals and oxidative stress. Am J Med 2000;108:652–9.

[32] Panes J, Granger DN. Leukocyte-endothelial cell interactions: molecular mechanisms and implications in gastrointestinal disease. Gastroenterology 1998;114:1066–90.

[33] Ishikawa M, Zhang JH, Nanda A, et al. Inflammatory responses to ischemia and reperfusion in the cerebral microcirculation. Front Biosci 2004;9:1339–47.

[34] McGown AD, Makker H, Elwell C, et al. Measurement of changes in cytochrome oxidase redox state during obstructive sleep apnea using near-infrared spectroscopy. Sleep 2003;26: 710–6.

[35] Findley LJ, Boykin M, Fallon T, et al. Plasma adenosine and hypoxemia in patients with sleep apnea. J Appl Physiol 1988;64:556–61.

[36] McKeon JL, Saunders NA, Murree-Allen K, et al. Urinary uric acid: creatinine ratio, serum erythropoietin, and blood 2,3-diphosphoglycerate in patients with obstructive sleep apnea. Am Rev Respir Dis 1990;142:8–13.

[37] Braghiroli A, Sacco C, Erbetta M, et al. Overnight urinary uric acid: creatinine ratio for detection of sleep hypoxemia. Validation study in chronic obstructive pulmonary disease and obstructive sleep apnea before and after treatment with nasal continuous positive airway pressure. Am Rev Respir Dis 1993;148:173–8.

[38] Sahebjani H. Changes in urinary uric acid excretion in obstructive sleep apnea before and after therapy with nasal continuous positive airway pressure. Chest 1998;113: 1604–8.

[39] Lassegue B, Griendling KK. Reactive oxygen species in hypertension; an update. Am J Hypertens 2004;17:852–60.

[40] Schulz R, Mahmoudi S, Hattar K, et al. Enhanced release of superoxide from poly-morphonuclear neutrophils in obstructive sleep apnea. Impact of continuous positive airway pressure therapy. Am J Respir Crit Care Med 2000;162(2 Pt 1):566–70.

[41] Dyugovskaya L, Lavie P, Lavie L. Increased adhesion molecules expression and production of reactive oxygen species in leukocytes of sleep apnea patients. Am J Respir Crit Care Med 2002;165:934–9.

[42] Chin K, Nakamura T, Shimizu K, et al. Effects of nasal continuous positive airway pressure on soluble cell adhesion molecules in patients with obstructive sleep apnea syndrome. Am J Med 2000;109:562–7.

[43] Ohga E, Nagase T, Tomita T, et al. Increased levels of circulating ICAM-1, VCAM-1, and L-selectin in obstructive sleep apnea syndrome. J Appl Physiol 1999;87:10–4.

[44] Lavie L, Vishnevsky A, Lavie P. Evidence for lipid peroxidation in obstructive sleep apnea. Sleep 2004;27:123–8.

[45] Christou K, Moulas AN, Pastaka C, et al. Antioxidant capacity in obstructive sleep apnea patients. Sleep Med 2003;4:225–8.

[46] Mackness MI, Arrol S, Abbott C, et al. Protection of low-density lipoprotein against oxidative modification by high-density lipoprotein associated paraoxonase. Atherosclerosis 1993;104:129–35.

[47] Aviram M, Rosenblat M, Bisgaier CL, et al. Paraoxonase inhibits high-density lipoprotein oxidation and preserves its functions. A possible peroxidative role for paraoxonase. J Clin Invest 1998;101:1581–90.

[48] Durrington PN, Mackness B, Mackness MI. Paraoxonase and atherosclerosis. Arterioscler Thromb Vasc Biol 2001;21:473–80.

[49] Ishikawa M, Cooper D, Russell J, et al. Molecular determinants of the prothrombogenic and inflammatory phenotype assumed by the postischemic cerebral microcirculation. Stroke 2003;34:1777–82.

[50] Ishikawa M, Cooper D, Arumugam TV, et al. Platelet-leukocyte-endothelial cell inter-actions after middle cerebral artery occlusion and reperfusion. J Cereb Blood Flow Metab 2004;24:907–15.

[51] Dyugovskaya L, Lavie P, Lavie L. Phenotypic and functional characterization of blood gamma-delta T cells in sleep apnea. Am J Respir Crit Care Med 2003;168:242–9.

[52] Dyugovskaya L, Lavie P, Hirsh M, et al. Activated CD8 T-lymphocytes in obstructive sleep apnoea. Eur Respir J 2005;25(5):820–8.

[53] Dyugovskaya L, Lavie P, Lavie L. Lymphocyte activation as a possible measure of atherosclerotic risk in sleep apnea patients. Autoimmunity. NY Acad Sci 2005;1051:340–50.

[54] Granger DN, Vowinkel T, Petnehazy T. Modulation of the inflammatory response in cardiovascular disease. Hypertension 2004;43:924–31.

[55] Willerson JT, Ridker PM. Inflammation as a cardiovascular risk factor. Circulation 2004; 109(21 Suppl 1):II2–10.

[56] Bokinsky G, Miller M, Ault K, et al. Spontaneous platelet activation and aggregation during obstructive sleep apnea and its response to therapy with nasal continuous positive airway pressure. A preliminary investigation. Chest 1995;108:625–30.

[57] Geiser T, Buck F, Meyer BJ, et al. In vivo platelet activation is increased during sleep in patients with obstructive sleep apnea syndrome. Respiration (Herrlisheim) 2002;69: 229–34.

[58] Eisensehr I, Ehrenberg BL, Noachtar S, et al. Platelet activation, epinephrine, and blood pressure in obstructive sleep apnea syndrome. Neurology 1998;51:188–95.

[59] Hui DS, Ko FW, Fok JP, et al. The effects of nasal continuous positive airway pressure on platelet activation in obstructive sleep apnea syndrome. Chest 2004;125:1768–75.

[60] Hoffstein V, Herridge M, Mateika S, et al. Hematocrit levels in sleep apnea. Chest 1994;106: 787–91.

[61] Nobili L, Schiavi G, Bozano E, et al. Morning increase of whole blood viscosity in obstructive sleep apnea syndrome. Clin Hemorheol Microcirc 2000;22:21–7.

[62] El-Solh AA, Mador MJ, Sikka P, et al. Adhesion molecules in patients with coronary artery disease and moderate-to-severe obstructive sleep apnea. Chest 2002;121:1541–7.

[63] Campbell DJ, Woodward M, Chalmers JP, et al. Prediction of heart failure by amino terminal-pro-B-type natriuretic peptide and C-reactive protein in subjects with cerebrovascular disease. Hypertension 2005;45:69–74.

[64] Cojocaru IM, Cojocaru M, Musuroi C, et al. Study of some markers of inflammation in atherothrombotic pathogenesis of acute ischemic stroke. Rom J Intern Med 2002;40:103–16.

[65] Pasceri V, Willerson JT, Yeh ET. Direct proinflammatory effect of C-reactive protein on human endothelial cells. Circulation 2000;102:2165–8.

[66] Nakajima T, Schulte S, Warrington KJ, et al. T-cell-mediated lysis of endothelial cells in acute coronary syndromes. Circulation 2002;105:570–5.

[67] Shamsuzzaman AS, Winnicki M, Lanfranchi P, et al. Elevated C-reactive protein in patients with obstructive sleep apnea. Circulation 2002;105:2462–4.

[68] Yokoe T, Minoguchi K, Matsuo H, et al. Elevated levels of C-reactive protein and interleukin-6 in patients with obstructive sleep apnea syndrome are decreased by nasal continuous positive airway pressure. Circulation 2003;107:1129–34.

[69] Guilleminault C, Kirisoglu C, Ohayon MM. C-reactive protein and sleep-disordered breathing. Sleep 2004;27:1507–11.

[70] Meier-Ewert HK, Ridker PM, Rifai N, et al. Effect of sleep loss on C-reactive protein, an inflammatory marker of cardiovascular risk. J Am Coll Cardiol 2004;43:678–83.

[71] Haddad JJ. Pharmaco-redox regulation of cytokine-related pathways: from receptor signaling to pharmacogenomics. Free Radic Biol Med 2002;33:907–26.

[72] Terkeltaub RA. IL-10: an "immunologic scalpel" for atherosclerosis? Arterioscler Thromb Vasc Biol 1999;19:2823–5.

[73] Haddad JJ, Fahlman CS. Redox- and oxidant-mediated regulation of interleukin-10: an anti-inflammatory, antioxidant cytokine? Biochem Biophys Res Commun 2002;297:163–76.

[74] Barath P, Fishbein MC, Cao J, et al. Detection and localization of tumor necrosis factor in human atheroma. Am J Cardiol 1990;65:297–302.

[75] Vgontzas AN, Papanicolaou DA, Bixler EO, et al. Elevation of plasma cytokines in disorders of excessive daytime sleepiness: role of sleep disturbance and obesity. J Clin Endocrinol Metab 1997;82:1313–6.

[76] Vgontzas AN, Papanicolaou DA, Bixler EO, et al. Sleep apnea and daytime sleepiness and fatigue: relation to visceral obesity, insulin resistance, and hypercytokinemia. J Clin Endocrinol Metab 2000;85:1151–8.

[77] Ohga E, Tomita T, Wada H, et al. Effects of obstructive sleep apnea on circulating ICAM-1, IL-8, and MCP-1. J Appl Physiol 2003;94:179–84.

[78] Nakamura K, Ueno T, Yamamoto H, et al. Relationship between cerebral injury and inflammatory responses in patients undergoing cardiac surgery with cardiopulmonary bypass. Cytokine 2005;29:95–104.

[79] Lavie L. Sleep apnea syndrome, endothelial dysfunction, and cardiovascular morbidity. Sleep 2004;27:1053–5.

[80] Schulz R, Schmidt D, Blum A, et al. Decreased plasma levels of nitric oxide derivative in obstructive sleep apnoea: response to nCPAP therapy. Thorax 2000;55:1046–51.

[81] Lavie L, Hefetz A, Luboshitzky R, et al. Plasma levels of nitric oxide and l-arginine in sleep apnea patients: effects of nCPAP treatment. J Mol Neurosci 2003;21:57–64.

[82] Carlson J, Hedner J, Patterson A. Increased plasma concentration of ADMA a naturally occurring nitric oxide synthesis inhibitor in OSA patients. Am J Respir Crit Care Med 1997;155:A869.

[83] Saarelainen S, Hasan J. Circulating endothelin-1 and obstructive sleep apnoea. Eur Respir J 2000;16:794–5.

[84] Schulz E, Anter E, Keaney JF Jr. Oxidative stress, antioxidants, and endothelial function. Curr Med Chem 2004;11:1093–104.

[85] Kraiczi H, Caidahl K, Samuelsson A, et al. Impairment of vascular endothelial function and left ventricular filling: association with the severity of apnea-induced hypoxemia during sleep. Chest 2001;119:1085–91.

[86] Ip MS, Tse HF, Lam B, et al. Endothelial function in obstructive sleep apnea and response to treatment. Am J Respir Crit Care Med 2004;169:348–53.

[87] Cosentino F, Volpe M. Hypertension, stroke, and endothelium. Curr Hypertens Rep 2005;7: 68–71.

ELSEVIER
SAUNDERS

NEUROLOGIC
CLINICS

Neurol Clin 23 (2005) 1077–1106

Non–Rapid Eye Movement Sleep Parasomnias

Mark W. Mahowald, MD[a,b,d,*], Carlos H. Schenck, MD[a,c,d]

[a]Minnesota Regional Sleep Disorders Center, Minneapolis, MN, USA
[b]Department of Neurology, Hennepin County Medical Center, Minneapolis, MN, USA
[c]Department of Psychiatry, Hennepin County Medical Center, Minneapolis, MN, USA
[d]University of Minnesota Medical School, Minneapolis, MN, USA

Parasomnias are unpleasant or undesirable behavioral or experiential phenomena that occur predominately or exclusively during the sleep period. Once believed to unitary phenomena, related to psychiatric disorders, it is now clear that parasomnias are the result of several completely different phenomena and usually are not related to psychiatric conditions. Parasomnias may be categorized conveniently as primary (disorders of the sleep states per se) and secondary (disorders of other organ systems that manifest themselves during sleep). The primary sleep parasomnias can be classified according to the sleep state of origin: rapid eye movement (REM) sleep, non-REM (NREM) sleep, or miscellaneous (ie, those not respecting sleep state). The secondary sleep parasomnias can be classified further by the organ system involved [1].

There is extensive reorganization of the central nervous system activity as the states of wakefulness, NREM sleep, and REM sleep appear. Most portions of the central nervous system are active across all three states of being, but active in a different mode. Parasomnias are clinical phenomena that appear as the brain becomes reorganized across states; therefore, they are particularly apt to occur during the transition periods from one state to another. In view of (1) the large number of neural networks, neurotransmitters, and other state-determining substances that must be recruited synchronously for full state declaration and (2) the frequent transitions among states during the sleep-wake cycle, it is surprising that errors in state

* Corresponding author. Minnesota Regional Sleep Disorders Center, Hennepin County Medical Center, 701 Park Avenue, Minneapolis, MN 55415.
E-mail address: mahow002@umn.edu (M.W. Mahowald).

declaration do not occur more frequently. Fig. 1 portrays a simplified conceptualization of the overlapping nature of the various parasomnias. Box 1 lists the various primary and secondary parasomias.

Primary sleep phenomena

The concepts that sleep and wakefulness are not invariably mutually exclusive states and that the various state-determining variables of wakefulness, NREM sleep, and REM sleep may occur simultaneously or oscillate rapidly are key to understanding the primary sleep parasomnias. The admixture of wakefulness and NREM sleep would explain confusional arousals (sleep drunkenness), automatic behavior, or microsleeps [2–5]. The tonic and phasic components of REM sleep may become dissociated, intruding or persisting into wakefulness, explaining cataplexy, wakeful dreaming, lucid dreaming, and the persistence of motor activity during REM sleep behavior disorder [6]. (See the article by Schenck and Mahowald elsewhere in this issue for discussion of REM sleep parasomnias.)

Non–rapid eye movement sleep phenomena—normal

Neurologists should be aware of several normal NREM phenomena that may result in clinical symptoms or complaints, often resulting in neurologic consultation.

Hypnagogic imagery

Dreaming is not confined to REM sleep but occurs throughout all stages of sleep. Prominent vivid dream-like mentation may occur at sleep onset,

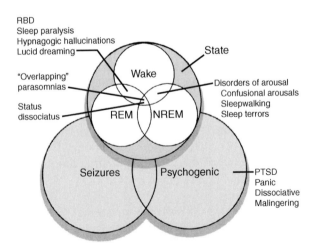

Fig. 1. The overlapping nature of state and conditions associated with parasomnias.

Box 1. Non–rapid eye movement sleep parasomnias

1. Primary sleep phenomena
   a. NREM sleep phenomena—normal
      1. Hypnagogic imagery
      2. Sleep starts (hypnic jerks)
   b. NREM phenomena—abnormal
      Disorders of arousal
      Confusional arousals
         Sleepwalking
         Sleep terror
         Sleep-related eating disorder
         Sleepsex (sexsomnia)
   c. Miscellaneous primary sleep parasomnias
      Nocturnal groaning (catathrenia)
      Bruxism
      Enuresis
      Rhythmic movement disorder
      Propriospinal myoclonus
      Post-traumatic stress disorder
      Somniloquy (sleep talking)
2. Secondary sleep phenomena
   a. Central nervous system parasomnias
      Seizures
      Headaches
         "Vascular" headaches
         Nonvascular headances
         Exploding head syndrome
         Hypnic headache
   b. Cardiopulmonary parasomnias
      Cardiac arrhythmias
      Nocturnal angina pectoris
      Nocturnal asthma
      Respiratory dyskinesias
      Sleep hiccup
      Sleep-related dyspnea, choking, and expiratory groaning
   c. Gastrointestinal parasomnias
      Gastroesophageal reflux
      Diffuse esophageal spasm
      Abnormal swallowing
   d. Miscellaneous secondary parasomnias
      Tinnitus
      Nocturnal panic attacks
      Psychogenic dissociative states

Functional disorders: malingering or Munchausen syndrome
Nocturnal muscle cramps
Nocturnal pruritus
Night sweats
Miscellaneous
    Tongue biting
    Sleep-onset syncope
    Intractable cough associated with the supine position

during light NREM sleep, and even during relaxed wakefulness [7]. Therefore, the report of dream-like experiences occurring at sleep onset does not necessarily imply REM-onset sleep and should not be used as a clinical marker for narcolepsy.

Sleep starts (hypnic jerks)

Sleep starts (hypnic jerks) are experienced by many individuals during the transition between wake and sleep. The most common are motor sleep starts, sudden jerks of all or part of the body, occasionally awakening victims or bed-partners. These are so prevalent as to result rarely in neurologic consultation [8]. Variations, however, may result in neurologic consultation. These include visual (flashes of light or fragmentary visual hallucinations), auditory (loud bangs or snapping noises), or somesthetic (pain, floating, or something flowing through the body) sleep starts. These sensory phenomena may occur without a body jerk [9–12]. Sleep starts represent a normal (although not understood) physiologic event and should not be confused with seizures or other neurologic conditions. Explosive tinnitus, characterized by a loud crashing or banging noise occurring during sleep, most likely represents an auditory sleep start [13]. Sleep starts may be repetitive and should not be confused with epileptic phenomena [14,15]. Familiarity with nonmotor sleep starts should eliminate unnecessary testing and pharmacologic treatment [16]. It is likely that the exploding head syndrome (see later discussion) is a variant of a sensory sleep start.

Non–rapid eye movement phenomena—abnormal

Disorders of arousal

Disorders of arousal are the most impressive and most frequent of the NREM sleep phenomena. They share common features: they tend to arise from slow wave sleep (stages 3 and 4 of NREM sleep), therefore occur usually in the first third of the sleep cycle (and rarely during naps); and they are common in childhood, usually decreasing in frequency with increasing age [16–18]. There often is a family history of arousal disorders; however, this association recently has been questioned. Although they occur most frequently during stages 3 and 4 of NREM sleep (slow wave sleep), disorders of arousal may occur during any stage of NREM sleep and may occur late in the sleep period [19]. Disorders of arousal occur on a broad spectrum ranging from confusional arousals to somnambulism (sleep walking) to sleep terrors (also termed pavor nocturnus and, erroneously, incubus or succubus). Some take the form of "specialized" behaviors (discussed later), such as sleep-related eating and sleep-related sexual activity, without conscious awareness.

Confusional arousals. Confusional arousals often are seen in children and are characterized by movements in bed, occasional thrashing about, or inconsolable crying [20]. Sleep drunkenness probably is a variation on this theme [21]. The prevalence of confusional arousals in adults is approximately 4% [22].

Sleepwalking. Sleepwalking is prevalent in childhood (1%–17%), peaking at 11 to 12 years of age, and is more common in adults (nearly 4%) than generally acknowledged [22–25]. Sleepwalking may be either calm or agitated, with varying degrees of complexity and duration.

Sleep terrors. Sleep terrors are the most dramatic disorder of arousal. They frequently are initiated by a loud, blood-curdling scream associated with extreme panic, followed by prominent motor activity such as hitting the wall, running around or out of the bedroom or even out of the house, and result in bodily injury or property damage. A universal feature is inconsolability. Although victims seem to be awake, they usually misperceive the environment, and attempts at consolation are fruitless and may serve only to prolong or even intensify the confusional state. Some degree of perception may be evident, for example running for and opening a door or window. Complete amnesia for the activity is typical but may be incomplete [17,18,26]. The intense endogenous arousal and exogenous unarousability constitute a curious paradox. As with sleepwalking, sleep terrors are more prevalent in adults than generally acknowledged (4%–5%) [27]. Although usually benign, these behaviors may be violent, resulting in considerable injury to the victim or others or damage to the environment, occasionally with forensic implications [28]. Rarely, sleep terrors may be associated with neurologic lesions [29].

Disorders of arousal may be triggered by febrile illness, alcohol, prior sleep deprivation, physical activity, or emotional stress [21,30]. Medication-induced cases are reported with sedative/hypnotics, neuroleptics, minor tranquilizers, stimulants, and antihistamines, often in combination with each other [21,31–33]. Disorders of arousal may be exacerbated by pregnancy or menstruation, suggesting hormonal factors [34–36]. Such precipitants should be considered triggering events in susceptible individuals, not causal.

Many other sleep disorders, which result in arousals (obstructive sleep apnea [37], nocturnal seizures, or periodic limb movements) may provoke these disorders. Sleep-disordered breathing is more common in children who have disorders of arousal [38]. The combination of frequent arousals and sleep deprivation seen in these other sleep disorders provides fertile ground for the appearance of disorders of arousal. These represent a sleep disorder within a sleep disorder—the clinical event is a disorder of arousal, but the true culprit is a different, unrelated sleep disorder. It is common clinical experience to observe an improvement in disorders of arousal after effective treatment of obstructive sleep apnea. Conversely, effective treatment of obstructive sleep apnea with nasal continuous positive airway pressure (PAP) may result in disorders of arousal, presumably associated with deep NREM sleep rebound [39,40].

Persistence of these behaviors beyond childhood or their development in adulthood often is taken as an indication of significant psychopathology [41,42]. Many studies have dispelled this myth, indicating that significant psychopathology usually is not present in adults who have disorders of arousal [43–45]. The mechanism of these disorders is not clear, but genetic [46] and environmental factors are operant. It is suggested that sleep terrors may be the manifestation of anomalous REM sleep admixed with NREM sleep [47].

Locomotor centers may play a role in the disorders of arousal, which represent motor activity that is dissociated from waking consciousness [48–51]. These areas project to the central pattern generator of the spinal cord, which itself is able to produce complex stepping movements in the absence of supraspinal influence [52]. This accounts for the fact that decorticate experimental and barnyard animals are capable of performing complex, integrated motor acts [53]. A biologic substrate is supported further by the similarity between spontaneously occurring sleep terrors in humans and sham rage induced in animals [54–56]. Human neuropathology may result in similar behaviors [57–61]. Dissociation of the locomotor centers from the parent state of NREM sleep would explain the presence of complex motor behavior seen in disorders of arousal. Spontaneous locomotion after decerebration in cats indicates that such centers, if dysfunctional, release motor activity into the sleeping state [62,63]. Single proton emission computed tomography study of a sleepwalker suggests activation of thalamocingulate pathways and persisting deactivation of other thalamo-cortical arousal systems, resulting in a dissociation between body sleep and mind sleep [64].

The cyclic alternating pattern (CAP) also may play a role in causing disorders of arousal. CAP is a physiologic component of NREM sleep and functionally is correlated with long-lasting arousal oscillations. CAP is a measure of NREM instability with high level of arousal oscillation [65]. There is no difference in the macrostructural sleep parameters between patients who have disorders of arousal and controls. More sophisticated monitoring techniques, such as topographic electroencephalographic (EEG) mapping suggests that there may be more delta EEG activity before the onset of sleep terrors [66]. Patients who have disorders of arousal, however, are found to have increases in CAP rate, in number of CAP cycles, and in arousals with EEG synchronization. An increase in sleep instability and in arousal oscillation is a typical microstructural feature of slow wave sleep-related parasomnias and may play a role in triggering abnormal motor episodes during sleep in these patients [67,68]. Microarousals preceded by EEG slow wave synchronization during NREM sleep are more frequent in patients who have sleepwalking and sleep terrors than in controls. This supports the existence of an arousal disorder in these individuals [67]. Although some investigators report hypersynchronous delta activity on polysomnograms of young adults who sleepwalk [69], this is not the experience of others [70,71]. EEG spectral analysis studies indicate that patients who sleepwalk demonstrate instability of slow wave sleep, particularly in the early portion of the sleep period [72]. As discussed previously, the transition from sleep to wakefulness may be protracted and may play a role in the susceptibility to disorders of arousal [73]. A typical polysomnographic example of a disorder of arousal is shown in Fig. 2.

These arousals may not be the culmination of ongoing psychologically significant mentation, in that somnambulism can be induced in normal children by standing them up during slow wave sleep [41,74] and sleep terrors can be triggered precipitously in susceptible individuals by auditory stimuli during slow wave sleep [75].

Given the high prevalence of these disorders in normal individuals, formal sleep center evaluation should be confined to those cases in which the behaviors potentially are injurious or violent, are extremely bothersome to other household members, result in symptoms of excessive daytime sleepiness, or have unusual clinical characteristics.

Treatment often is not necessary. Reassurance of their typically benign nature, lack of psychologic significance, and tendency to diminish over time often is sufficient. The tricyclic antidepressants and benzodiazepines may be effective and should be administered if the behaviors are dangerous to person or property or extremely disruptive to family members [21]. Paroxetine and trazodone are reported effective in isolated cases of disorders of arousal [76,77]. Nonpharmacologic treatment, such as psychotherapy [75], progressive relaxation [78], or hypnosis [79–81], is recommended for long-term management. Anticipatory awakening is reported effective in treating sleepwalking in children [82]. The avoidance of precipitants, such as drugs, alcohol, and sleep deprivation, also is important.

"Specialized" forms of disorders of arousal

Sleep-related eating disorder. The sleep-related eating disorder, characterized by frequent episodes of nocturnal eating, generally without full

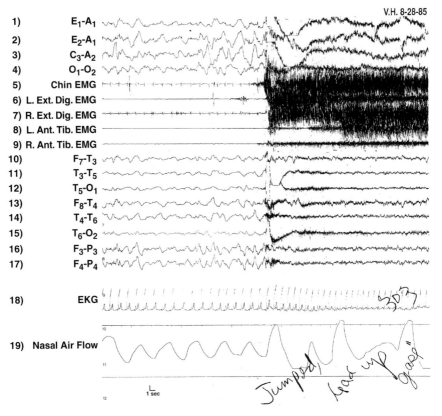

Fig. 2. Polysomnogram correlate of somnambulism. For the initial half of the tracing, there is well-established slow wave (delta) sleep; then, a precipitous arousal occurs, characterized by agitated behavior accompanied by sustained tachycardia (channel 18). Technologist remarks: 3:03 AM—jumped, head up, "gasp." Ant. Tib., anterior tibialis; Ext. Dig., extensor digitorum; L, left, R, right. (*From* Schenck CH, Mahowald MW. Polysomnographic, neurologic, psychiatric, and clinical outcome report on 70 consecutive cases with REM sleep behavior disorder (RBD): sustained clonazepam efficacy in 89.5% of 57 treated patients. Cleve Clin J Med 1990;7(Suppl):S9–23; with permission.)

conscious awareness, usually is not associated with waking eating disorders and likely represents a specialized form of disorder of arousal. This condition often responds to treatment with a combination of dopaminergic and opiate agents. D-fenfluramine, which is no longer available, is reported to be effective [83]. Formal sleep studies are indicated, as sleep-related eating may be the manifestation of other sleep disorders, such as restless legs syndrome, periodic limb movements of sleep, or obstructive sleep apnea, all of which predispose to arousal [84–88]. Nocturnal binging may be induced by benzodiazepine medication [89], and sleep-related eating is associated with zolpidem administration [90]. The sleep-related eating disorder is distinct from the night-eating syndrome, characterized by morning anorexia, evening hyperphagia (while awake), and insomnia, and is associated with hypothalamic-pituitary axis abnormalities [91,92].

Sleepsex. Inappropriate sexual behaviors occurring during the sleep state without conscious awareness, presumably the result of an admixture of wakefulness and sleep, are reported [93–100]. Such behaviors may result in feelings of guilt, shame, or depression and may have medical legal implications [101].

Miscellaneous primary sleep parasomnias

There remain several primary sleep phenomena that are understood poorly and seem not to respect sleep stages.

Nocturnal groaning (catathrenia)

Expiratory groaning, seen during NREM or REM sleep, is described but understood poorly. This may be socially disruptive. The cause is unknown, and no effective treatments are proposed [102–104].

Bruxism (teeth grinding)

Intermittent grinding or clenching of the teeth during sleep may occur at any age with an incidence of 15% to 22% in the general population (up to 88% in children) [105] and appears during any stage of sleep [106,107]. Bruxism is not associated with any specific mentation. The force of nocturnal bruxing may exceed that possible with conscious clenching [108] and, in severe cases, may result in damage to the teeth and surrounding structures [109]. There seems to be a strong genetic influence [110]. Bruxism may represent a symptom of several different disorders, including simple bruxism, orofacial dyskinesia, mandibular dystonia, and tremor [111]. Recently, criteria for the diagnosis of bruxism have been proposed [112,113].

Bruxism may be induced by medications, such as selective serotonin reuptake inhibitors, [114,115] and may be the manifestation of neuroleptic-induced movement disorders [116].

Proposed treatments for bruxism are legion and usually lack scientifically validated objective results. These include occlusal adjustment and splints, psychotherapy, and medications, without predictable or significant improvement [117,118]. The response to interocclusal appliances is variable, with a greater subjective than objective response. Other treatment options include nonsteroidal anti-inflammatory agents, stress management (such as diurnal and nocturnal biofeedback, counseling, avoidance conditioning, hypnosis and progressive relaxation, and occupational and lifestyle changes), physical therapy, muscle relaxants (such as diazepam), and suggestive hypnotherapy [105]. L-dopa or propranolol may be effective [119]. Malocclusion seems to have no role in bruxism; therefore, there is no scientifically valid reason to use early treatment of occlusal conditions to prevent bruxism [120]. Formal sleep studies to rule out nocturnal seizures may be indicated in individuals who experience significant oral damage [121].

Enuresis

Enuresis formerly was classified as a disorder of arousal, implying a relationship with NREM sleep [74]. Enuresis may occur during either NREM or REM sleep, however, and the sleep of enuretic children is normal [122–125]. Enuresis is frequent in childhood and is more prevalent in adolescence and adulthood than generally appreciated (1% to 2% of 18 year olds and 2.3% of adults) [126–128]. Many causes are suggested, including genetic [129], behavioral, and psychologic causes, bladder size or reactivity abnormalities, and delayed development [122,130]. Despite considerable literature, the causes of enuresis remain enigmatic [131]. Local urologic abnormalities account for only 2% to 4% of pediatric cases [132,133]. No specific psychopathology is identified, and there is overwhelming evidence that enuretic children have no more behavioral or psychologic problems than nonenuretic children and that genetic factors are important [123,134–136].

Formal urologic evaluation usually is not indicated, and simple reassurance and understanding on the part of the child and parents often are sufficient. Conditioning with a bell-and-pad device is effective but may be transient [134,137,138]. Psychotherapy generally is ineffective and indicated only if obvious psychopathology is present [126,131]. Tricyclic antidepressants (imipramine or desipramine) are effective and may be used for short-term treatment, but long-term pharmacologic treatment is discouraged. Their mechanism of action is not known but seem not to involve peripheral anticholinergic effects [139]. Desmopressin, an intranasally administered vasopressin analog, reportedly is beneficial [140].

Enuresis may be the sole manifestation of nocturnal seizures and may accompany obstructive sleep apnea [37,141–143]. Formal polysomnographic study with a full-seizure montage and enuresis detector is indicated in those cases with atypical histories or failure to respond to conventional therapy.

Rhythmic movement disorder

Rhythmic movement disorder (RMD), formerly termed *jactatio capitis nocturna*, refers to a group of behaviors characterized by stereotyped movements (rhythmic oscillation of the head or limbs, head-banging, or body-rocking during sleep) seen most frequently in childhood [144]. Its persistence into adulthood is not uncommon [145,146]. It may be familial in some cases. RMD may arise in all stages of sleep, including REM sleep [147,148], and may occur in the transition from wake to sleep. In some cases, RMD may be related temporally to the A phase of the CAP [149]. Significant injury from repetitive pounding may result [150]. The onset of persistent RMD is coincident with recurrent and severe otitis media in childhood [151].

The cause of RMD is unknown, and no systematic studies of pharmacologic or behavioral treatment are reported, although tricyclic antidepressants and benzodiazepines, particularly clonazepam, may be effective [152–155]. Preliminary data suggest that the use of a waterbed may improve the rhythmic behaviors [156]. Hypnosis has been effective in a single case [157]. An isolated case of nonepileptic, post-traumatic RMD responsive to imipramine is described [158]. Post-traumatic cases involving only the foot are reported [159]. Rarely, RMD may be the sole manifestation of a seizure [37].

Propriospinal myoclonus

Propriospinal myoclonus is a spinal cord–mediated movement disorder, occasionally associated with acquired spinal cord lesions. The movements may appear during relaxation and may result in severe insomnia, particularly at sleep onset [160]. Clonazepam or anticonvulsant medications may be effective in alleviating these movements [161]. Propriospinal myoclonus may be related to segmental myoclonus, spinal and palatal [162–164].

Post-traumatic stress disorder

Post-traumatic stress disorder (PTSD) often is associated with subjective sleep complaints, including nightmares and sleep terror–like experiences [165]. Any extraordinary emotional trauma, not just combat situations, may result in PTSD. Objective sleep abnormalities in PTSD are uncommon. Recent detailed objective studies of sleep in PTSD sufferers generally are strikingly unremarkable, suggesting a discrepancy between subjective sleep perception and objective sleep evaluation in those individuals [166–169]. Untreated obstructive sleep apnea may present as PTSD, with resolution after effective treatment of the apnea [170]. Treatment may be difficult and includes counseling. Imipramine or alprazolam may be effective [1].

Somniloquy (sleeptalking)

Sleeptalking is common in the general population, may have a genetic component [171], and may occur in REM or NREM sleep [172,173]. Most cases are not associated with serious psychopathology [174].

Secondary sleep phenomena

The secondary phenomena are those parasomnias representing either abnormal or excessive autonomic or physiologic events arising from specific organ systems and occurring preferentially during the sleep period. These can be categorized by organ system.

Central nervous system parasomnias

Headaches

"Vascular" headaches. The headache symptoms of cluster headache, chronic paroxysmal hemicrania, and possibly migraines, in some cases, tend to be REM sleep related, explaining the common report of sleep-related headaches in these conditions [175–179]. This fact explains the worsening of these symptoms after the discontinuation of REM sleep–suppressing agents (resulting in a rebound of REM sleep), such as tricyclic antidepressants, monoamine oxidase inhibitors, clonidine, alcohol, and amphetamines [180–182]. Circadian rhythm abnormalities may play a role in cluster headache and chronic paroxysmal hemicrania [183,184]. Episodic paroxysmal hemicrania may respond to calcium channel blockers [185].

Nonvascular headaches. Sleep-related headaches are not more common in conventional obstructive sleep apnea than in the general population [186]. In some susceptible individuals, however, obstructive sleep apnea may trigger cluster headaches, which are responsive to bilevel PAP [187]. Headaches associated with sleep-disordered breathing are seen more commonly in patients who have neuromuscular disease and who experience REM sleep–related hypoventilation, with hypercapnia-induced migraines arising from the sleep period. Carbon monoxide poisoning must not be forgotten as a cause of morning headaches.

Exploding head syndrome. Exploding head syndrome is characterized by abrupt arousal, usually occurring in the transition from wake to sleep, with the sensation of a loud sound, like an explosion or a sensation of bursting of the head [188,189]. Most reported cases occur in the twilight state of sleep onset, but polysomnographic recording documents their occurrence during wakefulness and well-declared REM sleep [190,191]. These events may represent a variant of sleep starts [192] and usually are benign [193]; however, similar phenomena may represent the sole manifestation of a seizure [194]. Clomipramine or nifedipine may be effective, however, not indicated in most cases because of the benign nature of the condition [190,195].

Hypnic headache. The hypnic headache syndrome is described in older patients who have regular awakenings from sleep at a consistent time of night (usually between 4 and 6 hours after sleep onset), occasionally during a dream with a diffuse headache generally lasting 30 to 60 minutes associated with nausea but no autonomic symptoms. The headaches usually are generalized but may be unilateral [196]. This condition is believed to be a benign sleep-related headache syndrome affecting the elderly. These headaches may arise from REM or NREM sleep, may represent a circadian phenomenon, and may respond to lithium, indomethacin, prednisone, flunarizine, gabapentin, or caffeine administered before bedtime [197–205].

Cardiopulmonary parasomnias

Cardiac arrhythmias

Cardiac arrhythmias occurring during sleep have been studied extensively. In large groups of individuals, any relationship between sleep in general and sleep stage specifically to arrhythmias is variable and unpredictable [206]. Dramatic anecdotal exceptions include REM sleep–related asystole [207], sound-induced ventricular fibrillation [208], and other dramatic state-dependent cardiac arrhythmias in young, otherwise healthy individuals [209–211]. The autonomic nervous system changes during REM sleep may predispose to cardiac events, as exemplified by the fact that relative risk for sudden death during REM sleep may be has high as 1.2 times that during wakefulness [212–214].

Nocturnal angina pectoris

As with sleep-related arrhythmias, there may be a correlation between angina and sleep or sleep stage in certain individuals, but no generalizations are possible [215–224]. Nocturnal angina may be associated with obstructive sleep apnea [225].

Nocturnal asthma

Sleep-related exacerbation is a common complaint in patients who are asthmatic. No predictable sleep-stage relationship is identified [226–230], and multiple circadian factors including sleep and endocrine and body temperature may play a role [231]. There may be a causal relationship between nocturnal asthma and sleep-disordered breathing [232], and there is some evidence that in individuals who have sleep apnea and asthma, the asthma is less symptomatic after effective treatment of the sleep apnea by nasal continuous PAP [233].

Respiratory dyskinesias

There are many respiratory dyskinesias that may occur or persist during the sleep period. These include segmental myoclonus, such as palatal myoclonus [234,235] or diaphragmatic flutter [236–238], and paroxysmal dystonia [239]. Respiratory dyskinesias also may be the manifestation of neuroleptic-induced dyskinesias and may or may not persist during sleep [240–243]. These should be differentiated from unusual nocturnal seizures that present with primarily or exclusively respiratory symptoms [244–246].

Sleep hiccup

Persistent hiccup may continue during all stages of sleep, but its appearance during sleep in individuals who have chronic hiccup is variable [247]. The frequency diminishes during sleep, more so in REM than NREM sleep. Interestingly, sleep hiccups rarely are associated with arousals [248,249].

Miscellaneous cardiopulmonary

Isolated cases of sleep-related dyspnea and choking are reported; cause and treatment are unclear [102]. Paroxysmal choking may be the sole manifestation of nocturnal seizures [250]. Phantom shocks from implantable cardioverter-defibrillators are reported. Patients are awakened from a sound sleep with the sensation of having received a defibrillator discharge. These were not associated with dream recall. By observation, there was a motor "jolt" associated with crying out, as though an actual shock was administered. Review of the counters indicate that no shock was delivered. These phantom shocks should be identified before medical treatment or device reprogramming is prescribed [251].

Gastrointestinal parasomnias

Many gastrointestinal events may result in paroxysmal arousals during sleep, often mimicking disorders of other organ systems. These include gastroesophageal reflux, diffuse esophageal spasm, and abnormal swallowing.

Gastroesophageal reflux

During sleep, gastroesophageal reflux may present as abrupt awakenings, associated with a choking sensation, dyspnea, chest pain, and severe anxiety. Gastroesophageal reflux may result in prolonged laryngospasm [252–254] or stridor [254]. Gastroesophageal reflux may exacerbate bronchial asthma or result in pulmonary aspiration [255]. The diagnosis may be difficult if the symptoms are exclusively nocturnal and may require continuous polygraphic recording with esophageal pH monitoring [256,257]. Medical treatment is the same as for diurnal gastroesophageal reflux [258]. Obstructive sleep apnea, which predisposes to nocturnal gastroesophageal reflux, always should be ruled out [259,260].

Diffuse esophageal spasm

Nocturnal diffuse esophageal spasm simulates nocturnal cardiac disease, occasionally even resulting in arrhythmias [261,262]. Diagnosis may be made with esophageal manometric monitoring. Treatment includes the administration of anticholinergics, nitrates, or calcium antagonists [263].

Abnormal swallowing

Abnormal swallowing during sleep may cause arousals induced by coughing, aspiration, or choking. Polysomnographic studies show brief episodes of coughing and gagging [264]. Cause and treatment are unknown.

Miscellaneous secondary parasomnias

Tinnitus

Tinnitus may persist during sleep, resulting in sleep complaints in up to 50% of patients [265,266]. The sleep complaints are not associated with mood or emotional distress [267]. Subjective improvement in sleep follows use of an electrical tinnitus suppressor [268]. In another study, nortriptyline decreased depression, functional disability, and loudness of tinnitus, but sleep was not mentioned [269]. This condition is understood poorly and requires more systematic study before any conclusions may be reached. Evidence exists that tinnitus may be mediated centrally [270]. The term, explosive tinnitus, most likely refers to an auditory sleep start [13].

Nocturnal panic attacks

Sleep-related panic attacks may occur in many (30% to 50%) patients who have diurnal panic, may precede the appearance of diurnal panic, or may be exclusively nocturnal in nature [271–276]. Panic disorder can begin in childhood and adolescence and may masquerade as a wide variety of neurologic syndromes [277,278]. Subjective sleep complaints are common in patients who have panic disorder (up to 70%) and include insomnia, nocturnal panic attacks, or fear of going to bed or falling asleep [279]. Formal sleep studies may be unremarkable, with no abnormalities of sleep macrostructure or excessive arousability, but suggest that nocturnal panic is a NREM phenomenon [280,281]. It is easy to understand how nocturnal panic and other sleep disorders characterized by precipitous arousals (particularly sleep apnea or gastroesophageal reflux) may be confused [282]. The striking similarity of the symptoms of dream anxiety attacks, sleep terrors, nocturnal seizures, sleep apnea, and nighttime panic urges caution in diagnosis [272,282–287].

Psychogenic dissociative states

Complex, potentially injurious behavior, occasionally confined to the sleep period, may be the manifestation of a psychogenic dissociative state [288,289]. A history of childhood physical or sexual abuse almost always is present (but may be difficult to elicit) [290,291]. In this condition (and malingering), unlike in other parasomnias, the complex behavior during polysomnographic monitoring is seen to arise from well-developed EEG-determined wakefulness [292]. The term, pseudoparasomnia, is proposed for this condition [293].

Functional disorders: malingering or Munchausen syndrome

These disorders may present to a sleep specialist as sleep-related stridor, asthma, upper airway obstruction, sleep-related violent behaviors in adults [294–299], or sleep apnea (Munchausen syndrome by proxy) in children [300–304]. Cyclic hypersomnia also is reported as a manifestation of a factitious disorder [305].

Nocturnal muscle cramps

The complaint of muscle cramping, frequently nocturnal, is common but understood poorly. The true incidence and cause are unknown and there is no systematic study of nocturnal muscle cramps. A subjective response to quinine sulfate, magnesium, vitamin E, gabapentin, or verapamil is reported as is an isolated case responding to transcutaneous nerve stimulation [306–311].

Nocturnal pruritus

Patients who have a variety of dermatologic disorders associated with pruritus may demonstrate recurrent episodes of scratching during sleep, resulting in sleep disruption [312–314]. These scratching episodes occur during all stages of sleep, most frequently during light NREM, intermediately during REM, and least often during slow wave sleep [315,316]. The duration of scratching episodes is the same in the sleep stages [317]. Such scratching may interfere with treatment and may play a role in factitious dermatoses [318].

Night sweats

Night sweats are common but tend not to be reported to physicians [319]. Night sweats (unrelated to infectious, endocrine, or malignant conditions) may be associated with several unrelated conditions, including obstructive sleep apnea [320], spinal syringomyelia [321], medications [319], gastroesophageal reflux [322], and autonomic seizures [323]. Night sweats also may appear around the time of menopause [324,325]. There is no known effective treatment.

Miscellaneous

Tongue biting during sleep is reported as a manifestation of several unrelated conditions, including myoclonic activity, nocturnal seizures, disorder of arousal, or RMD [326–331].

A single case of sleep-onset syncope, attributed to sleep-onset fluctuation in vagal tone, is reported in a patient who had nasopharyngeal carcinoma [332].

Intractable cough associated with the supine position, presumably the result of position-related collapse of the upper airway, responsive to nasal continuous PAP, is reported [333,334].

Evaluation of parasomnias

Isolated, often bizarre, sleep-related events may be experienced by otherwise healthy people, and most do not warrant further extensive or expensive evaluation. The initial approach to complaints of an unusual sleep-related behavior is to determine if further evaluation is necessary. Patients should be queried regarding the exact nature of the events. Because many of these episodes may be associated with partial or complete amnesia, additional descriptive information from a bed partner or other observer may prove invaluable. Home videotapes of the clinical event may be helpful. In general, indications for formal evaluation of parasomnias include behaviors that [1]

- Are potentially violent or injurious
- Are extremely disruptive to other household members
- Result in the complaint of excessive daytime sleepiness
- Are associated with medical, psychiatric, or neurologic symptoms or findings

Serious attention should be paid to such parasomnia complaints under these circumstances. Formal polysomnographic studies, appropriately performed, provide direct or indirect diagnostic information in the majority of cases. This is of more than academic interest, as most of these conditions readily are treatable. Emphasis must be placed on the types of studies required; routine polysomnograms performed for conventional sleep disorders are inadequate. In addition to the physiologic parameters monitored in the standard polysomnogram, there must be an expanded EEG montage and there must be continuous audiovisual monitoring [69,335]. Experienced technologist observation is invaluable. Multiple night studies may be required to capture an event. Interpretation should be made by a polysomnographer experienced in these disorders. Unattended studies have no role in the evaluation of parasomnias [336].

References

[1] Mahowald MW, Ettinger MG. Things that go bump in the night—the parasomnias revisited. J Clin Neurophysiol 1990;7:119–43.
[2] Niedermeyer E, Singer HS, Folstein SE, et al. Hypersomnia with simultaneous waking and sleep patterns in the electroencephalogram. J Neurol 1979;221:1–13.
[3] Roth B, Nevsimalova S, Rechtschaffen A. Hypersomnia with "sleep drunkenness." Arch Gen Psychiatry 1972;26:456–62.
[4] Zorick FJ, Salis PJ, Roth T, et al. Narcolepsy and automatic behavior: a case report. J Clin Psychiatry 1979;40:194–7.
[5] Roth B, Nevsimalova S, Sagova V, et al. Neurological, psychological and polygraphic findings in sleep drunkenness. Archives Suisses de Neurologie. Neurochirg Psychiatrie 1981;129:209–22.
[6] Mahowald MW, Cramer-Bornemann MA. NREM sleep parasomnias. In: Kryger MH, Roth T, Dement WC, editors. Principles and practice of sleep medicine. 4th edition. Philadelphia: Elsevier/Saunders; 2005. p. 889–96.
[7] Nielsen TA. Cognition in REM and NREM sleep; A review and possible reconciliation of two models of sleep mentation. Behav Brain Sci 2000;23:851–66.
[8] Parkes JD. The parasomnias. Lancet 1986;2:1021–5.
[9] Oswald I. Sudden bodily jerks on falling asleep. Brain 1959;82:92–103.
[10] Dagnino N, Loeb C, Massazza G, et al. Hypnic physiological myoclonus in man: an EEG-EMG study in normals and neurological patients. Eur Neurol 1969;2:47–58.
[11] Lugaresi E, Coccagna G, Cirignotta F. Phenomena occurring during sleep onset in man. In: Popoviciu L, Asgian B, Badiu G, editors. Sleep 1978. Fourth European Congress on Sleep Research, Tirgu-Mures. Basel: S. Karger; 1980. p. 24–7.
[12] Gastaut H, Broughton R. A clinical and polygraphic study of episodic phenomena during sleep. Recent Adv Biol Psychiatry 1967;7:197–221.

[13] Teixido MT, Connolly K. Explosive tinnitus: an underrecognized disorder. Otolaryngol Head Neck Surg 1998;118:108–9.

[14] Fusco L, Pachatz C, Cusmai R, et al. Repetitive sleep starts in neurologically imparied children: an unusual non-epileptic manifestation in otherwise epileptic subjects. Epileptic Disord 1999;1:63–7.

[15] Kotagal P, Costa M, Wyllie E, et al. Paroxysmal nonepileptic events in children and adolescents. Pediatrics 2002;110:e46.

[16] Sander HW, Geisse H, Quinto C, et al. Sensory sleep starts. J Neurol Neurosurg Psychiatry 1998;64:690.

[17] Fisher C, Kahn E, Edwards A, et al. A psychophysiological study of nightmares and night terrors. I. Physiological aspects of the stage 4 night terror. J Nerv Ment Dis 1973; 157:75–98.

[18] Fisher C, Kahn E, Edwards A, et al. A psychophysiological study of nightmares and night terrors. III. Mental content and recall of stage 4 night terrors. J Nerv Ment Dis 1974;158: 174–88.

[19] Naylor MW, Aldrich MS. The distribution of confusional arousals across sleep stages and time of night in children and adolescents with sleep terrors. Sleep Res 1991;20:308.

[20] Rosen G, Mahowald MW, Ferber R. Sleepwalking, confusional arousals, and sleep terrors in the child. In: Ferber R, Kryger M, editors. Principles and practice of sleep medicine in the child. Philadelphia: Saunders; 1995. p. 99–106.

[21] Nino-Murcia G, Dement WC. Psychophysiological and pharmacological aspects of somnambulism and night terrors in children. In: Meltzer HY, editor. Psychopharmacology: the third generation of progress. New York: Raven Press; 1987. p. 873–9.

[22] Ohayon M, Guilleminault C, Priest RG. Night terrors, sleepwalking, and confusional arousal in the general population: their frequency and relationship to other sleep and mental disorders. J Clin Psychiatry 1999;60:268–76.

[23] Hublin C, Kaprio J, Partinen M, et al. Prevalence and genetics of sleepwalking; a population-based twin study. Neurology 1997;48:177–81.

[24] Klackenberg G. Somnambulism in childhood—prevalence, course and behavior correlates. A prospective longitudinal study (6–16 years). Acta Paediatr Scand 1982;71:495–9.

[25] Bixler EO, Kales A, Soldatos CR, et al. Prevalence of sleep disorders in the Los Angeles metropolitan area. Am J Psychiatry 1979;136:1257–62.

[26] Kahn E, Fisher C, Edwards A. Night terrors and anxiety dreams. In: Ellman SD, Antrobus JS, editors. The mind in sleep: psychology and psychophysiology. 2nd edition. New York: John Wiley & Sons; 1991. p. 437–47.

[27] Crisp AH. The sleepwalking/night terrors syndrome in adults. Postgrad Med J 1996;72: 599–604.

[28] Mahowald MW, Schenck CH. Violent parasomnias: forensic medicine issues. In: Kryger MH, Roth T, Dement WC, editors. Principles and practice of sleep medicine. 4th edition. Philadelphia: Elsevier/Saunders; 2005. p. 960–8.

[29] Di Gennaro G, Autret A, Mascia A, et al. Night terrors associated with thalamic lesion. Clin Neurophysiol 2004;115:2489–92.

[30] Vela Bueno A, Blanco BD, Cajal FV. Episodic sleep disorder triggered by fever - a case presentation. Waking Sleeping 1980;4:243–51.

[31] Warnes H, Osivka S, Montplaisir J. Somnambulistic like behavior induced by lithium-neuroleptic treatment. Sleep Res 1993;22:287.

[32] Mendelson WB. Sleepwalking associated with zolpidem. J Clin Psychopharmacol 1994;14: 150.

[33] Harazin J, Berigan TR. Zolpidem tartrate and somnambulism. Mil Med 1999;164:669–70.

[34] Schenck CH, Mahowald MW. Two cases of premenstrual sleep terrors and injurious sleep-walking. J Psychosom Obstet Gynecol 1995;16:79–84.

[35] Snyder S. Unusual case of sleep terror in a pregnant patient. Am J Psychiatry 1986;143:391.

[36] Berlin RM. Sleepwalking disorder during pregnancy: a case report. Sleep 1988;11:298–300.

[37] Guilleminault C. Sleeping and waking disorders: indications and techniques. Menlo Park (CA): Addison-Wesley; 1982.

[38] Goodwin JL, Kaemingk KL, Fregosi Rf, et al. Parasomnias and sleep disordered breathing in Caucasian and Hispanic children—the Tucson children's assessment of sleep apnea study. Available at: www.biomedcentral.com/1741-7015/2. Accessed July 23, 2005.

[39] Millman RP, Kipp GR, Carskadon MA. Sleepwalking precipitated by treatment of sleep apnea with nasal CPAP. Chest 1991;99:750–1.

[40] Fietze I, Warmuth R, Witt C, Baumann G. Sleep-related breathing disorder and pavor nocturnus. Sleep Res 1995;24A:301.

[41] Kales A, Jacobson A, Paulson MJ, et al. Somnambulism: psychophysiological correlates. I. All-night EEG studies. Arch Gen Psychiatry 1966;14:586–94.

[42] Soldatos CR, Kales A. Sleep disorders: research in psychopathology and its practical implications. Acta Psychiatr Scand 1982;65:381–7.

[43] Schenck CH, Hurwitz TD, Bundlie SR, et al. Sleep-related injury in 100 adult patients: a polysomnographic and clinical report. Am J Psychiatry 1989;146:1166–73.

[44] Guilleminault C, Moscovitch A, Leger D. Forensic sleep medicine: nocturnal wandering and violence. Sleep 1995;18:740–8.

[45] Llorente MD, Currier MB, Norman S, et al. Night terrors in adults: phenomenology and relationship to psychopathology. J Clin Psychiatry 1992;53:392–4.

[46] Hori A, Hirose G. Twin studies on parasomnias. Sleep Res 1995;24A:324.

[47] Arkin AM. Night-terrors as anomalous REM sleep component manifestation in slow-wave sleep. Waking Sleeping 1978;2:143–7.

[48] Mori E, Yamadori A. Acute confusional state and acute delirium. Occurrence after infarction in the right middle cerebral artery territory. Arch Neurol 1987;44:1139–43.

[49] Grillner S, Dubic R. Control of locomotion in vertebrates: spinal and supraspinal mechanisms. Adv Neurol 1988;47:425–53.

[50] Berntson GG, Micco DJ. Organization of brainstem behavioral systems. Brain Res Bull 1976;1:471–83.

[51] Mogenson GJ. Limbic-motor integration. Progr Psychobiol Physiol Psychology 1986;12:117–70.

[52] Mori S, Nishimura H, Aoki M. Brain stem activation of the spinal stepping generator. In: Hobson JA, Brazier MAB, editors. The reticular formation revisited. New York: Raven Press; 1980. p. 241–59.

[53] Rossignol S, Dubuc R. Spinal pattern generation. Curr Opin Neurol 1994;4:894–902.

[54] Elliott FA. Neuroanatomy and neurology of aggression. Psychiatr Ann 1987;17:385–8.

[55] Siegel A, Pott CB. Neural substrates of aggression and flight in the cat. Prog Neurobiol 1988;31:261–83.

[56] Bandler R. Brain Mechanisms of aggression as revealed by electrical and chemical stimulation: suggestion of a central role for the midbrain periaqueductal region. Prog Psychobiol Physiol Psychol 1988;13:67–154.

[57] Kelts KA, Hoehn MM. Hypothalamic atrophy. J Clin Psychiatry 1978;39:357–8.

[58] Kelleffer FA, Stern WE. Chronic effects of hypothalamic injury. Arch Neurol 1970;22:419–29.

[59] Reeves AG. Hyperphagia, rage, and dementia accompanying a ventromedial hypothalamic neoplasm. Arch Neurol 1969;20:616–24.

[60] Haugh RM, Markesbery WR. Hypothalamic astrocytoma. Syndrome of hyperphagia, obesity, and disturbances of behavior and endocrine and autonomic function. Arch Neurol 1983;40:560–3.

[61] Sano K, Mayanagi Y. Postermedial hypothalamotomy in the treatment of violent, aggressive behavior. Acta Neurochir (Wien) 1988;44(Suppl):145–51.

[62] Lai YY, Siegel JM. Brainstem-mediated locomotion and myoclonic jerks. II. Pharmacological effects. Brain Res 1997;745:265–70.

[63] Lai YY, Siegel JM. Brainstem-mediated locomotion and myoclonic jerks. I. Neural substrates. Brain Res 1997;745:257–64.

[64] Bassetti C, Vella S, Donati F, et al. SPECT during sleepwalking. Lancet 2000;356:484–5.

[65] Terzano MG, Parrino L, Piroli A, et al. Comparison of cyclic alternating pattern (CAP) parameters in normal sleep of young and aged adults. In: Koella WP, Obal F, Schulz H, Visser P, editors. Sleep '86. Stuttgart (Germany): Gustav Fischer Verlag; 1988. p. 290–2.

[66] Zadra AL, Nielsen TA. Topographical EEG mapping in a case of recurrent sleep terrors. Dreaming 1998;8:67–74.

[67] Halasz P, Ujszaszi J, Gadoros J. Are microarousals preceded by electroencephalographic slow wave synchronization precursors of confusional awakenings? Sleep 1985;8: 231–8.

[68] Zuccone M, Oldani A, Ferini-Strambi L, et al. Arousal fluctuations in non-rapid eye movement parasomnias: the role of cyclic alternating pattern as a measure of sleep instability. J Clin Neurophysiol 1995;12:147–54.

[69] Blatt I, Peled R, Gadoth N, et al. The value of sleep recording in evaluating somnambulism in young adults. EEG Clin Neurophysiol 1991;78:407–12.

[70] Schenck CH, Pareja JA, Patterson AL, et al. An analysis of polysomnographic events surrounding 252 slow-wave sleep arousals in 38 adults with injurious sleepwalking and sleep terrors. J Clin Neurophysiol 1998;15:159–66.

[71] Pressman MR. Hypersynchronous delta sleep EEG activity and sudden arousals from slow-wave sleep in adults without a history of parasomnias: clinical and forensic implications. Sleep 2004;27:706–10.

[72] Guilleminault C, Poyares D, Abat F, et al. Sleep and wakefulness in somnambulism. A spectral analysis study. J Psychosom Res 2001;51:411–6.

[73] Horner RL, Sanford LD, Pack AI, et al. Activation of a distinct arousal state immediately after spontaneous awakening from sleep. Brain Res 1997;778:127–34.

[74] Broughton RJ. Sleep disorders: disorders of arousal? Science 1968;159:1070–8.

[75] Kales JD, Cadieux RJ, Soldatos CR, et al. Psychotherapy with night-terror patients. Am J Psychother 1982;36:399–407.

[76] Lillywhite AR, Wilson SJ, Nutt DJ. Successful treatment of night terrors and somnambulism with paroxetine. Br J Psychiatry 1994;164:551–4.

[77] Balon R. Sleep terror disorder and insomnia treated with trazodone: a case report. Ann Clin Psychiatry 1994;6:161–3.

[78] Kellerman J. Behavioral treatment of night terrors in a child with acute leukemia. J Nerv Ment Dis 1979;167:182–5.

[79] Gutnik BD, Reid WH. Adult somnambulism: two treatment approaches. Nebr Med J 1982; 67:309–12.

[80] Reid WH, Ahmed I, Levie CA. Treatment of sleepwalking: a controlled study. Am J Psychother 1981;35:27–37.

[81] Hurwitz TD, Mahowald MW, Schenck CH, et al. A retrospective outcome study and review of hypnosis as treatment of adults with sleepwalking and sleep terror. J Nerv Ment Dis 1991;179:228–33.

[82] Tobin JDJ. Treatment of somnambulism with anticipatory awakening. J Pediatr 1993;122: 426–7.

[83] Mancini MC, Aloe F. Nocturnal eating syndrome: a case report with therapeutic response to dexfenfluramine. Sao Paulo Med J 1994;112:569–71.

[84] Schenck CH, Hurwitz TD, O'Connor KA, et al. Additional categories of sleep-related eating disorders and the current status of treatment. Sleep 1993;16:457–66.

[85] Schenck CH, Mahowald MW. Review of nocturnal sleep-related eating disorders. Int J Eat Disord 1994;15:343–56.

[86] Manni R, Ratti MT, Tartara A. Nocturnal eating: prevalence and features in 120 insomniac referrals. Sleep 1997;20:734–8.

[87] Winkelman JW, Herzog DB, Fava M. The prevalence of sleep-related eating disorder in psychiatric and non-psychiatric populations. Psychol Med 1999;29:1461–6.

[88] Winkelman JW. Treatment of nocturnal eating syndrome and sleep-related eating disorder with topiramate. Sleep Med 2003;4:243–6.

[89] Menkes DB. Triazolam-induced nocturnal bingeing with amnesia. Aust N Z J Psychiatry 1992;26:320–1.

[90] Morgenthaler TI, Silber MH. Amnestic sleep-related eating disorder associated with zolpidem. Sleep Med 2002;3:323–7.

[91] Birketvedt GS, Florholmen J, Sundsfjord J, et al. Behavioral and neuroendocrine characteristics of the night-eating syndrome. JAMA 1999;282:657–63.

[92] Birketvedt GS, Sundsfjord J, Florholmen JR. Hypothalamic-pituitary-adrenal axis in the night eating syndrome. Am J Physiol Endocrinol Metab 2001;282:E366–9.

[93] Wong KE. Masturbation during sleep—a somnambulistic variant? Singapore Med J 1986; 27:542–3.

[94] Shapiro CM, Fedoroff JP, Trajanovic NN. Sexual behavior in sleep: a newly described parasomnia. Sleep Res 1996;25:367.

[95] Shapiro CM, Trajanovic NN, Fedoroff JP. Sexsomnia—a new parasomnia? Can J Psychiatry 2003;48:311–7.

[96] Hurwitz TD, Mahowald MW, Schenck CH, et al. Sleep-related sexual abuse of children. Sleep Res 1989;18:246.

[97] Buchanan A. Sleepwalking and indecent exposure. Med Sci Law 1991;31:38–40.

[98] Fenwick P. Sleep and sexual offending. Med Sci Law 1996;36:122–34.

[99] Alves R, Aloe F, Tavares S,et al. Sexual behavior in sleep, sleepwalking and possible REM behavior disorder: a case report. Sleep Res Online 1999;3:71–2. Available at: www.sro.org/bin/article.dll?Paper&1603&0&0. Accessed July 23, 2005.

[100] Rosenfeld DS, Elhajjar AJ. Sleepsex: a variant of sleepwalking. Arch Sex Behav 1998;27: 269–78.

[101] Guilleminault C, Moscovitch A, Yuen K, et al. Atypical sexual behavior during sleep. Psychosom Med 2002;64:328–36.

[102] DeRoeck J, Van Hoof E, Cluydts R. Sleep-related expiratory groaning: a case report. Sleep Res 1983;12:237.

[103] Pevernagie DA, Boon PA, Mariman AN, et al. Vocalization during episodes of prolonged expiration: a parasomnia related to REM sleep. Sleep Med 2001;2:19–30.

[104] Vetrugno R, Provini F, Plazzi G, et al. Catathrenia (nocturnal groaning): a new type of parasomnia. Neurology 2001;56:681–3.

[105] Attanasio R. Nocturnal bruxism and its clinical management. Dent Clin North Am 1991; 35:245–52.

[106] Glaros AG. Incidence of diurnal and nocturnal bruxism. J Prosthet Dent 1981;45:545–9.

[107] Rugh JD, Harlan J. Nocturnal bruxism and temporomandibular disorders. Adv Neurol 1988;49:329–41.

[108] Clarke NG, Townsend GC, Carey SE. Bruxing patterns in man during sleep. J Oral Rehab 1984;11:123–7.

[109] Ware JC, Rugh JD. Destructive bruxism: sleep stage relationship. Sleep 1988;11:172–81.

[110] Hublin C, Kaprio J, Partinen M, et al. Sleep bruxism based on self-report in a nationwide twin cohort. J Sleep Res 1998;7:61–7.

[111] Clarke GT, Koyano K, Browne PA. Oral motor disorders in humans. Calif Dent Assoc J 1993;21:19–30.

[112] Ikeda T, Nishigawa K, Kondo K, et al. Criteria for the detection of sleep-associated bruxism in humans. J Orofac Pain 1996;10:270–82.

[113] Lavigne GJ, Rompre PH, Montplaisir JY. Sleep bruxism: validity of clinical research diagnostic criteria in a controlled polysomnographic study. J Dent Res 1996;75:546–52.

[114] Ellison JM, Stanziani P. SSRI-associated nocturnal bruxism in four patients. J Clin Psychiatry 1993;54:432–4.

[115] Romanelli F, Adler DA, Bungay KM. Possible paroxetine-induced bruxism. Ann Pharmacother 1996;30:1246–8.

[116] Micheli F, Pardal MF, Gatto M, et al. Bruxism secondary to chronic antidopaminergic drug exposure. Clin Neuropharmacol 1993;16:315–23.

[117] Nadler SC. Bruxism, a classification: critical review. J Am Dent Assoc 1957;54:615–22.

[118] Gallagher SJ. Diagnosis and treatment of bruxism: a review of the literature. Gen Dent 1980;28:62–5.

[119] Lavigne GJ, Manzini C, Bruxism. In: Kryger MH, Roth T, Dement WC, editors. Principles and practice of sleep medicine. 3rd edition. Philadelphia: W.B. Saunders; 2000. p. 773–85.

[120] Vanderas A. Relationship between malocclusion and bruxism in children and adolescents: a review. Pediatr Dent 1995;17:7–12.

[121] Meletti S, Cantalupo G, Volpi L, et al. Rhythmic teeth grinding induced by temporal lobe seizures. Neurology 2004;62:2306–9.

[122] Gillin JC, Rapoport JL, Mikkelsen EJ, et al. EEG sleep patterns in enuresis: a further analysis and comparison with normal controls. Biol Psychiatry 1982;17:947–53.

[123] Mikkelsen EJ, Rapoport JL, Nee L, et al. Childhood enuresis. I. Sleep patterns and psychopathology. Arch Gen Psychiatry 1980;37:1139–44.

[124] Hunsballe JM, Rittig S, Djurhuus JC. Sleep and arousal in adolescents and adults with nocturnal enuresis. Scand J Urol Nephrol 1995;173(Suppl):59–61.

[125] Bader G, Neveus T, Kruse S, et al. Sleep of primary enuretic children and controls. Sleep 2002;25:579–83.

[126] Burke EC, Stikler GB. Enuresis—is it being overtreated? Mayo Clin Proc 1980;55:118–9.

[127] Hirasing RA, van Leerdam FJM, Bolk-Bennink L, et al. Enuresis nocturnal in adults. Scand J Urol Nephrol 1997;31:533–6.

[128] Yeung CK, Sihoe JDY, Sit FKY, et al. Characteristics of primary nocturnal enuresis in adults: an epidemiological study. BJU Int 2004;93:341–5.

[129] Bakwin H. The genetics of enuresis. In: Kolvin I, MacKeith S, Meadow R, editors. Bladder control and enuresis. London: Lavenham Press; 1973.

[130] Robert M, Averous M, Besset A, et al. Sleep polygraphic studies using cystomanometry in twenty patients with enuresis. Eur Urol 1993;24:97–102.

[131] Fritz GK, Armbrust J. Enuresis and encopresis. Psychiatr Clin North Am 1982;5:283–96.

[132] Fritz GK, Anders TF. Enuresis: the clinical application of an etiologically based classification system. Child Psychiatry Hum Dev 1979;10:103–13.

[133] Hallgren B. Nocturnal enuresis: etiologic aspects. Acta Pediatr 1958;118(Suppl):66.

[134] Werry J, Coharssen J. Enuresis: an etiologic and therapeutic study. J Pediatr 1965;67: 423–31.

[135] Lund S. Primary nocturnal enuresis in children. Background and treatment. Scand J Urol Nephrol 1994;156(Suppl):1–48.

[136] Hublin C, Kaprio J, Partinen M, Koskenvuo M. Nocturnal enuresis in a nationwide twin cohort. Sleep 1998;21:579–85.

[137] Sireling LI, Crisp AH. Sleep and the enuresis alarm device. J R Soc Med 1983;76:131–3.

[138] Alon US. Nocturnal enuresis. Pediatr Nephrol 1995;9:94–103.

[139] Rapoport JL, Mikkelsen EJ, Zavadi A, et al. Childhood enuresis. II. Psychopathology, tricyclic concentration in plasma, and antidiuretic effect. Arch Gen Psychiatry 1980;37: 1146–52.

[140] Post EM, Richman RA, Blackett PR, et al. Desmopressin response of enuretic children. Am J Dis Child 1983;137:962–3.

[141] Fermaglich JL. Electroencephalographic study of enuretics. Am J Dis Child 1969;118: 473–7.

[142] Arguner A, Baybas S, Gozukirmizi E, et al. Focal and generalized abnormalities during sleep in cases of enuresis nocturna. In: Popoviciu L, Asgian B, Badiu G, editors. Sleep 1978. Fourth European Congress on Sleep Research, Tirgu-Mures. Basel: Karger; 1980. p. 717–20.

[143] Everaert K, Pevernagie D, Oosterlinck W. Nocturnal enuresis provoked by an obstructive sleep apnea syndrome. J Urol 1995;153:1236.

[144] Hoban TF. Rhythmic movement disorder in children. CNS Spectr 2003;8:135–8.

[145] Happe S, Ludemann P, Ringelstein EB. Persistence of rhythmic movement disorder beyond childhood: a videotape demonstration. Mov Disord 2000;15:1296–7.

[146] Kohyama J, Masukura F, Kimura K, et al. Rhythmic movement disorder: polysomnographic study and summary of reported cases. Brain Dev 2002;24:33–8.

[147] Kempenaers C, Bouillon E, Mendlewicz E. A rhythmic movement disorder in REM sleep: a case report. Sleep 1994;17:274–9.

[148] Gagnon P, De Koninck J. Repetitive head movements during REM sleep. Biol Psychiatry 1985;20:176.

[149] Manni R, Terzaghi M, Sartori I, et al. Rhythmic movement disoder and cyclic alternating pattern during sleep: a video-polysomnographic study in a 9-year old boy. Mov Disord 2004;19:1186–90.

[150] Whyte J, Kavey NB, Gidro-Frank S. A self-destructive variant of jactatio capitis nocturna. J Nerv Mental Disord 1991;179:49.

[151] Bramble D. Two cases of severe head-banging parasomnias in peripuberal males resulting from otitis media in toddlerhood. Child: care, health, and development 1995; 21:247–53.

[152] Thorpy MJ. Rhythmic movement disorder. In: Thorpy MJ, editor. Handbook of sleep disorders. New York: Marcel Dekker; 1990. p. 609.

[153] Manni R, Tartara A. Clonazepam treatment of rhythmic movement disorders. Sleep 1997; 20:812.

[154] Chisholm T, Morehouse RL. Adult headbanging: sleep studies and treatment. Sleep 1996; 19:343–6.

[155] Hashizume Y, Yoshijima H, Uchimura N, et al. Case of headbanging that continued to adolescence. Psychiatry Clin Neurosci 2002;56:255–6.

[156] Garcia J, Rosen G, Mahowald M. Waterbeds in treatment of rhythmic movement disorders: experience with two cases. Sleep Res 1996;25:243.

[157] Rosenberg C. Elimination of a rhythmic movement disorder with hypnosis—a case report. Sleep 1995;18:608–9.

[158] Drake MEJ. Jactatio nocturna after head injury. Neurology 1986;36:867–8.

[159] Broughton R. Pathological fragmentary myoclonus, intensified hypnic jerks and hypnagogic foot tremor: three unusual sleep-related movement disorders. In: Koella WP, Obal F, Schulz H, Visser P, editors. Sleep '86. Stuttgart: Gustav Fischer Verlag; 1988. p. 240–3.

[160] Vetrugno R, Provini F, Meletti S, et al. Propriospinal myoclonus at the sleep-wake transition: a new type of parasomnia. Sleep 2001;24:835–43.

[161] Montagna P, Provini F, Plazzi G, et al. Propriospinal myoclonus upon relaxation and drowsiness: a cause of severe insomnia. Mov Disord 1997;12:66–72.

[162] Jankovic J, Pardo R. Segmental myoclonus: clinical and pharmacologic study. Arch Neurol 1986;43:1025–31.

[163] Hoehn MM, Cherington M. Spinal myoclonus. Neurology 1977;27:942–6.

[164] Bauleo S, De Mitri P, Coccagna G. Evolution of segmental myoclonus during sleep: polygraphic study of two cases. Ital J Neurol Sci 1996;17:227–32.

[165] American Psychiatric Association. Diagnostic and statistical manual of mental disorders. 3rd edition. Washington, DC: American Psychiatric Association; 1987.

[166] Dagan Y, Zinger Y, Lavie P. Actigraphic sleep monitoring in posttraumatic stress disorder (PTSD) patients. J Psychosom Res 1997;42:577–81.

[167] Hurwitz TD, Mahowald MW, Kuskowski M, et al. Polysomnographic sleep is not clinically impaired in Vietnam combat veterans with chronic posttraumatic stress disorder. Biol Psychiatry 1998;44:1066–73.

[168] Pillar G, Malhotra A, Lavie P. Post-traumatic stress disorder and sleep—what a nightmare! Sleep Med Rev 2000;4:183–200.

[169] Klein E, Koren D, Arnon I, et al. Sleep complaints are not corroborated by objective sleep measures in post-traumatic stress disorder: a 1-year prospective study in survivors of motor vehicle crashes. J Sleep Res 2003;12:35–41.

[170] Youakim JM, Doghramji K, Schutte SL. Posttraumatic stress disorder and obstructive sleep apnea syndrome. Psychosomatics 1998;39:168–71.

[171] Abe K, Shimakawa M. Genetic and developmental aspects of sleeptalking and teeth-grinding. Acta Paedopsychiatr 1966;33:339–44.

[172] Arkin AM, Toth MF, Baker J, et al. The frequency of sleep talking in the laboratory among chronic sleep talkers and good dream recallers. J Nerv Ment Dis 1970;151:369–74.

[173] Arkin AM, Toth MG, Baker J, et al. The degree of concordance between the content of sleep talking and mentation recalled in wakefulness. J Nerv Ment Dis 1970;151:375–93.

[174] Hublin C, Kaprio J, Partinen M, et al. Sleeptalking in twins: epidemiology and psychiatric comorbidity. Behav Genet 1998;28:289–98.

[175] Dexter JD, Weitzman ED. The relationship of nocturnal headaches to sleep stage patterns. Neurology 1970;20:513–8.

[176] Dexter JD, Riley TL. Studies in nocturnal migraine. Headache 1975;15:51–62.

[177] Kayed K, Godtlibsen OB, Sjaastad O. Chronic paroxysmal hemicrania. IV. "REM sleep locked" nocturnal headache attacks. Sleep 1978;1:91–5.

[178] Pfaffenrath V, Pollmann W, Ruther E, et al. Onset of nocturnal attacks of chronic cluster headache in relation to sleep stages. Acta Neurol Scand 1986;73:403–7.

[179] Sahota PK, Dexter JD. Sleep and headache syndromes: a clinical review. Headache 1990;30:80–4.

[180] Kay DC, Blackburn AB, Buckingham JA, et al. Human pharmacology of sleep. In: Williams RL, Karacan I, editors. Pharmacology of sleep. New York: Wiley; 1976. p. 83–210.

[181] Jarrott B, Lewis S, Conway EL, et al. The involvement of central alpha adrenoreceptors in the antihypertensive actions of methyldopa and clonidine in the rat. Clin Exp Hypertens 1984;61:387–400.

[182] Autret A, Minz M, Beillevaire T, Cathala H-P, et al. Effect of clonidine on sleep patterns in man. Eur J Clin Pharmacol 1977;12:319–22.

[183] Micieli G, Cavallini A, Facchinetti F, et al. chronic paroxysmal hemicrania: a chronobiological study (case report). Cephalalgia 1989;9:281–6.

[184] Bono G, Micieli G, Manzoni GC, et al. Chronobiological basis for the management of periodic headaches. In: Rose C, editor. Migraine. Proceedings of the 5th International Migraine Symposium, London 1984. Basel: Karger; 1985. p. 206–17.

[185] Coria F, Claveria LE, Jimenez-Jimenez FJ, et al. Episodic paroxysmal hemicrania responsive to calcium channel blockers. J Neurol Neurosurg Psychiatry 1992;55:166.

[186] Aldrich MS, Chauncey JB. Are morning headaches part of the obstructive sleep apnea syndrome? Arch Intern Med 1990;150:1265–7.

[187] Buckle P, Kerr P, Kryger M. Nocturnal cluster headache associated with sleep apnea. A case report. Sleep 1993;16:487–9.

[188] Declerck AC, Arends JB. An exceptional case of parasomnia: the exploding head syndrome. Sleep-Wake Res Neth 1994;5:41–3.

[189] Pearce JMS. Clinical features of the exploding head syndrome. J Neurol Neurosurg Psychiatry 1989;52:907–10.

[190] Sachs C, Svanborg E. The exploding head syndrome: polysomnographic recordings and therapeutic suggestions. Sleep 1991;14:263–6.

[191] Walsleben JA, O'Malley EB, Freeman J, et al. Polysomnographic and topographic mapping of EEG in the exploding head syndrome. Sleep Res 1993;22:284.

[192] Pearce JMS. Exploding head syndrome. Headache 2001;41:602–3.

[193] Green MW. The exploding head syndrome. Curr Pain Headache Rep 2001;5:279–80.

[194] Fornazzari L, Farcnik K, Smith I, et al. Violent visual hallucinations and aggression in frontal lobe dysfunction: clinical manifestations of deep orbitofrontal foci. J Neuropsychiatry Clin Neurosci 1992;4:42–4.

[195] Jacome DE. Exploding head syndrome and idiopathic stabbing headache relieved by nifedipine. Cephalalgia 2001;21:617–8.

[196] Gould JD, Silberstein SD. Unilateral hypnic headache: a case study. Neurology 1997;49: 1749–51.

[197] Raskin NH. The hypnic headache syndrome. Headache 1988;28:534–6.

[198] Newman LC, Lipton RB, Solomon S. The hypnic headache syndrome: a benign headache disorder of the elderly. Neurology 1990;40:1904–5.

[199] Dodick DW, Mosek AC, Campbell JK. The hypnic ("alarm clock") headache syndrome. Cephalalgia 1998;18:152–6.

[200] Ivanez V, Soler R, Barreiro P. Hypnic headache syndrome: a case with good response to indomethacin. Cephalalgia 1998;18:225–6.

[201] Relja G, Zorzon M, Locatelli L, et al. Hypnic headache: rapid and long-lasting response to prednisone in two new cases. Cephalalgia 2002;222:157–9.

[202] Vieira-Dias M, Esperanca P. Hypnic headache: report of two cases. Headache 2001;41: 726–7.

[203] Patsouros N, Laloux P, Ossemann M. Hypnic headache: a case report with polysomnography. Acta Neurol Belg 2004;104:37–40.

[204] Manni R, Sances G, Terzaghi M, et al. Hypnic headache. PSG evidence of both REM- and NREM-related attacks. Neurology 2004;62:1411–3.

[205] Cohen AS, Kaube H. Rare nocturnal headaches. Curr Opin Neurol 2004;17:295–9.

[206] Motta J, Guilleminault C. Cardiac dysfunction during sleep. Ann Clin Res 1985;17: 190–8.

[207] Guilleminault C, Pool P, Motta J, et al. Sinus arrest during REM sleep in young adults. N Engl J Med 1984;311:1106–10.

[208] Wellens HJJ, Vermeulen A, Durrer D. Ventricular fibrillation occurring on arousal from sleep by auditory stimuli. Circulation 1972;46:661–5.

[209] Pressman MR, Greenspon AJ, Greenspon LW, et al. 1,665 episodes of sinus arrest and AV block in a single night of sleep in a nonapneic, otherwise healthy 21 yrs. old athlete. Sleep Res 1992;21:40.

[210] Tobe TJM, de Langen CDJ, Bink-Boelkens MT-E, et al. Late potentials in a bradycardia-dependent long QT syndrome associated with sudden death during sleep. J Am Coll Cardiol 1992;19:541–9.

[211] Rattenborg NC, Lindblom S, Best J, et al. REM sleep-related asystole associated with unusual polysomnographic features: a case history. Sleep Res 1995;24:324.

[212] Verrier RL, Muller JE, Hobson JA. Sleep, dreams, and sudden death: the case for sleep as an autonomic stress test for the heart. Cardiovasc Res 1996;31:181–211.

[213] Lavery CE, Mittleman MA, Cohen MC, et al. Nonuniform nighttime distribution of acute cardiac events. A possible effect of sleep states. Circulation 1997;96:3321–7.

[214] Bassetti C, Jung HH, Hess CW. Near cardiac death with onset in REM sleep: a polysomnographic case report. J Sleep Res 1997;6:57–8.

[215] Nowlin JB, Troyer W Jr, Collins WS, et al. The association of nocturnal angina pectoris with dreaming. Ann Intern Med 1965;63:1040–6.

[216] Murao S, Shimomura K, Yoshimoto N, et al. Nocturnal angina pectoris. Comparison between angina with ST segment elevation and depression documented by continuous orthogonal ECG recording. Jpn Heart J 1980;21:607–19.

[217] King MJ, Zir LM, Kaltman AJ, et al. Variant angina associated with angiographically demonstrated coronary artery spasm and REM sleep. Am J Med Sci 1973;265:419–22.

[218] Shappel SD, Orr WC. Variant angina and sleep: a case report with therapeutic considerations. Dis Nerv Syst 1975;36:295–8.

[219] Maggini C, Guazzelli M, Mauri M. Sleep and hemodynamic patterns in nocturnal angina. In: Koella WP, Levin P, editors. Sleep 1976. Third European Congress sleep research (Montpellier). Basel: Karger; 1977. p. 955–68.

[220] Figueras J, Singh BN, Ganz W, et al. Mechanism of rest and nocturnal angina: observations during continuous hemodynamic and electrocardiographic monitoring. Circulation 1979; 59:955–68.

[221] Murao S, Harumi K, Katayama S, et al. All-night polygraphic studies of nocturnal angina pectoris. Jpn Heart J 1972;13:295–306.

[222] Quyyumi AA, Wright CA, Mockus LT, et al. Mechanisms of nocturnal angina pectoris: importance of increased myocardial oxygen demand in patients with severe coronary artery disease. Lancet 1984;1:1207–9.

[223] Waters DD, Miller DD, Bouchard A, et al. Circadian variation in variant angina. Am J Cardiol 1984;54:61–4.

[224] Tamada K, Ito Y, Fukuzaki H. Autonomic hyperactivity in patients with vasospastic angina. Jpn Heart J 1985;26:715–26.

[225] Franklin KA, Nilsson JB, Sahlin C, et al. Sleep apnoea and nocturnal angina. Lancet 1995; 345:1085–7.

[226] Kales A, Beall GN, Bajor GF, et al. Sleep studies in asthmatic adults: relationship of attacks to sleep stage and time of night. J Allergy Clin Immunol 1968;41:164–73.

[227] Smith TF, Huggel DW. Arterial oxygen desaturation during sleep in children with asthma and its relation to airway obstruction and ventilatory drive. Pediatrics 1980;66:746–51.

[228] Montplaisir J, Walsh J, Malo JL. Nocturnal asthma: features of attacks, sleep and breathing patterns. Am Rev Respir Dis 1982;125:18–22.

[229] Catterall JR, Douglas NJ, Calverley PMA, et al. Irregular breathing and hypoxaemia during sleep in chronic stable asthma. Lancet 1982;1:301–4.

[230] Issa FG, Sullivan CE. Respiratory muscle activity and thoracoabdominal motion during acute episodes of asthma during sleep. Am Rev Respir Dis 1985;132:999–1004.

[231] Barnes PJ. Circadian variation in airway function. Am J Med 1985;79:5–9.

[232] Bohadana AB, Hannhart B, Teculescu DB. Nocturnal worsening of asthma and sleep-disordered breathing. J Asthma 2002;39:85–100.

[233] Ciftci TU, Ciftci B, Guven SF, et al. Effect of nasal continuous positive airway pressure in uncontrolled nocturnal asthmatic patients with obstructive sleep apnea syndrome. Respir Med 2005;99:529–34.

[234] Jankovic J, Pardo R. Segmental myoclonus. Arch Neurol 1986;43:1025–31.

[235] Lapresle J. Palatal myoclonus. Adv Neurol 1986;43:265–73.

[236] Iliceto G, Thompson BL, Day JC, et al. Diaphragmatic flutter, the moving umbilicus syndrome, and "belly dancer's" dyskinesia. Mov Disord 1990;1:15–22.

[237] Phillips JR, Eldridge FL. Respiratory myoclonus (Leeuwenhoek's disease). N Engl J Med 1973;289:1390–5.

[238] Corbett CL. Diaphragmatic flutter. Postgrad Med J 1977;53:399–402.

[239] Sethi KD, Hess DC, Huffnagle VH, et al. Acetazolamide treatment of paroxysmal dystonia in central demyelinating disease. Neurology 1992;42:919–21.

[240] Weiner WJ, Goetz CG, Nausieda PA, et al. Respiratory dyskinesias: extrapyramidal dysfunction and dyspnea. Ann Intern Med 1978;88:327–31.

[241] Kuna ST, Awan R. The irregularly irregular pattern of respiratory dyskinesia. Chest 1986; 90:779–81.

[242] Wilcox PG, Bassett A, Jones B, et al. Respiratory dysrhythmias in patient with tardive dyskinesias. Chest 1994;105:203–7.

[243] Rich MW, Radwany SM. Respiratory dyskinesia. An underrecognized phenomenon. Chest 1994;105:1826–32.

[244] Wantanabe K, Hara K, Hakamada S, et al. Seizures with apnea in children. Pediatrics 1982; 70:87–90.

[245] Thach BT. Sleep apnea in infancy and childhood. Med Clin North Am 1985;6:1289–315.

[246] Walls TJ, Newman PK, Cumming WJK. Recurrent apnoeic attacks as a manifestation of epilepsy. Postgrad Med J 1981;57:575–6.

[247] Lanouis S, Bizec JL, Whitelaw WA, et al. Hiccup in adults: an overview. Eur Respir J 1993; 6:563–75.

[248] Arnulf I, Boisteanu D, Whitelaw WA, et al. Chronic hiccups and sleep. Sleep 1995;19: 227–31.

[249] Askenasy JJM. Sleep hiccup. Sleep 1988;11:187–94.

[250] Brown LW, Fry JM. Paroxysmal nocturnal choking: a newly described manifestation of sleep-related epilepsy. Sleep Res 1988;17:153.

[251] Kowey PR, Mainchak RA, Rials SJ. Things that go bang in the night. N Engl J Med 1992; 327:1884.

[252] Guilleminault C, Miles L. Differential diagnosis of obstructive sleep apnea syndrome: the abnormal esophageal reflux and laryngospasm during sleep. Sleep Res 1980;9: 200.

[253] Thurnheer R, Henz S, Knoblauch A. Sleep-related laryngospasm. Eur Respir J 1997;10: 2084–6.

[254] Orenstein SR, Orenstein DM, Whitington PF. Gastroesophageal reflux causing stridor. Chest 1983;84:301–2.

[255] Orr WC. Clinical implications of nocturnal gastroesophageal reflux. Pract Gastroenterol 1994;13:28a [e, f, h.].

[256] Dent J, Dodds WJ, Friedman RH, et al. Mechanism of gastroesophageal reflux in recumbent asymptomatic human subjects. J Clin Invest 1980;65:256–67.

[257] DeMeester TR, Wang C, Wernly JA, et al. Technique, indications, and clinical use of 24 hour esophageal pH monitoring. J Thorac Cardiovasc Surg 1980;79:656–70.

[258] Castell DO. Medical therapy for reflux esophagitis: 1986 and beyond. Ann Intern Med 1986;104:112–4.

[259] Green BT, Broughton WA, O'Connor B. Marked improvement in nocturnal gastroesophageal reflux in a large cohort of patients with obstructive sleep apnea treated with continuous positive airway pressure. Arch Intern Med 2003;163:41–5.

[260] Valipour A, Makker H, Hardy R, et al. Symptomatic gastroesophageal reflux in subjects with a breathing sleep disorder. Chest 2002;121:1748–53.

[261] Fontan JP, Heldt GP, Heyman MB, et al. Esophageal spasm associated with apnea and bradycardia in an infant. Pediatrics 1984;73:52–5.

[262] Bortolotti M, Cirignotta F, Labo G. Atrioventricular block induced by swallowing in a patient with diffuse esophageal spasm. JAMA 1982;248:2297–9.

[263] Traube M, McCallum RW. Primary oesophageal motility disorders. Current therapeutic concepts. Drugs 1985;30:66–77.

[264] Guilleminault C, Raynal D, Takahashi S, et al. Evaluation of short-term and long-term treatment of the narcolepsy syndrome with clomipramine hydrochloride. Acta Neurol Scand 1976;54:71–87.

[265] Altster J, Shemesh Z, Ornan M, et al. Sleep disturbance associated with chronic tinnitus. Biol Psychiatry 1993;34:84–90.

[266] Folmer RL, Griest SE. Tinnitus and insomnia. Am J Otolaryngol 2000;21:287–93.

[267] Hallum RS. Correlates of sleep disturbance in chronic distressing tinnitus. Scand Audiol 1996;25:263–6.

[268] Matsushima J, Sakai N, Sakajiri M, et al. An experience of the usage of electrical tinnitus suppressor. Artif Organs 1996;20:955–8.

[269] Sullivan M, Katon W, Russo J, et al. A randomized trial of nortriptyline for severe chronic tinnitus. Arch Intern Med 1993;153:2251–9.

[270] Plewnia C, Bartels M, Gerloff C. Transient suppression of tinnitus by transcranial magnetic stimulation. Ann Neurol 2002;53:263–6.

[271] Mellman TA, Uhde TW. Sleep panic attacks: new clinical findings and theoretical implications. Am J Psychiatry 1989;146:1204–7.

[272] Mellman TA, Uhde TW. Electroencephalographic sleep in panic disorder. Arch Gen Psychiatry 1989;46:178–84.

[273] Mellman TA, Uhde TW. Patients with frequent sleep panic: clinical findings and response to medication treatment. J Clin Psychiatry 1990;51:513–6.

[274] Rosenfield DS, Furman Y. Pure sleep panic: two case reports and a review of the literature. Sleep 1994;17:462–5.

[275] Craske MG, Rowe MK. Nocturnal panic. Clin Psychol Sci Pract 1997;4:153–74.

[276] Craske MG, Kreuger MT. Prevalence of nocturnal panic in a college population. J Anxiety Disord 1990;4:125–39.

[277] Herskowitz J. Neurologic presentations of panic disorder in childhood and adolescence. Dev Med Child Neurol 1986;28:617–23.

[278] Black B, Robbins DR. Panic disorder in children and adolescents. J Am Acad Child Adolesc Psychiatry 1990;29:36–44.

[279] Lepola U, Koponen H, Leinonen E. Sleep in panic disorders. J Psychosom Res 1994; 38(Suppl 1):105–11.

[280] Stein MB, Enns MW, Kryger MH. Sleep in nondepressed patients with panic disorder: II. Polysomnographic assessment of sleep architecture and sleep continuity. J Affect Disord 1993;28:1–6.

[281] Landry P, Marchand L, Mainguy N, et al. Electroencephalography during sleep of patients with nocturnal panic disorder. J Nerv Ment Dis 2002;190:559–62.

[282] Edlund MJ, McNamara ME, Millman RP. Sleep apnea and panic attacks. Compr Psychiatry 1991;32:130–2.

[283] Lesser IM, Poland RE, Holcomb C, et al. Electroencephalographic study of nighttime panic attacks. J Nerv Ment Dis 1985;173:744–6.

[284] Grunhaus L, Birmaher B. The clinical spectrum of panic attacks. J Clin Psychopharmacol 1985;5:93–9.

[285] Hauri P, Friedman M, Ravaris CL. Sleep in patients with spontaneous panic attacks. Sleep 1989;12:323–37.

[286] McNamara ME. Absence seizures associated with panic attacks initially misdiagnosed as temporal lobe epilepsy: the importance of prolonged EEG monitoring in diagnosis. J Psychiatry Neurosci 1993;18:46–8.

[287] Wall M, Tuchman M, Mielke D. Panic attacks and temporal lobe seizures associated with a right temporal lobe arteriovenous malformation: case report. J Clin Psychiatry 1985;46: 143–5.

[288] Agargun MY, Kara H, Ozer OA, et al. Characteristics of patients with nocturnal dissociative disorders. Sleep Hypnosis 2001;3:131–4.

[289] Agargun MY, Kara H, Ozer OA, et al. Sleep-related violence, dissociative experiences, and childhood traumatic events. Sleep Hypnosis 2002;4:52–7.

[290] Chu JA, Dill DL. Dissociative symptoms in relation to childhood physical and sexual abuse. Am J Psychiatry 1990;147:887–92.

[291] Putnam FW, Guroff JJ, Silberman EK, et al. The clinical phenomenology of multiple personality disorder: review of 100 recent cases. J Clin Psychiatry 1986;47:285–93.

[292] Schenck CS, Milner DM, Hurwitz TD, et al. Dissociative disorders presenting as somnambulism: polysomnographic, video, and clinical documentation (8 cases). Dissociation 1989;4:194–204.

[293] Molaie M, Deutsch GK. Psychogenic events presenting as parasomnia. Sleep 1997;20: 402–5.

[294] Mahowald MW, Schenck CH, Rosen GR, et al. The role of a sleep disorders center in evaluating sleep violence. Arch Neurol 1992;49:604–7.

[295] Baker CE, Major E. Munchausen's syndrome. A case presenting as asthma requiring ventilation. Anaesthesia 1994;49:1050–1.

[296] Elshami AA, Tino G. Coexistent asthma and functional upper airway obstruction. Case reports and review of the literature. Chest 1996;110:1358–61.

[297] Walker EA. Murder or epilepsy? J Nerv Ment Dis 1961;133:430–7.

[298] Butani L, O'Connell EJ. Functional respiratory disorders. Ann Allergy Asthma Immunol 1997;79:91–101.

[299] Goldman J, Muers M. Vocal cord dysfunction and wheezing. Thorax 1991;46:401–4.

[300] Light MJ, Sheridan MS. Munchausen syndrome by proxy and sleep apnea. Clin Pediatr 1990;29:162–8.

[301] Griffith JC, Slovik LS. Munchausen by proxy and sleep disorders medicine. Sleep 1989;12: 178–83.

[302] Skau K, Mouridsen SE. Munchausen syndrome by proxy: a review. Acta Paediatr 1995;84: 977–82.

[303] Samuels MP, McClaughlin W, Jacobson RR, et al. Fourteen cases of imposed upper airway obstruction. Arch Dis Child 1992;67:162–70.

[304] Byard RW, Beal SM. Munchausen syndrome by proxy: repetitive infantile apnoea and homicide. J Paediatr Child Health 1993;29:77–9.

[305] Feldman MD, Russell JL. Factitious cyclic hypersomnia: a new variant of factitious disorder. South Med J 1991;84:1991.

[306] Weiner IH, Weiner HL. Nocturnal leg muscle cramps. JAMA 1980;244:2332–3.

[307] Baltodano N, Gallo BV, Weidler DJ. Verapamil vs. quinine in recumbent nocturnal leg cramps in the elderly. Arch Intern Med 1988;148:1969–70.

[308] Mills KR, Newham DJ, Edwards RHT. Severe muscle cramps relieved by trans-cutaneous nerve stimulation: a case report. J Neurol Neurosurg Psychiatry 1982;45: 539–42.

[309] Connolly PS, Shirley EA, Wasson JH, et al. Treatment of nocturnal leg cramps. A crossover trial of quinine vs. vitamin E. Arch Intern Med 1992;152:1877–80.

[310] Serrao M, Rossi P, Cardinali P, et al. Gabapentin treatment for muscle cramps: an open-label trial. Clin Neuropharmacol 2000;23:45–9.

[311] Kannan N, Sawaya R. Nocturnal leg cramps: clinically mysterious and painful—but manageable. Geriatrics 2001;56:34–42.

[312] Bender BG, Leung SB, Lueng DYM. Actigraphic assessment of sleep disturbance in patients with atopic dermatitis: an objective life quality measure. J Allergy Clin Immunol 2003;111:598–602.

[313] Yosipovitch G, Ansari N, Goon A, et al. Clinical characteristics of pruritus in chronic idiopathic urticaria. Br J Dermatol 2002;147:32–6.

[314] Stores G, Burrows A, Crawford C. Physiological sleep disturbance in children with atopic dermatitis: a case control study. Pediatr Dermatol 1998;15:264–8.

[315] Aoki T, Kushimoto H, Hishikawa Y, et al. Nocturnal scratching and its relationship to the disturbed sleep of itchy subjects. Clin Exp Dermatol 1991;16:268–72.

[316] Monti JM, Vignale R, Monti D. Sleep and nighttime pruritus in children with atopic dermatitis. Sleep 1989;12:309–14.

[317] Savin JA, Paterson WD, Oswald I, et al. Further studies of scratching during sleep. Br J Dermatol 1975;93:297–302.

[318] Brodland DG, Staats BA, Peters MS. Factitial leg ulcers associated with an unusual sleep disorder. Arch Dermatol 1989;125:1115–8.

[319] Mold JW, Mathew MK, Shuaib B. et al. revalence of night sweats in primary care patients: an OKPRN and TAFP-Net collaborative study. J Fam Pract 2002;51:452–6.

[320] Duhon DR. Night sweats: two other causes [letter]. JAMA 1994;271:1577.

[321] Gordon D. Night sweats: two other causes [letter]. JAMA 1994;271:1577.

[322] Reynolds WA. Are night sweats a sign of esophageal reflux? [letter]. J Clin Gastroenterol 1989;11:590–1.

[323] Solomon GE. Diencephalic autonomic epilepsy caused by a neoplasm. J Pediatr 1973;83: 277–80.

[324] Woodward S, Freedman RR. The thermoregulatory effects of menopausal hot flashes on sleep. Sleep 1994;17:497–501.

[325] Kronenberg F. Menopausal hot flashes: randomness or rhythmicity. Chaos 1991;1:271–8.

[326] Johnson LF, Kinsbourne M, Renuart AW. Hereditary chin-trembling with nocturnal myoclonus and tongue-biting in dizygous twins. Dev Med Child Neurol 1971;13:726–9.

[327] Vasiknanonte P, Kuasirikul S, Vasiknanonte S. Two faces of nocturnal tongue biting. J Med Assoc Thai 1997;80:500–6.

[328] Tuxhorn I, Hoppe M. Parasomnia with rhythmic movements manifesting as nocturnal tongue biting. Neuropediatrics 1993;24:167–8.

[329] Edwards JC, Dinner DS, Gordon PH. Violent tongue biting as a parasomnia. Sleep Res 1997;26:358.

[330] Aguglia U, Gambardella A, Quattrone A. Sleep-induced masticatory myoclonus: a rare parasomnia associated with insomnia. Sleep 1991;14:80–2.

[331] Vetrugno R, Provini F, Plazzi G, et al. Familial nocturnal facio-mandibular myoclonus mimicking sleep bruxism. Neurology 2002;58:644–7.

[332] Atsuumi T, Maehara K, Saito T, et al. Syncope at sleep onset in a patient with nasopharyngeal carcinoma. Heart Vessels 1997;12:203–5.

[333] Bonnet R, Jorres R, Downey R, et al. Intractable cough associated with the supine body position. Effective therapy with nasal CPAP. Chest 1995;108:581–5.

[334] Teng AY, Sullivan CE. Nasal mask continuous positive airway pressure in the treatment of chronic nocturnal cough in a young child. Respirology 1997;2:131–4.

[335] Aldrich MS, Jahnke B. Diagnostic value of video-EEG polysomnography. Neurology 1991;41:1060–6.

[336] Mahowald MW, Schenck CS. Parasomnia purgatory—the epileptic/non-epileptic interface. In: Rowan AJ, Gates JR, editors. Non-epileptic seizures. Boston: Butterworth-Heinemann; 1993. p. 123–39.

ELSEVIER
SAUNDERS

Neurol Clin 23 (2005) 1107–1126

NEUROLOGIC
CLINICS

Rapid Eye Movement Sleep Parasomnias

Carlos H. Schenck, MD[a,b,d,*],
Mark W. Mahowald, MD[a,c,d]

[a]Minnesota Regional Sleep Disorders Center, Minneapolis, MN, USA
[b]Department of Psychiatry, Hennepin County Medical Center, Minneapolis, MN, USA
[c]Department of Neurology, Hennepin County Medical Center, Minneapolis, MN, USA
[d]University of Minnesota Medical School, Minneapolis, MN, USA

Classification of the parasomnias includes primary and secondary sleep phenomena that can emerge throughout the sleep cycle. Rapid eye movement (REM) sleep behavior disorder (RBD) is the REM sleep parasomnia that is of greatest relevance and interest to neurologists. This article, therefore, focuses primarily on this recently identified syndrome that has a corresponding animal model. Other REM sleep parasomnias also are described briefly.

Rapid eye movement sleep behavior disorder

Although various polysomnographic (PSG) and clinical components of RBD have been identified by European, Japanese and American investigators since 1966 [1–5], RBD was not recognized formally and named until 1985–1987 [6,7], and it was incorporated within the International Classification of Sleep Disorders in 1990 [8]. A typical clinical presentation is described from the authors' index case [6]:

> A 67-year-old dextral man was referred because of violent behavior during sleep…He had slept uneventfully through adolescence in a small room with three brothers. But on his wedding night, his wife was "scared with surprise" over his sleep talking, groaning, tooth grinding, and minor body movements. This persisted without consequence for 41 years until one night, 4 years before referral, when he experienced the first "physically moving dream" several hours after sleep onset; he found himself out of bed attempting to carry out a dream. This episode signaled the onset of an

---

* Corresponding author. Minnesota Regional Sleep Disorders Center, Hennepin County Medical Center, 701 Park Avenue South, Minneapolis, MN 55415.
 E-mail address: schen010@umn.edu (C.H. Schenck).

0733-8619/05/$ - see front matter © 2005 Elsevier Inc. All rights reserved.
doi:10.1016/j.ncl.2005.06.002   *neurologic.theclinics.com*

increasingly frequent and progressively severe sleep disorder; he would punch and kick his wife, fall out of bed, stagger about the room, crash into objects, and injure himself...his wife began to sleep in another room 2 years before referral. They remain happily married, believing that these nocturnal behaviors are out of his control and discordant with his waking personality.

A description of oneirism (dream-enacting behavior) in this patient is as follows:

I was on a motorcycle going down the highway when another motorcyclist comes up alongside me and tries to ram me with his motorcycle. Well, I decided I'm going to kick his motorcycle away and at that point my wife woke me up and said, "What in heavens are you doing to me?" because I was kicking the hell out of her.

I was a halfback playing football, and after the quarterback received the ball from the center he lateraled it sideways to me and I'm supposed to go around end and cut back over tackle and—this is very vivid—as I cut back over tackle there is this big 280-pound tackle waiting, so I, according to football rules, was to give him my shoulder and bounce him out of the way, and when I came to I was standing in front of our dresser and I had knocked lamps, mirrors, and everything off the dresser, hit my head against the wall and my knee against the dresser.

The patient sustained ecchymoses and lacerations during these recurrent nocturnal episodes. Fig. 1 shows how another patient who had RBD chose to protect himself during sleep every night before presenting to the authors' center. RBD often is misdiagnosed as a nocturnal seizure disorder, a psychiatric disorder, or an unusual or severe form of obstructive sleep apnea.

Animal model of rapid eye movement sleep behavior disorder: paradox lost

REM sleep in mammals involves a highly energized state of brain activity, with tonic (ie, continuous) and phasic (ie, intermittent) activations occurring across a spectrum of physiologic parameters [3]. Sleep neuro-physiologists refer to REM sleep as active sleep because of the high level of brain activity (measured electrophysiologically and by cerebral blood flow, oxygen consumption, and glucose use) and as paradoxic sleep because there is a virtual absence of skeletal muscle activity despite a highly activated brain state. Generalized skeletal muscle atonia (REM atonia) is one of the three defining features of mammalian REM sleep (besides REMs and a desynchronized electroencephalogram [EEG]) (Fig. 2A). Thus, the paradox of REM sleep resides in the absence of overt motor expression during an active brain and mind (dream) state. The loss of this customary paradox in RBD bears serious clinical consequences: paradox lost means loss of safe sleep. Serious injuries, including subdural hematomas, may result from dream-enacting behaviors [9,10].

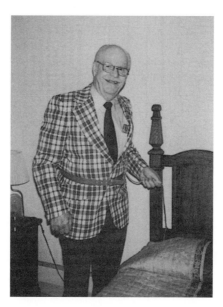

Fig. 1. Photograph of a 70-year-old man who had RBD and who for 6 years tethered himself to bed with a rope and belt in an effort to prevent injury from leaping out of bed during attempted dream enactments. (*From* Schenck CH. REM sleep behavior disorder. In: Carskadon M, editor. Encyclopedia of sleep and dreaming. New York: Macmillan; 1993. p. 499; with permission.)

In 1965, Jouvet and Delorme [11] reported that experimentally induced, bilateral, symmetric, dorsolateral pontine tegmental lesions in cats resulted in continuous and permanent loss of REM atonia, whereas lesions in other brainstem structures had no effect on REM sleep. These cats displayed de novo hallucinatory-type behaviors during REM sleep that strongly resembled oneirism. The oneiric behaviors in these cats always occurred during unequivocal REM sleep, and REM sleep retained all of its identifying features (apart from loss of REM atonia): periodic cycling with non-REM (NREM) sleep; cortical EEG activation; rapid, microvoltaic electrical activity of the olfactory bulb; pontogeniculooccipital waves; pronounced myosis; relaxation of the nictitating membranes; and unresponsiveness to environmental stimuli. Thus, the mechanisms responsible for the oneiric behaviors were postulated to originate in the brain and be dependent on the internal neural organization of REM sleep.

Further work by Jouvet's group on "paradoxical sleep without atonia" [12,13] revealed that a restricted, stereotypic repertoire of behaviors is displayed spontaneously during REM sleep, in the absence of any environmental stimulation, with attack the most common behavior and sexual or feeding activity never observed. Also, these cats never were inappropriately aggressive while awake.

Morrison's group [14–16], in addition to Jouvet's group, identified four categories of oneiric RBD behaviors. The appearance of each behavioral

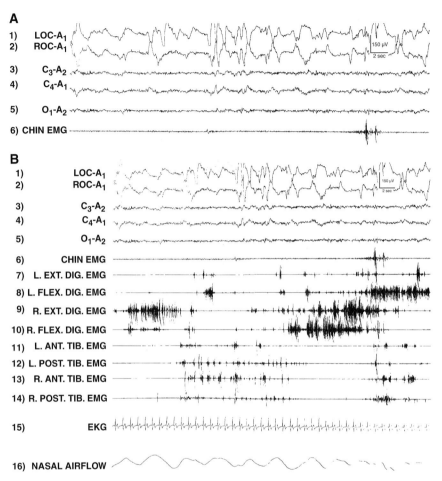

Fig. 2. REM sleep PSGs demonstrating the necessity of extensive extremity EMG monitoring in documenting RBD. (*A*) Customary REM sleep, with its distinct electrophysiologic profile: the triad of dense, high-voltage REMs [1–2], activated EEG [3–5], and chin EMG atonia with one minor burst of phasic twitching [6]. Channels 1–6 are sufficient for scoring sleep stages throughout the night, according to the standard methods and criteria of Rechtschaffen and Kales. (*B*) Identical channels 1–6 to those in Fig. 2A reveal that extensor and flexor EMGs of the four limbs have excessive twitching. EKG rate 15 remains constant and respirations 16 are mildly irregular. (*Adapted from* Mahowald MW, Schenck CH. REM-sleep behavior disorder. In: Thorpy MJ, editor. Handbook of sleep disorders. New York: Marcel Dekker; 1990. p. 567; with permission.)

category is dependent on the location and size of the pontine tegmental lesions [14]: (1) a minimal syndrome of generalized limb or truncal twitching and jerking, which at times becomes prominent and violent; (2) orienting and exploratory behaviors, involving staring, head raising, head turning, reaching, grasping, or searching; (3) stalking imaginary prey and episodic attack behavior; and (4) locomotion.

These experiments show that loss of REM atonia alone is insufficient to generate RBD. There also must be disinhibition of motor pattern generators in the mesencephalic locomotor region to result in overexcitation of phasic motor activity with behavioral release during REM sleep [14,16]. Recent studies of dogs by Lai and Siegel reveal a colocalization of the atonia and locomotor systems of REM sleep in the pons, providing an anatomic basis for the simultaneous dysregulation of these two systems in RBD [17].

The supraspinal mechanisms responsible for REM atonia [18,19] originate in the perilocus coeruleus (LC)-alpha nucleus in the pons that sends excitatory projections to the nucleus reticularis magnocellularis in the medulla, which then transmit descending inhibitory projections—more powerful than the competing descending excitatory projections—to the spinal alpha motoneurons, resulting in hyperpolarization and, hence, muscle atonia. Therefore, REM atonia results from an active process involving specific neuronal circuitry and is not the result of passive cessation of muscle tone. Finally, the motor system in normal REM sleep is shut down at the level of the spinal motoneurons; otherwise, the motor system at higher levels of the neuraxis is quite activated.

Human rapid eye movement sleep behavior disorder: diagnostic methods in the clinical evaluation

At the authors' center, the evaluation of injurious or disruptive nocturnal behaviors consists of the following:

1. Clinical sleep-wake interview, with review of physician referral information and past medical records and with review of a completed, structured, patient questionnaire, covering sleep-wake, medical, psychiatric, and alcohol or substance use history (including family history), and review of systems.
2. Psychiatric and neurologic interviews and examinations.
3. Extensive overnight PSG monitoring with continuous videotaping. Fig. 2A, B depicts the PSG monitoring montage that includes an electrooculogram, expanded electroencephalogram (EEG: only 3 of a total 8 channels are shown), chin and four-limb electromyograms (EMG), EKG, and airflow. Urine toxicology screening is performed whenever indicated.
4. Daytime multiple sleep latency testing (MSLT), if there is a complaint or suspicion of daytime sleepiness or fatigue.
5. If RBD is diagnosed, then neuropsychometric testing [20] should be performed because parkinsonism is prevalent in RBD, and dementia is common in parkinsonism; also, RBD can be associated closely with dementia with Lewy body disease [21]. Also, a brain imaging study, preferably a magnetic resonance scan, may be indicated, depending on findings elicited from the clinical history or neurologic examination.

Minimum diagnostic criteria of rapid eye movement sleep behavior disorder

These criteria are [3,8]

1. PSG abnormality during REM sleep: elevated submental EMG tone or excessive phasic submental or limb EMG twitching.
2. Documentation of abnormal REM sleep behaviors during PSG studies (prominent limb or truncal jerking; complex, vigorous, or violent behaviors) or a history of injurious or disruptive sleep behaviors.
3. Absence of EEG epileptiform activity during REM sleep.

Clinical characteristics of rapid eye movement sleep behavior disorder

RBD is more common above age 50, and 80% to 90% of affected patients are men, but the disorder may begin at any age [22,23]. It presents most frequently with the complaint of dramatic, violent, potentially injurious motor activity during sleep. These behaviors include talking, yelling, swearing, grabbing, punching, kicking, jumping, or running out of the bed. Injuries are not uncommon and include ecchymoses, lacerations, or fractures involving the individual or bed partner. The reported motor activity usually correlates with remembered dream mentation, leading to the complaint of "acting out my dreams." In some cases, bruxism, somniloquy, or periodic limb movements of sleep may be the heralding or primary manifestation of this disorder. The duration of behaviors is brief, and on awakening from an episode, there usually is rapid return of alertness and orientation. Some patients adopt extraordinary measures to prevent injury during sleep: they may tether themselves to the bed with a rope or belt, sleep in sleeping bags, or sleep on a mattress on the floor in a room devoid of furniture.

The frequency of the episodes ranges from once every few weeks to multiple nightly episodes [24]. Despite the impressive behavioral and EMG motor activity, few patients who have RBD complain of excessive sleep disruption and daytime fatigue. The MSLT rarely documents daytime somnolence, apart from cases in which RBD is associated with narcolepsy.

Acute rapid eye movement sleep behavior disorder

Acute onset of RBD almost always is induced by medications (tricyclic antidepressants, monoamine oxidase inhibitors, serotonin-specific reuptake inhibitors, bisoprolol, selegiline, or cholinergic treatment for Alzheimer's disease) or associated with their withdrawal (alcohol, barbiturate, or meprobamate) [25–30]. Caffeine and chocolate abuse is implicated in causing or unmasking RBD [31]. RBD may be triggered by selegiline prescribed as treatment for Parkinson's disease and by cholinergic agents prescribed for patients who have Alzheimer's disease [25,27,32]. Drug-induced (in particular selective serotinin reuptake inhibitor medication) RBD increasingly is common.

Chronic rapid eye movement sleep behavior disorder

The chronic form of RBD is idiopathic in 25% to 60% of occurrences [22,23,33]. The remaining cases are associated with various degenerative neurologic disorders (discussed later). All PSG and behavioral features of RBD are indistinguishable across subgroups, irrespective of gender, age, or the presence or absence of a neurologic disorder [34]. This suggests the presence of a final common pathway in RBD that can be accessed by a variety of pathologic states. Figs. 2, 3, 4, and 5 depict a range of common PSG findings in RBD. One finding that deserves particular emphasis— a finding not predicted by the animal model of RBD—is that loss of submental (ie, background) EMG atonia is necessary neither for the release of excessive phasic EMG twitching during REM sleep nor for the expression of RBD behaviors. Fig. 2B illustrates this important point. The authors also have analyzed quantitatively the EMGs during REM sleep in 17 older males who had idiopathic RBD and found that submental EMG atonia was

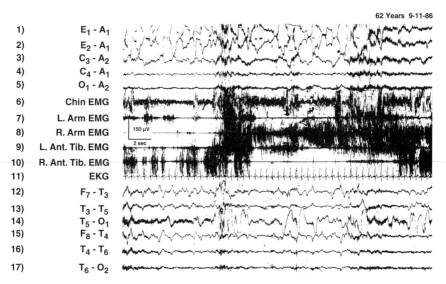

Fig. 3. PSG correlates of dream-enacting behaviors in RBD. REM sleep contains dense, high-voltage REM activity 1–2, and there is a fast-frequency, low-voltage, desyncronized EEG 3–5, 12–17 characteristic of REM sleep. The submental EMG muscle tone is increased 6, often seen with RBD. The arms 7–8 and legs 9–10 show bursts of intense twitching, which accompany observable behaviors noted by the technician. The EKG 11 shows a constant rate of 64 per minute, despite the vigorous movements, which is consistent with maintenance of REM sleep and inconsistent with an abrupt awakening. This sequence culminates in a spontaneous awakening, when the man reports a dream of running down a hill in Duluth, Minnesota, and taking shortcuts through backyards, and he suddenly finds himself on a barge that is rocking back and forth. He feels "haunted" and holds desperately onto anything to prevent falling into the cargo hold, where there are skeletons awaiting him. (*From* Mahowald MW, Schenck CH. REM sleep behavior disorder. In: Kryger MH, Roth T, Dement WC, editors. Principles and practice of sleep medicine, 2nd edition. Philadelphia: WB Saunders; 1994. p. 574.)

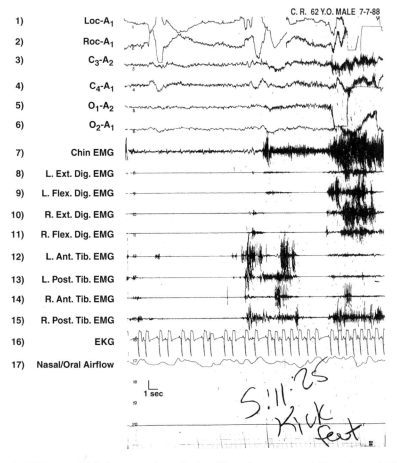

Fig. 4. REM-sleep PSG demonstrating selective bilateral extensor and flexor leg twitching 12–15, which corresponds to the technician's simultaneous observation that the patient is kicking his feet. REMs 1–2 and tonic-phasic chin EMG activity appear in conjunction with these vigorous behaviors. EKG 16 is abnormal and reflects a chaotic atrial rhythm, which is present throughout the night. EEG 3–6 is activated and respirations are irregular 17. (*From* Mahowald MW, Schenck CH. REM-sleep behavior disorder. In: Thorpy MJ, editor. Handbook of sleep disorders. New York: Marcel Dekker; 1990. p. 567; with permission.)

preserved in 54% of all 7.5-second time bins containing bursts of phasic limb twitching [35].

RBD behaviors occur within REM sleep, often without associated tachycardia, and not during arousals from REM sleep. Complex RBD behaviors generally are aggressive or exploratory and never appetitive (feeding or sexual). There is an almost inextricable link between altered dreams and dream-enacting behaviors, suggesting a mutual pathophysiology: patients do not enact their customary dreams, rather they enact distinctly altered dreams, usually involving confrontation, aggression, and violence.

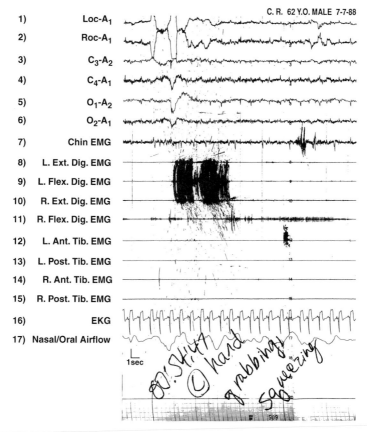

Fig. 5. REM-sleep PSG (same patient and same night as in Fig. 4), revealing selective, dense, high-voltage left flexor arm EMG twitching 9 in conjunction with observed grabbing and squeezing behaviors of the left hand. A burst of REMs 1–2 precedes these gross behaviors. The EEG 3–6 is activated, the chin EMG [7] has minimal tone with occasional twitching, and the leg EMGs 12–15 are completely inactive. (*From* Mahowald MW, Schenck CH. REM-sleep behavior disorder. In: Thorpy MJ, editor. Handbook of sleep disorders. New York: Marcel Dekker; 1990. p. 567; with permission.)

Treatment of rapid eye movement sleep behavior disorder

Clonazepam is a remarkably effective treatment of human RBD in controlling the behavioral and the dream-disordered components of RBD [34]. Treatment usually is immediately effective at a dose of 0.5 to 1.0 mg at bedtime (range, 0.25–4.0 mg). Prompt relapse of RBD occurs whenever patients fail to take clonazepam on a given night. The mechanism of therapeutic action is shown by Lapierre and Montplaisir to involve suppression of phasic EMG activity during REM sleep rather than restoration of REM atonia [36]. The long-term efficacy and safety of chronic, nightly clonazepam treatment of RBD and other parasomnias at the authors' center recently has been reported [37]. Adjunctive or alternative treatments for the few patients who have RBD and who do not respond fully to clonazepam or who develop daytime somnolence from this agent include the following: desipramine or imipramine, carbamazepine. clonidine, carbidopa/L-dopa, L-tryptophan, or gabapentin [3]. Recently, melatonin (in relatively high doses: 6 mg–12 mg at bedtime) [38–40] or pramipexole [41,42] reportedly are effective.

World literature on rapid eye movement sleep behavior disorder

The literature contains hundreds of cases of RBD [22,43]. Increasingly, chronic, "idiopathic" RBD is associated with neurologic disorders, but there is great diversity in category and location. Three pertinent comments are warranted. First, neurodegenerative disorders and narcolepsy are the most common neurologic disorders associated with RBD. Second, the pons rarely are grossly involved, as ascertained by clinical neuroanatomic and neurophysiologic testing, which stands in contrast to the animal model of RBD. Third, a variety of neurologic conditions also can manifest REM sleep without atonia or excessive phasic EMG twitching in REM sleep, as an isolated PSG observation but without the clinical emergence of RBD—in other words, various preclinical forms of RBD can be found in the same neurologic disorders that are associated with RBD but also in individuals who have no apparent neurologic disease [3,28,44–46]. Sleep bruxism, in one case, is reported to be a subclinical manifestation of RBD [47].

Recent findings in rapid eye movement sleep behavior disorder

Association with parkinsonism

Recent findings from the authors' center [48] and other centers [21,49–51] suggest that first, parkinsonism may be quite prevalent in RBD; second, RBD may be the initial manifestation of a parkinsonian disorder in a substantial number of RBD cases initially considered idiopathic (there also is a case report of RBD as the herald of Shy-Drager syndrome [52]); and, third, a high percentage of parkinsonian patients who have no sleep complaints may have either preclinical or clinical RBD.

As more patients who have idiopathic RBD are followed carefully over time, it is becoming clear that the majority eventually will develop neurodegenerative disorders, most notably the synucleinopathies (Parkinson's disease; multiple system atrophy, including olivopontocerebellar degeneration and Shy-Drager syndrome; or dementia with Lewy body disease). RBD also is described in association with progressive supranuclear palsy (a tauopathy) [53] and Parkinson's disease associated with *parkin* mutations [54]. RBD may be the first manifestation of these conditions and may precede any other manifestation of the underlying neurodegenerative process by more than 10 years [21,48,51,55–57]. There is growing evidence of more widespread subtle clinical and neurophysiologic abnormalities present in patients who have RBD [58–62].

Association with narcolepsy

An association of RBD and narcolepsy is described in detail in two reports [4,63]. Combined narcolepsy-RBD was documented in a series of 10 cases (80% male); mean age of narcolepsy onset was 22.8 ($\pm$15.1) years (range 12–59), and mean age of RBD onset was 28.4 ($\pm$17.3) years [4]. RBD emerged in tandem with narcolepsy in five cases and early in the course of narcolepsy in three cases. Treatment of cataplexy (with tricyclic antidepressants) either induced or aggravated RBD in three cases. There was strong expression of the narcolepsy tetrad in all 10 patients. In the second report [63], records of 14 narcoleptic patients who had RBD were analyzed retrospectively in a controlled design, and the (testable) suggestion was made that sleep motor dyscontrol in narcolepsy may start as a NREM sleep parasomnia in childhood and then "the onset of narcolepsy might represent the turning point for its intrusion into REM sleep."

Association of rapid eye movement sleep behavior disorder with specific HLA haplotypes

Narcolepsy, like RBD, is a prominent disorder of REM sleep dysregulation [64]. Narcolepsy has a strong association with HLA class II genes, with the DQB1*0602 (DQw1 group) allele expressed in nearly all cases. In an effort to understand RBD better, the authors performed HLA class II antigen phenotyping in a group of 25 white males who had RBD but not narcolepsy: 84% (N = 21) were DQw1 (DQB1*05,06) positive (28% [N = 7] were DR2-positive); DQB1*0501 (N = 9) and DQB1*0602 (N = 7) were the most common phenotypes. The 84% DQw1 rate in RBD was significantly greater ($P = .015$) than the 56% DQw1 rate in a local white comparison group (N = 66), and was greater than the 39% to 66% DQw1 rates in 12 published white groups (N = 40–418 per group). In contrast to the nearly 100% DQw1-DR2 linkage in narcolepsy, only 28% of patients who had RBD in this report were DR2 positive. The strong dissociation between DQw1 and DR2 in RBD can be contrasted with the strong DQw1-DR2 association in narcolepsy. Narcolepsy and RBD, therefore, have strikingly convergent (DQw1) and divergent (DR2) HLA findings.

Postmortem brain findings in rapid eye movement sleep behavior disorder

Uchiyama and colleagues published the first extensive description of postmortem brain findings in RBD [65]. Upon death, an 84-year-old man who had idiopathic RBD for 20 years was found to have severe depletion of monoaminergic neurons in the locus ceruleus, associated with extensive Lewy body disease. The investigators postulated that because the nor-adrenergic LC exerts an inhibitory influence on the cholinergic brainstem nuclei, then RBD could result from disinhibition of brainstem cholinergic (pedunculopontine and laterodorsal tegmental) nuclei secondary to LC cell loss. There is growing evidence that RBD is highly associated with the synucleinopathies [21]. Further research on postmortem brain findings in RBD is needed.

Association of rapid eye movement sleep behavior disorder with psychiatric disorders and stress

Less than 8% of the patients who have RBD at the authors' center have psychiatric disorders that are linked causally with RBD, and prominent organic factors seem to play crucial roles in the genesis of RBD in all but two cases: during fluoxetine treatment of obsessive-compulsive disorder [28] or after cessation of use or abuse of REM-suppressing agents (ethanol, amphetamine, cocaine, or imipramine), presumably inducing a persistent and intense REM rebound disorder [7]. In two cases, major stress (divorce or automobile accident) precipitated RBD [7,66]. There are two other published cases of stress-related RBD, one a 20-year-old survivor of a sea disaster [67] and the other a 22-year-old teacher who was subjected to public humiliation [68]. The phenomenon of stress-related RBD may be explained in part by experience-mediated changes in cortical organization and in synaptic transmission that reflect an impressive plasticity within the central nervous system [69–71].

Rapid eye movement sleep behavior disorder variations

Parasomnia overlap syndrome:

The authors have identified a subgroup of patients who have RBD with PSG-documented overlapping NREM-REM sleep motor parasomnias consisting of sleepwalking, sleep terrors, and RBD [72]. Two other overlap parasomnia cases are reported [73,74]. These cases demonstrate motor–behavioral dyscontrol extending across NREM and REM sleep. The authors also report a family in which three adult first-degree relations are documented to have RBD, sleepwalking, sleep terrors, narcolepsy, and periodic/aperiodic limb movements of NREM sleep in various combina-tions, thus revealing an expanded spectrum of intrafamilial REM-NREM sleep motor dyscontrol [75].

Status dissociatus

Status dissociatus is the most extreme form of RBD and seems to represent the complete breakdown of state-determining boundaries [75,76].

Clinically, these patients seem to be either awake or "asleep"; however, their "sleep" is atypical, characterized by frequent muscle twitching, vocalization, and reports of dream-like mentation upon spontaneous or forced awakening. Polygraphically, there are no features of conventional REM or NREM sleep; rather, there is the simultaneous admixture of elements of wakefulness, REM sleep, and NREM sleep. "Sleep" often is perceived as normal and restorative, despite the nearly continuous motor and verbal behaviors and absence of PSG-defined REM or NREM sleep. Conditions associated with status dissociatus include protracted withdrawal from alcohol abuse, narcolepsy, olivopontocerebellar degeneration, and prior open heart surgery. The authors also have documented an AIDS-related case with prominent brainstem involvement. Similar signs and symptoms can be seen in fatal familial insomnia, a prion disease associated with preferential thalamic degeneration [77,78]. The abnormal motor and verbal nocturnal behaviors of status dissociatus may respond to treatment with clonazepam.

Agrypnia excitata

This recently described condition is characterized by generalized overactivity associated with loss of slow wave sleep, mental oneiricism (inability to initiate and maintain sleep with wakeful dreaming), and marked motor and autonomic sympathetic activation seen in such diverse conditions as delirium tremens, Morvan's fibrillary chorea, and fatal familial insomnia [79–81]. Oneirism dementia likely is a related condition [82].

Differential diagnosis

RBD is one of several disorders that can manifest as violent sleep- and dream-related behaviors with forensic implications [83,84]. Other disorders include disorders of arousal (confusional arousals, sleepwalking, and sleep terrors); nocturnal seizures, including hypnogenic paroxysmal dystonia; obstructive sleep apnea (with agitated arousals); rhythmic movement disorders of NREM and REM sleep, including rhythmic movement disorder (jactatio capitis nocturna); psychogenic dissociative disorders; and malingering [3,85]. This broad differential diagnosis mandates formal sleep studies in suspected RBD.

Other rapid eye movement sleep parasomnias

Nightmares

Nightmares are defined as frightening dreams that usually awaken the sleeper from REM sleep [8]. Behavioral activation (such as talking, screaming, thrashing about, or ambulation) rarely occurs and helps distinguish nightmares from RBD, sleep terrors, and sleepwalking. Nightmares can occur at any age after early childhood and can affect either gender, although in adults, women are affected more than men. There are many predisposing factors, including medical and psychiatric disorders and the treatment of such disorders (L-dopa treatment of parkinsonism, propranolol treatment of migraines, imipramine or fluoxetine treatment of depression, and so forth). It is important to consider nocturnal complex partial seizures in the differential diagnosis of nightmares.

The relationship of nightmares with specific personality profiles and with psychiatric disorders is controversial. Most reported nightmare sufferers, however, do not have a formal psychiatric history. Furthermore, whereas nightmare distress may be linked with psychopathology, nightmare frequency is not [86]. Nightmare frequency also is unrelated to self-reported levels of anxiety [87]. Frequent nightmare sufferers have a nonpsychotic profile on psychometric testing [88].

Treatment involves, first, the control of any underlying medical or psychiatric disorder—or the cessation or adjustment of the treatment of any medical or psychiatric disorder—that is believed to be responsible for the nightmares. Second, for chronic nightmares unrelated to any medical or psychiatric disorder, or else unresponsive to treatment of such disorders, successful cognitive-behavioral therapies are reported [89,90], as are pharmacologic treatments, such as cyproheptadine (a serotonin inhibitor), 4 to 24 mg at bedtime [91,92].

Rapid eye movement sleep–related sinus arrest

REM sleep–related sinus arrest was described first by Guilleminault and coworkers in 1984 [93]; it is a cardiac rhythm disorder that affects otherwise healthy young adults of either gender and is characterized by sinus arrest during REM sleep, usually in clusters, with periods of asystole lasting up to 9 seconds [8]. In one case, vocalizations occurred during periods of REM sleep asystole, with a loud scream and a sensation of being shocked (but without chest pain or related symptoms) associated with the longest asystole [94].

Periods of asystole do not occur during NREM sleep and are not associated with sleep apnea. Some patients experience faintness, light-headedness, and blurred vision during abrupt awakenings, and syncope can occur during ambulation after an awakening. Also, there may be complaints of vague chest pain or tightness or intermittent palpitations during the daytime. Daytime EKG (including Holter monitoring) usually is normal, however, and angiography, when performed, is unremarkable. The underlying pathophysiology, therefore, seem to be autonomic dysfunction. The clinical course is unknown. Complications include loss of consciousness and even cardiac arrest from prolonged asystole. This condition must be considered in cases of sudden, unexplained death during sleep. Treatment usually is not indicated, although prophylactic intervention includes a ventricular-inhibited pacemaker with a low rate limit.

Impaired sleep-related penile erections

Impaired sleep-related penile erections is defined as the inability to sustain a penile erection during sleep that would be sufficiently large or rigid enough to engage in sexual intercourse [8]. The manifestation of naturally occurring penile erectile cycles depends on the quality and quantity of sleep, particularly REM sleep, when most nocturnal erections occur. Substantial reduction or absence of sleep-related penile erections, in the presence of reasonably intact sleep architecture, usually indicates an organic cause of the impotence, such as hypertension (and its treatment), diabetes mellitus, heart or renal disease, urogenital disorders, alcoholism, drug abuse, or virtually any condition that affects normal vascular, neural, and endocrine functioning. Major depression can be associated with abnormal erectile patterns during sleep, albeit in the context of disturbed sleep architecture. Therefore, a history of depression should be elicited in the evaluation of all patients complaining of impotence. The prevalence of impotence in the United States is estimated to be approximately 10%, with two thirds of affected males having an organic cause of their impotence. The monitoring procedures and diagnostic criteria are well described [95]. Treatment is beyond the scope of this article.

Sleep-related painful erections

Sleep-related painful erections are characterized by penile pain with erections that occur typically during REM sleep [8]. Middle-aged or older males typically are affected; they complain of recurrent awakenings with partial or full erections and pain. The cumulative effects of nightly sleep disruption and sleep loss can result in the additional complaints of insomnia, irritability, anxiety, and daytime somnolence. There usually is a history of normal erections during wakefulness. Pathology of the penis usually is not found. Although the course is not well known, this condition can become more severe over time. Successful treatment has yet to be identified.

Summary

The recognition of RBD has shed additional scientific light on the "bumps in the night"; expanded knowledge of states of being and state dissociation; opened up new areas of research on brain and mind dysfunction during sleep; expanded knowledge of various neurologic disorders, particularly narcolepsy and parkinsonism; and reaffirmed the vital link between basic research and clinical medicine. Moreover, the safe and effective treatment of RBD with clonazepam is especially gratifying.

References

[1] Hayashi M, Inoue Y, Iwakawa Y, et al. REM sleep abnormalities in severe athetoid cerebral palsy. Brain Dev 1990;12:494–7.

[2] Hishikawa Y, Shimizu T, Tachibana N, et al. Oneiric behavior during REM sleep without muscle atonia in patients with neurologic disease and some withdrawal delirium. Sleep Research 1991;20A:425.

[3] Mahowald MW, Schenck CH. REM sleep parasomnias. In: Kryger MH, Roth T, Dement WC, editors. Principles and practice of sleep medicine. 4th edition. Philadelphia: Elsevier/Saunders; 2005. p. 897–916.

[4] Schenck CH, Mahowald MW. Motor dyscontrol in narcolepsy: rapid-eye-movement (REM) sleep without atonia and REM sleep behavior disorder. Ann Neurol 1992;32:3–10.

[5] Shimizu T, Sugita Y, Teshima Y, et al. Sleep study in patients with spinocerebellar degeneration and related diseases. In: Koella WP, editor. Sleep 1980. Basel: S. Karger; 1980. p. 435.

[6] Schenck CH, Bundlie SR, Ettinger MG, et al. Chronic behavioral disorders of human REM sleep: a new category of parasomnia. Sleep 1986;9:293–308.

[7] Schenck CH, Bundlie SR, Patterson AL, et al. REM sleep behavior disorder: a treatable parasomnia affecting older adults. JAMA 1987;257:1786–9.

[8] American Academy of Sleep Medicine. The International Classification of Sleep Disorders, 2nd edition. Diagnostic and coding manual. Westchester (IL): American Academy of Sleep Medicine; 2005.

[9] Dyken ME, Lin-Dyken DC, Seaba P, et al. Violent sleep-related behavior leading to subdural hemorrhage. Arch Neurol 1995;52:318–21.

[10] Gross PT. REM sleep behavior disorder causing bilateral subdural hematomas. Sleep Research 1992;21:204.

[11] Jouvet M, Delorme F. Locus coeruleus et sommeil paradoxal. CR Soc Biol 1965;159:895–9.

[12] Jouvet M, Sastre J-P, Sakai K. Toward an etho-ethnology of dreaming. In: Karacan I, editor. Psychophysiological aspects of sleep. Park Ridge (NJ): Noyes Medical Publishers; 1981.

[13] Sastre J-P, Jouvet M. Le comportement onirique du chat. Physiol Behav 1979;22:979.

[14] Hendricks JC, Morrison AR, Mann GL. Different behaviors during paradoxical sleep without atonia depend upon lesion site. Brain Res 1982;239:81–105.

[15] Henly K, Morrison AR. A re-evaluation of the effects of lesions of the pontine tegmentum and locus coeruleus on phenomena of paradoxical sleep in the cat. Acta Neurobiol Exp 1974; 34:215–32.

[16] Morrison AR. Brain-stem regulation of behavior during sleep and wakefulness. In: Sprague JM, Epstein AN, editors. Progress in psychobiology and physiological psychology. New York: Academic Press; 1979. p. 91.

[17] Lai YY, Siegel JM. Muscle tone suppression and stepping produced by stimulation of midbrain and rostral pontine reticular formation. J Neurosci 1990;10:2727–34.

[18] Pompeiano O. Mechanisms responsible for spinal inhibition during desynchronized sleep: experimental study. In: Guilleminault C, Dement WC, Passouant P, editors. Advances in sleep research, vol. 3. Narcolepsy. New York: Spectrum Press; 1976. p. 411.

[19] Sakai K, Sastre J-P, Kanamori N, et al. State-specific neurons in the ponto-medullary reticular formation with special reference to the postural atonia during paradoxical sleep in the cat. In: Pompeiano O, Ajmone Marsan C, editors. Brain mechanisms and perceptual awareness. New York: Raven Press; 1981. p. 405–29.

[20] Cox S, Risse G, Hawkins J, et al. Neuropsychological data in 34 patients with REM sleep behavior disorder (RBD). Sleep Res 1990;19:206.

[21] Boeve BF, Silber MH, Parisi JE, et al. Synucleinopathy pathology and REM sleep behavior disorder plus dementia or parkinsonism. Neurology 2003;61:40–5.

[22] Olson EJ, Boeve BF, Silber MH. Rapid eye movement sleep behaviour disorder: demographic, clinical and laboratory findings in 93 cases. Brain 2000;123:331–9.

[23] Schenck CH, Hurwitz TD, Mahowald MW. REM sleep behavior disorder: a report on a series of 96 consecutive cases and a review of the literature. J Sleep Res 1993;2: 224–31.

[24] Mahowald MW. REM sleep behavior disorder. In: Gilman S, editor. Neurobase. San Diego (CA): Arbor; 1999. p. CD ROM.

[25] Carlander B, Touchon J, Ondze B, et al. REM sleep behavior disorder induced by cholinergic treatment in Alzheimer's disease. J Sleep Res 1996;5(Suppl 1):28.

[26] Iranzo A, Santamaria J. Bisoprolol-induced rapid eye movement sleep behavior disorder. Am J Med 1999;107:390–2.

[27] Louden MB, Morehead MA, Schmidt HS. Activation by selegiline (Eldepryle) of REM sleep behavior disorder in parkinsonism. W V Med J 1995;91:101.

[28] Schenck CH, Mahowald MW, Kim SW, et al. Prominent eye movements during NREM sleep and REM sleep behavior disorder associated with fluoxetine treatment of depression and obsessive-compulsive disorder. Sleep 1992;15:226–35.

[29] Schutte S, Doghramji K. REM behavior disorder seen with venlafaxine (Effexor). Sleep Res 1996;25:364.

[30] Silber MH. REM sleep behavior disorder associated with barbiturate withdrawal. Sleep Res 1996;25:371.

[31] Stolz SE, Aldrich MS. REM sleep behavior disorder associated with caffeine abuse. Sleep Res 1991;20:341.

[32] Ross LL, Yu D, Kropla WC. Stereotyped behavior in developmentally delayed or autistic populations. Rhythmic or nonrhythmic? Behav Modif 1998;22:321–34.

[33] Sforza E, Krieger J, Petiau C. REM sleep behavior disorder: clinical and physiopathological findings. Sleep Med Rev 1997;1:57–69.

[34] Schenck CH, Mahowald MW. Polysomnographic, neurologic, psychiatric, and clinical outcome report on 70 consecutive cases with REM sleep behavior disorder (RBD): sustained clonazepam efficacy in 89.5% of 57 treated patients. Cleve Clin J Med 1990; 57(Suppl):S9–23.

[35] Schenck CH, Hopwood J, Duncan E, et al. Preservation and loss of REM-atonia in human idiopathic REM sleep behavior disorder (RBD): quantitative polysomnographic (PSG) analyses in 17 patients. Sleep Res 1992;21:16.

[36] Lapierre O, Montplaisir J. Polysomnographic features of REM sleep behavior disorder: development of a scoring method. Neurology 1992;42:1371–4.

[37] Schenck CH, Mahowald MW. Long-term, nightly benzodiazepine treatment of injurious parasomnias and other disorders of disrupted nocturnal sleep in 170 adults. Am J Med 1996; 100:333–7.

[38] Kunz D, Bes F. Effects of exogenous melatonin on periodic limb movement disorder: an open pilot study. Sleep 1999;22:S162.

[39] Boeve BF, Silber MH, Ferman JT. Melatonin for treatment of REM sleep behavior disorder in neurologic disorders: results in 14 patients. Sleep Med 2003;4:281–4.

[40] Takeuchi N, Uchimura N, Hashizume Y, et al. Melatonin therapy for REM sleep behavior disorder. Psychiatry Clin Neurosci 2001;55:267–9.

[41] Fantini ML, Gagnon J-F, Filipini D, et al. The effects of pramipexole in REM sleep behavior disorder. Neurology 2003;61:1418–20.

[42] Tan A, Salgado M, Fahn S. Rapid eye movement sleep behavior disorder preceding Parkinson's disease with therapeutic response to levodopa. Mov Disord 1996;11: 214–6.

[43] Schenck CH, Mahowald MW. REM sleep behavior disorder: clinical, developmental, and neuroscience perspectives 16 years after its formal identification in *Sleep*. Sleep 2002;25: 120–30.

[44] Schenck CH, Mahowald MW. Pre-clinical tonic and phasic REM motor disturbances in 19 patients. Sleep Res 1991;20:322.

[45] Tachibana N, Kimura K, Kitajima K, et al. REM sleep motor dysfunction in multiple system atrophy. Sleep Res 1995;24A:415.

[46] Tachibana N, Sugita Y, Tachibana N, et al. Sleeptalking in REM sleep could be the prodromal symptom of REM sleep behavior disorder. Sleep Res 1995;24A:242.

[47] Tachibana N, Yamanaka K, Kaji R, et al. Sleep bruxism as a manifestation of subclinical rapid eye movement sleep behavior disorder. Sleep 1994;17:555–8.

[48] Schenck CH, Bundlie SR, Mahowald MW. Delayed emergence of a parkinsonian disorder in 38% of 29 older men initially diagnosed with idiopathic rapid eye movement sleep behavior disorder. Neurology 1996;46:388–93.

[49] Gagnon J, Bedard M, Fantini ML, et al. REM sleep behavior disorder and REM sleep without atonia in Parkinson's disease. Neurology 2002;59:585–9.

[50] Comella CL, Tanner CM, Ristanovic RK. Polysomnographic sleep measures in Parkinson's disease patients with treatment-induced hallucinations. Ann Neurol 1993;34:710–4.

[51] Boeve BF, Silber MH, Parisi JE, et al. Synuceinopathy pathology often underlies REM sleep behavior disorder and dementia or parkinsonism. Neurology 2003;61:40–5.

[52] Wright BA, Rosen JR, Buysse DJ, et al. Shy-Drager syndrome presenting as a REM behavior disorder. J Geriatr Psychiatry Neurol 1990;3:110–3.

[53] Arnulf I, Merino-Andreu M, Bloch F, et al. REM sleep behavior disorder and REM without atonia in patients with progressive supranuclear palsy. Sleep 2005;28:349–54.

[54] Kumru H, Santamaria J, Tolosa E, et al. Rapid eye movement sleep behavior disorder in Parkinsonism with *PARKIN* mutations. Ann Neurol 2004;56:599–603.

[55] Pareja JA, Caminero AB, Masa JF, et al. A first case of progressive supranuclear palsy and pre-clinical REM sleep behavior disorder presenting as inhibition of speech during wakefulness and somniloquy with phasic muscle twitching during REM sleep. Neurologia 1996;11:304–6.

[56] Boeve BF, Silber MH, Ferman JT, et al. Association of REM sleep behavior disorder and neurodegenerative disease may reflect an underlying synucleinopathy. Mov Disord 2001;16: 622–30.

[57] Montplaisir J, Petit D, Decary A, et al. Sleep and quantitative EEG in patients with progressive supranuclear palsy. Neurology 1997;49:999–1003.

[58] Fantini ML, Ferini-Strambi L, Montplaisir J. Idiopathic REM sleep behavior disorder. Toward a better nosologic definition. Neurology 2005;64:780–6.

[59] Fantini ML, Gagnon J-F, Petit D, Rompre S, et al. Slowing of electroencephalogram in rapid eye movement sleep behavior disorder. Ann Neurol 2003;53:774–80.

[60] Massicotte-Marquez J, Carrier J, Decary A, et al. Slow-wave sleep and delta power in rapid eye movement sleep behavior disorder. Sleep 2005;57:277–82.

[61] Stiasny-Kolster K, Doerr Y, Moller JC, et al. Combination of 'idiopathic' REM sleep behavior disorder and olfactory dysfunction as possible indicator for alpha-synucleinopathy demonstrated by dopamine transporter FP-CIT-SPECT. Brain 2005;128:126–37.

[62] Ferini-Strambi L, DeGioia MR, Castronovo VE, et al. Neuropsychological assessment in idiopathic REM sleep behavior disorder (RBD). Does the idiopathic form of RBD really exist? Neurology 2004;62:41–5.

[63] Mayer G, Meier-Ewert K. Motor dyscontrol in sleep of narcoleptic patients (a lifelong development?). J Sleep Res 1993;2:143.

[64] Schenck CH, Garcia-Rill E, Segall M, et al. HLA class II genes associated with REM sleep behavior disorder. Ann Neurol 1996;39:261–3.

[65] Uchiyama M, Isse K, Tanaka K, et al. Incidental Lewy body disease in a patient with REM sleep behavior disorder. Neurology 1995;45:709–12.

[66] Schenck CH, Hurwitz TD, Bundlie SR, et al. W. Sleep-related injury in 100 adult patients: a polysomnographic and clinical report. Am J Psychiatry 1989;146:1166–73.

[67] Hefez A, Metz L, Lavie P. Long-term effects of extreme situational stress on sleep and dreaming. Am J Psychiatry 1987;144:344–7.

[68] Sugita Y, Taniguchi M, Terashima K, et al. A young case of idiopathic REM sleep behavior disorder (RBD) specifically induced by socially stressful conditions. Sleep Res 1991;20A:394.

[69] Cohen LG, Roth BJ, Wassermann EM, et al. Magnetic stimulation of the human cortex, an indicator of reorganization of motor pathways in certain pathological conditions. J Clin Neurophysiol 1991;8:56–65.

[70] Kandel ER. Environmental determinants of brain architecture and of behavior: early experience and learning. In: Kandel ER, Schwartz JH, editors. Principles of neural science. New York: Elsevier/North Holland; 1981. p. 620–32.

[71] Pons TP, Garraghty PE, Ommaya K, et al. Massive cortical reorganization after sensory deafferentation in adult Macaques. Science 1991;252:1857–60.

[72] Schenck CH, Boyd JL, Mahowald MW. A parasomnia overlap disorder involving sleepwalking, sleep terrors, and REM sleep behavior disorder in 33 polysomnographically confirmed cases. Sleep 1997;20:972–81.

[73] Bokey K. Conversion disorder revisited: severe parasomnia discovered. Aust N Z J Psychiatry 1993;27:694.

[74] Kushida CA, Clerk AA, Kirsch CM, et al. Prolonged confusion with nocturnal wandering arising from NREM and REM sleep: a case report. Sleep 1995;18:757–64.

[75] Mahowald MW, Schenck CH. Dissociated states of wakefulness and sleep. Neurology 1992; 42:44–52.

[76] Mahowald MW, Schenck CH. Status dissociatus—a perspective on states of being. Sleep 1991;14:69–79.

[77] Medori R, Tritschler H-J, LeBlanc A, et al. Fatal familial insomnia, a prion disease with a mutation at codon 178 of the prion protein gene. N Engl J Med 1992;326:444.

[78] Tinuper P, Montagna P, Medori P, et al. The thalamus participates in the regulation of the sleep-waking cycle. A clinico-pathological study in fatal familial thalamic degeneration. EEG Clin Neurophysiol 1989;73:117–23.

[79] Lugaresi E, Provini F. Agrypnia excitata: clinical features and pathophysiological implications. Sleep Med Rev 2001;5:313–22.

[80] Montagna P, Lugaresi E. Agrypnia excitata: a generalized overactivity syndrome and a useful concept in the neurophysiology of sleep. Clin Neurophysiol 2002;113:552–60.

[81] Plazzi G, Montagna P, Meletti S, et al. Polysomnographic study of sleeplessness and onericisms in the alcohol withdrawal syndrome. Sleep Med 2002;3:279–82.

[82] Cibula JE, Eisenschenk S, Gold M, et al. Progressive dementia and hypersomnolence with dream-enacting behavior. Oneiric dementia. Arch Neurol 2002;59:630–4.

[83] Mahowald MW, Schenck CH. Violent parasomnias: forensic medicine issues. In: Kryger MH, Roth T, Dement WC, editors. Principles and practice of sleep medicine. 3rd edition. Philadelphia: W.B. Saunders; 2000. p. 786–95.

[84] Mahowald MW, Schenck CH. Violent parasomnias: forensic medicine issues. In: Kryger MH, Roth T, Dement WC, editors. Principles and practice of sleep medicine. 4th edition. Philadelphia: Elsevier/Saunders; 2005. p. 960–8.

[85] Iranzo A, Santamaria J. Severe obstructive sleep apnea/hypopnea mimicking REM sleep behavior disorder. Sleep 2005;28:203–6.

[86] Belicki K. Nightmare frequency versus nightmare distress: relations to psychopathology and cognitive style. J Abnorm Psychol 1992;101:592.

[87] Wood JM, Bootzin RR. The prevalence of nightmares and their independence from anxiety. J Abnorm Psychol 1990;99:64.

[88] Berquier A, Ashton R. Characteristics of the frequent nightmare sufferer. J Abnorm Psychol 1992;101:246.

[89] Eccles A, Wilde A, Marshall WL. In Vivo desensitization in the treatment of recurrent nightmares. J Behav Ther Exp Psychiat 1988;19:318.

[90] Matsumoto M, Mutoh F, Naoe H, et al. The effects of imipramine on REM sleep behavior disorder in 3 cases. Sleep Res 1991;20A:351.

[91] Brophy MH. Cyproheptadine for combat nightmares in post-traumatic stress disorder and dream anxiety disorder. Mil Med 1991;156:100.

[92] Harsch HH. Cyproheptadine for recurrent nightmares. Am J Psychiatry 1986;143:1491.

[93] Guilleminault C, Pool P, Motta J, et al. Sinus arrest during REM sleep in young adults. N Engl J Med 1984;311:1106–10.

[94] Rattenborg NC, Lindblom S, Best J, et al. REM sleep-related asystole associated with unusual polysomnographic features: a case history. Sleep Res 1995;24:324.

[95] Ware JC, Hirshkowitz M. Assessment of sleep-related erections. In: Kryger MH, Roth T, Dement WC, editors. Principles and practice of sleep medicine. 4th edition. Philadelphia: Elsevier Saunders; 2005. p. 1394–402.

ELSEVIER
SAUNDERS

NEUROLOGIC
CLINICS

Neurol Clin 23 (2005) 1127–1147

Sleep and Epilepsy

Beth A. Malow, MD, MS

Department of Neurology, Vanderbilt University School of Medicine,
2100 Pierce Avenue (Medical Center South), Room 352, Nashville, TN 37212, USA

Since Aristotle and Hippocrates noted the occurrence of epileptic seizures during sleep, the relationship between sleep and epilepsy has intrigued physicians and researchers. In the late nineteenth century, Gowers [1] commented on the relationship of seizures to the sleep-wake cycle. In 1929, Langdon-Down and Brain [2] observed that nocturnal seizures peaked approximately 2 hours after bedtime and between 4 AM and 5 AM, whereas daytime seizures were most prevalent in the first hour after waking. Berger's discovery of the electroencephalogram (EEG) in the 1920s provided a diagnostic tool for studies researching the interrelationship of sleep and epilepsy [3]. Gibbs and Gibbs [4] demonstrated that interictal epileptiform discharges were activated by sleep, and obtaining sleep during an EEG recording remains a standard activating procedure today. Janz [5] differentiated awakening, nocturnal, and diurnal/nocturnal epilepsies, and Niedermeyer [6] described the activating influence of arousal on epilepsy.

This review summarizes the basic mechanisms of epilepsy and the influence of sleep on epileptic seizures, highlights several epileptic syndromes that occur commonly during sleep, outlines the differential diagnosis of paroxysmal events and diagnostic tests for epilepsy, summarizes the evidence for sleep disorders in patients who have epilepsy, and discusses the management of sleep-related epilepsy.

Mechanisms

Epilepsy is a chronic disorder characterized by recurrent seizures. During seizures, abnormal electrical discharges are synchronized throughout a localized or distributed population of neurons in the brain [7]. Seizures may be partial, originating in a focal area of cortex, or generalized, arising diffusely from both hemispheres. Experimental models of partial and generalized epilepsy can be produced by applying chemicals, such as

E-mail address: beth.malow@vanderbilt.edu

penicillin, directly to cortical tissue or by electrical stimulation. In the generalized epilepsies, spike and wave discharges seen in the human surface EEG are generated by thalamocortic neurons, with excitatory action potentials alternating with periods of inhibition [8], although cortical mechanisms also seem to be involved [9]. In experimental models of the partial epilepsies, the cellular correlate of the interictal spike is the paroxysmal depolarizing shift (PDS), a prolonged high-amplitude depolarization followed by a hyperpolarization [7]. A large excitatory postsynaptic potential underlies the PDS. A variety of mechanisms (including membrane receptor alterations and neurochemical release) operating at local (eg, hippocampal) and more widespread (eg, thalamocortic) levels are implicated in amplifying excitatory postsynaptic potential enhancement and PDS generation. The onset of seizure activity seems to be linked to attenuation of the hyperpolarizing membrane potential.

Sleep is an example of a physiologic state capable of modulating seizures through the involvement of widespread circuits, including thalamocortic networks [10]. The influence of sleep on epilepsy is supported by observation that, in specific epileptic syndromes, seizures occur exclusively or primarily during non–rapid eye movement (NREM) sleep. In almost all epileptic syndromes, interictal epileptiform discharges are more prevalent during NREM sleep and less prevalent during rapid eye movement (REM) sleep. Neuronal synchronization within thalamocortic networks during NREM sleep results in enhanced neuronal excitability, leading to more diffuse distribution of focal discharges and facilitation of seizures and interictal epileptiform discharges in many persons who have partial epilepsy. Neuronal synchronization is disrupted on arousal or transition to REM sleep, and focal discharges become more localized [11]. The biochemical pharmacology of sleep and arousal is under intensive study; the involvement of a variety of neurotransmitters is likely. The preoptic area of the hypothalamus is a major sleep-promoting system that uses γ-aminobutyric acid (GABA) as a neurotransmitter. Sleep-active neurons in the preoptic area project to brainstem regions that contain neurons involved in arousal from sleep and, by inhibiting these regions, in turn promote sleep. These regions include the pedunculopontine and laterodorsal tegmental nuclei, the locus coeruleus, and the dorsal raphe [12].

Epileptic syndromes associated with sleep

The proportion of patients who have seizures that occur exclusively or predominantly during sleep ranges from 7.5% to 45% in several series studying sleep-related epilepsy [13,14]. This wide variation in prevalence may reflect differences in epileptic syndromes among patient populations, with seizures more likely to occur during sleep in certain epileptic syndromes. The 1989 Classification and Terminology of the International League Against Epilepsy [15], the most widely used classification of the epilepsies, distinguishes a variety of epileptic syndromes primarily on the basis of clinical characteristics, epidemiology, and EEG and neuroimaging studies.

A major discriminating factor is whether or not seizures originate in a group of neurons within one hemisphere (partial, focal, or localization related) or within neurons throughout both hemispheres (generalized). Specific partial and generalized epileptic syndromes associated with sleep are described in this article and outlined in Table 1. Two probable epileptic syndromes—paroxysmal nocturnal dystonia and epileptic arousals from sleep—also are discussed.

Partial seizures

Crespel and colleagues [16] found that frontal lobe seizures are more common during sleep and temporal lobe seizures more common during wakefulness. Herman and coworkers analyzed 613 seizures in 133 patients who had partial seizure and underwent video-EEG monitoring [17]. Forty-three percent of all partial seizures began during sleep, the majority during stages 1 and 2 sleep and none during REM sleep. Temporal lobe seizures were more likely to generalize secondarily during sleep than wakefulness compared with frontal lobe seizures, which were less likely to generalize secondarily during sleep. Frontal lobe seizures were most likely to occur during sleep, with temporal lobe seizures next, and occipital or parietal lobe seizures occurring rarely during sleep. Minecan and coworkers [18] show that seizures statistically were more common during NREM stages 1 and 2, at least for isolated seizures occurring in one night. Some seizures did occur during REM sleep, but this was the least frequent sleep stage for seizures to occur. Log delta power, an automated measure of sleep depth, increased in the 10 minutes before seizures, suggesting that seizures occur as sleep is deepening within NREM stages 1 and 2 sleep.

Temporal lobe epilepsy

Complex partial seizures that begin focally and impair consciousness are the predominant seizure type in temporal lobe epilepsy (TLE) [19]. Staring,

Table 1
Epilepsy syndromes associated with sleep-related seizures

Epilepsy syndrome	Age of onset
TLE	Late childhood to early adulthood
Frontal lobe epilepsy	Late childhood to early adulthood
Benign childhood epilepsy with centrotemporal spikes	3–13 y (peak 9–10 y)
Epilepsy with GTCS on awakening	6–25 y (peak 11–15 y)
Juvenile myoclonic epilepsy	12–18 y (peak 14 y)
Absence epilepsy	3–12 y (peak 6–7 y)
Lennox-Gastaut syndrome	1–8 y (peak 3–5 y)
Continuous spike and slow wave discharges during sleep	8 mo–11.5 y

orofacial or limb automatisms, and head and body movements occur frequently. The most common cause is idiopathic; trauma, tumor, stroke, and other focal lesions must be considered and are detectable with brain MRI. Idiopathic cases often show hippocampal sclerosis on MRI. Most patients continue to have seizures and require antiepileptic drug therapy; many patients, however, are controlled easily.

Because TLE is the most common type of partial epilepsy in adults, seizures during sleep commonly are of temporal lobe origin. In most patients who have TLE, however, seizures are more likely to occur during wakefulness than sleep. Bernasconi and colleagues [20] identified a group of 26 patient who had nonlesional refractory TLE and in whom seizures occurred exclusively or predominantly (>90%) after they fell asleep or before they awakened. These patients manifested the typical clinical manifestations of TLE, and in addition, some also exhibited sleepwalking as a manifestation of their seizure activity. Their prognosis for seizure freedom after epilepsy surgery was more favorable than in patients who had nonlesional TLE and seizures during wakefulness.

Although temporal lobe seizures occur more frequently during NREM than REM sleep [17], they may occur occasionally during REM sleep [18]. Interictal epileptiform activity is more common during NREM sleep than during wakefulness and REM sleep. Sammaritano and colleagues [21] found that 78% of subjects had increases in the frequency of spikes recorded by surface electrodes during NREM stages 3 and 4 and that the field of spiking increased in NREM sleep compared with wakefulness and REM sleep. Increased spiking during deep NREM sleep also was found in depth electrode studies [22,23]. Overnight sleep recordings may reveal interictal foci not present on routine EEGs, thus providing prognostic information for the epilepsy surgery evaluation, especially in cases where the interictal spiking remains unilateral [24]. Examples of interictal epileptiform activity are shown in Figs. 1 and 2.

Frontal lobe epilepsy

As with temporal lobe epilepsy, the most common cause of frontal lobe epilepsy is idiopathic, although focal lesions also may be the cause. As the clinical manifestations of nocturnal frontal lobe seizures often include prominent tonic or motor manifestations, they are more likely to be noticed by the patient or family than complex partial seizures of temporal lobe origin; however, the brevity, the minimal amount or lack of postictal confusion, the psychogenic-appearing features (including kicking, thrashing, and vocalizations), and the frequently normal interictal and ictal recordings may complicate diagnosis. Nocturnal episodes may suggest diagnoses of sleep terrors, REM sleep behavior disorder (RBD), psychogenic spells, or paroxysmal nocturnal dystonia (discussed later). Scheffer and colleagues [25] describe an autosomal dominant nocturnal frontal epilepsy syndrome

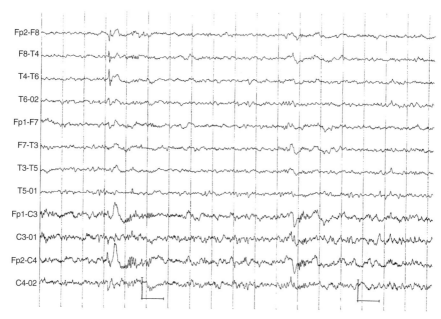

Fig. 1. Right anterior temporal interictal epileptiform discharge with phase reversal at F8 electrode during stage 2 NREM sleep. Calibration symbol: 150 μV, 1 s.

(ADNFLE) with clustering of nocturnal motor seizures documented by video-EEG monitoring. Many of the 39 individuals from six families had been misdiagnosed with nonepileptic disorders. This large Australian kindred showed a missense mutation in the alpha-4 subunit of the neuronal

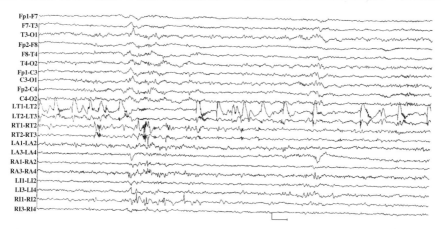

Fig. 2. Bilateral independent interictal epileptiform discharges from temporal depth electrode contacts RT1–RT2, RT2–RT3 (right anterior hippocampus) and LT1–LT2, LT2–LT3 (left anterior hippocampus). Note absence of interical epileptiform activity on simultaneously recorded scalp electrodes. Calibration symbols: 30 μV, 1 s (surface electrodes); 150 μV, 1 s (intracranial electrodes).

nicotinic acetylcholine receptor gene, located on chromosome 20q. This aberrant acetylcholine receptor may be related to the preferential occurrence of ADNFLE during sleep, in that physiologic sleep mechanisms are disrupted [26]. This model is complicated; independent investigators have determined that ADNFLE is a genetically heterogeneous disorder, however, with other families not showing linkage to chromosome 20q [27].

Frontal lobe seizures arise from a variety of structures, including the supplementary motor area; the cingulate gyrus; the anterior frontopolar, orbitofrontal, dorsolateral, and opercular regions; and the motor cortex. Correlation between anatomic location and clinical characteristics has limitations because of rapid propagation, although an anatomic classification still is used because of its simplicity. One example of frontal lobe epilepsy is the syndrome associated with supplementary sensorimotor area seizures that originate in or spread to involve area 6 on the medial surface of the cerebral hemisphere [28]. These seizures, which often occur in sleep, begin abruptly with tonic posturing of one or more extremities, sometimes followed by rhythmic or clonic movements. A sensation of pulling, pulsing, heaviness, numbness, or tingling may precede tonic posturing. The surface EEG often is normal, although interictal epileptiform activity or ictal patterns may occur in electrodes at or adjacent to the midline (ie, Cz). Seizures of sensorimotor area origin may be mistaken for psychogenic spells because of thrashing behavior, preservation of consciousness, absence of postictal confusion, and absence of interictal or ictal EEG activity. Diagnostic points supporting sensorimotor area seizures include (1) short duration (less than 30 seconds to a minute), (2) stereotyped nature, (3) tendency to occur predominantly or exclusively during sleep, and (4) tonic contraction of the arms in abduction. Psychogenic spells usually are longer in duration (1 to several minutes), are nonstereotypic, and occur in the awake or drowsy state [29]. Withdrawal of antiepileptic medications to promote generalized tonic-clonic seizures (GTCS) during in-patient evaluation with continuous video-EEG monitoring is a useful diagnostic maneuver [30].

Partial seizures with complex automatisms

Pedley and Guilleminault [31] describe six patients who had unusual sleepwalking episodes involving screaming or other vocalizations and complex, often violent automatisms. They distinguished these probable epileptic spells from NREM sleep confusional arousals (described previously) on the basis of several characteristics. Probable epileptic spells occurred in a slightly older age group (adolescents and young adults) in association with complex behaviors and complete unresponsiveness to the environment, with a family history for confusional arousals lacking. Epileptiform EEG abnormalities and responsiveness to antiepileptic medications also supported a diagnosis of epilepsy. Montagna and colleagues [32] performed EEG polysomnography in six patients who had complex arousals from NREM sleep characterized by wandering, motor agitation, and screaming. One patient experienced GTCS after an EEG arousal, and two responded to carbamazepine, supporting a diagnosis of epilepsy.

Benign epilepsy of childhood with centrotemporal spikes

Also known as benign rolandic epilepsy, this common childhood seizure disorder, which accounts for 15% to 20% of childhood epilepsy, responds favorably to antiepileptic medication [33,34]. The cause is idiopathic, with a genetic predisposition. Seizures occur predominantly during sleep. Oropharyngeal signs, including hypersalivation and guttural sounds, are the most common manifestations. Speech arrest, clonic jerks, tonic contraction of the mouth, and occasionally clonic jerks of the arm or leg also are common. Consciousness is preserved in most cases unless secondary generalization occurs. The EEG usually shows centrotemporal or rolandic spikes or sharp waves, reflecting the anatomic areas underlying the most common clinical manifestations (Fig. 3).

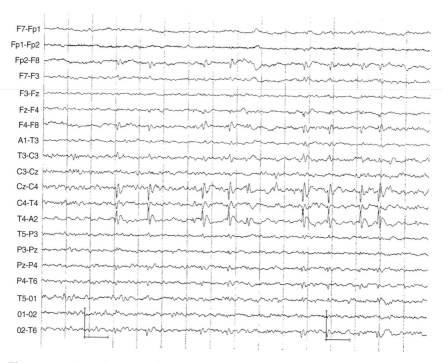

Fig. 3. Runs of interictal epileptiform with a centrotemporal dominance in benign rolandic epilepsy. Calibration symbol: 500 μV, 1 s.

Generalized seizures

Epilepsy with generalized tonic-clonic seizures on awakening

In this idiopathic syndrome, which most likely has a genetic basis, GTCS occur exclusively or predominantly (>90%) shortly after awakening (regardless of time of day) or in the evening period of relaxation [13]. Myoclonic or absence seizures may coexist. Photosensitivity is common, and sleep deprivation is a frequent precipitant. The EEG shows interictal generalized spike-wave activity. Complete seizure control with medication occurs in most patients, although most relapse if medication is withdrawn.

Juvenile myoclonic epilepsy is a related syndrome. It is one of the most common forms of idiopathic generalized epilepsy, and consists of a combination of myoclonic seizures that occur shortly after awakening, GTCS, and absence seizures [35]. When questioned, patients may report being clumsy and dropping items while carrying out their morning activities of daily living, including shaving, applying cosmetics, or preparing breakfast. Brain MRI and neurologic examination are normal. Interictal EEGs in untreated patients are characterized by diffuse polyspike and slow wave complexes of 4 to 6 Hz. Response to antiepileptic medications usually is excellent, although lifelong treatment often is necessary.

Absence epilepsy

Absence epilepsy is another genetically determined form of generalized epilepsy. Seizures are brief spells, usually lasting less than 10 seconds, characterized by the abrupt cessation of ongoing activity, a blank stare, and abrupt return to awareness with resumption of activity [36]. Mild clonic, atonic, or tonic components or automatisms may be associated. They often are precipitated by hyperventilation, photic stimulation, and drowsiness and are suppressed by attention. The brevity of the attacks and the lack of an aura or postictal confusion help to distinguish these spells from complex partial seizures [37]. The waking EEG correlate to absence seizures is the classical 3-second spike and wave discharge. Drowsiness and sleep activate spike and wave discharges, which are most marked during the first sleep cycle, maximal during NREM sleep, and rare or absent in REM sleep [38]. The morphology of spike and wave discharges also is affected by NREM sleep, with irregular polyspike-wave discharges predominating. Prognosis with treatment is excellent. The seizures decrease with advancing age, and medications can be withdrawn from most patients by late adolescence, although some patients continue to require treatment for life.

Lennox-Gastaut syndrome

This syndrome is characterized by generalized tonic, atonic, and atypical absence seizures, slow background on interictal EEG with slow (usually 2.0–2.5 Hz) spike and wave complexes, and mental retardation [39]. There are cryptogenic forms with no prior neurologic abnormality, normal development, and normal neuroimaging and symptomatic forms of other neurologic abnormalities, abnormal development, or abnormal neuro-imaging. NREM sleep is associated with increased spikes and rhythmic 10-Hz spikes that may be accompanied by tonic seizures.

Other epilepsies

In some epilepsy syndromes, it is uncertain if seizures are focal or generalized. Epilepsy with continuous spike-waves during slow wave sleep (CSWS) is one such syndrome, Patry and colleagues [40] described "subclinical" electrical status epilepticus induced by sleep in children with almost continuous spike and slow wave discharges during NREM sleep. The disorder affects only 0.5% of children with epilepsy, and its cause is unclear, although approximately one-third of children have neurologic abnormalities [41]. It is a striking form of epilepsy because of the markedly abnormal state dependent EEG: 2.0- to 2.5-Hz generalized spike and wave discharges occur during at least 85% of NREM sleep, whereas during REM sleep and wakefulness, spike-wave discharges are less continuous and more focal. Seizures are not universal, although they frequently occur in CSWS and may be manifested as nocturnal partial motor seizures or GTCS, atypical absence, or myoclonic jerks. Progressive behavioral disturbances are common. Although treatment of seizures is partially or completely effective, cognitive impairment usually persists.

Probable epileptic disorders

Nocturnal paroxysmal dystonia

This syndrome, initially termed hypnogenic paroxysmal dystonia and subsequently, nocturnal paroxysmal dystonia (NPD), is characterized by brief (15–45 seconds) stereotyped motor attacks consisting of dystonic posturing, ballistic or choreic dyskinesias, and vocalizations during NREM sleep without clear ictal or interictal EEG changes that are responsive to carbamazepine [42]. Although the lack of EEG changes might seem to make epilepsy an unlikely cause, the lack of surface EEG abnormalities does not exclude epilepsy; seizures originating in deep mesial frontal generators often lack interictal and ictal correlates and require invasive monitoring for definitive diagnosis. Tinuper and colleagues [43] report two patients who had "typical" NPD attacks that culminated in GTCS with electrographic ictal correlates. The attacks of NPD resemble frontal lobe seizures in their brevity and motor involvement. In evaluating a patient who has a history consistent with NPD, EEGs during wake and sleep should be performed. Additional supraorbital electrodes should be placed to increase frontal lobe coverage. Care should be taken to identify and differentiate central spikes from physiologic vertex sharp waves of sleep. Intracranial monitoring may be required for refractory cases in which there is a high suspicion of epilepsy.

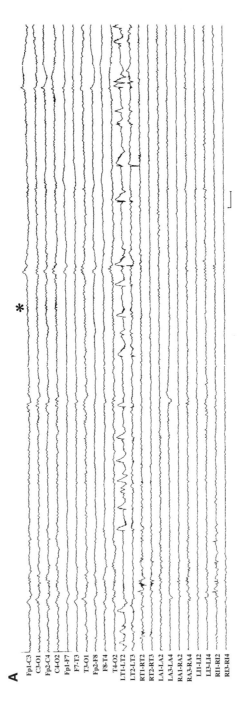

Fig. 4. Combined surface electrode (first 10 channels) and intracranial montage (last 12 channels). Calibration symbols: 30 μV, 1 s (surface electrodes); 150 μV, 1 s (intracranial channels). (*A*) Prior to seizure onset, sleep spindles (*asterisk*) are apparent in the surface electrodes, and frequent interictal epileptiform discharges are observed in the left and right temporal depth electrode contacts (RT1–RT2, RT2–RT2 and LT1–LT2, LT2–LT3). (*B*) At the open arrow, the earliest definite intracranial ictal discharge (spike and wave complex in the right temporal depth electrode contacts leading to rhythmic sinusoidal alpha frequency activity) is seen, preceding the clinical arousal from sleep (*solid arrow*, indicating myogenic activity) and the earliest definite scalp ictal discharge (*bracket*, indicating myogenic activity with emerging right temporal rhythmic theta activity). (*From* Malow BA, Varma NK. Seizures and arousals from sleep—which comes first? Sleep 1995;18:783–6; with permission.)

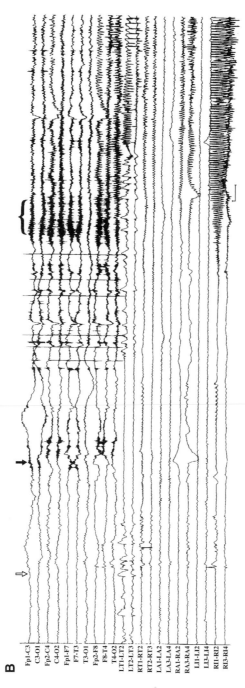

Fig. 4 (continued)

"Epileptic" arousals from sleep

Athough most arousals from sleep are not the result of epilepsy, epileptic seizures and interictal epileptiform activity sometimes may be associated with arousals and excessive daytime somnolence. In two of the epilepsy syndromes described previously—epilepsy with GTCS on awakening and juvenile myoclonic epilepsy—transition from the sleep to wake state is a clear precipitant. Peled and Lavie [44] describe 14 patients who had hypersomnolence and paroxysmal epileptic discharges during stages 2 and 3 of NREM sleep that were associated with arousals, fragmentation of sleep, and reduction in sleep efficiency, in particular REM sleep. Three of these patients responded to anticonvulsant agents with a clinical and polysomnographic improvement in sleep patterns.

It is important to recognize the shortcomings of surface EEG when investigating the relationship between arousals and seizures. In cases in which seizures seem to follow clinical arousals, the onset of ictal activity may be delayed on the surface EEG compared with the intracranial EEG [45]. Fig. 4 illustrates an example from combined surface intracranial monitoring in which the surface EEG does not demonstrate ictal activity until several seconds after a clinical arousal from sleep. The concomitant intracranial EEG reveals seizure onset just before the clinical arousal from sleep.

Differential diagnosis

The differentiation of nocturnal seizures from nonepileptic spells during sleep can be challenging for several reasons (Box 1). First, in partial seizures occurring during wakefulness, patients may report postictal confusion or recall the beginning of a seizure (aura) that precedes loss of consciousness. These elements of the history support the diagnosis of epilepsy and frequently are absent in seizures occurring during sleep. Second, nocturnal events may not be observed properly. Bed partners may not be present or, if present, may not be fully awake and coherent. Complex partial seizures of temporal lobe origin in particular may lack vigorous motor activity and may fail to wake the bed partner. Third, a variety of sleep disorders (discussed later) are characterized by vigorous movements and behaviors that mimic seizures. Finally, certain types of seizures, particularly those of frontal lobe origin, are manifested by bizarre movements suggestive of a psychiatric disorder, including kicking, thrashing, and vocalizations. These epilepsies may be associated with normal ictal and interictal EEGs and normal imaging studies, making definitive diagnosis difficult.

Non–rapid eye movement arousal disorders

NREM arousal disorders include a spectrum of confusional arousals, somnambulism (sleepwalking), and night terrors. These three disorders share

---

Box 1. Differential diagnosis of nocturnal spells

Epileptic seizures
Frontal lobe epilepsy
TLE
GTCS
Benign rolandic epilepsy

Probable epileptic seizures
NPD
Epileptic arousals from sleep

NREM arousal disorders
Confusional arousals
Night terrors
Somnambulism

REM sleep behavior disorder
Sleep-related movement disorder
PLMS
Sleep-onset myoclonus
Bruxism
Rhythmic movement disorder

Psychiatric disorders
Nocturnal panic disorder
Post-traumatic stress disorder
Psychogenic seizures

---

the following features: (1) they usually arise from NREM stages 3 or 4 sleep and, therefore, occur preferentially in the first third of the sleep cycle when NREM stages 3 and 4 are predominant; (2) they are more common in childhood; and (3) a positive family history frequently is elicited, suggesting a genetic component. Broughton [46] contrasted confusional arousals, characterized by body movement, autonomic activation, mental confusion and disorientation, and fragmentary recall of dreams with the nightmares of REM sleep, in which subjects became lucid almost immediately and usually recalled dreaming. Somnambulism is a related NREM arousal disorder in which patients may wander out of the bedroom or house during confusional episodes. Night terrors begin with an intense scream followed by vigorous motor activity. Children often are inconsolable and completely amnestic for the event. The subject appears to be awake but is unable to perceive the environment. If mental activity preceding the event is recalled, the images are simple (eg, face, animal, or fire) compared with the complex plots of REM nightmares. Patients often report an oppressive experience, such as being locked up in a tomb, or having rocks piled on their chests. Intense autonomic activation results in diaphoresis, mydriasis, tachycardia, hypertension, and tachypnea [47]. In contrast to seizures, NREM arousal disorders are less stereotyped and commonly occur in the first third of the night.

Rapid eye movement sleep behavior disorder

Patients who have this disorder often present with vigorous motor activity during sleep [48]. Patients may injure themselves or their bed partners. In RBD, the physiologic muscle atonia present during REM sleep is absent; persistence of muscle tone enables patients to act out their dreams. Episodes of RBD are less stereotyped, longer in duration, and more likely to begin after age 50 compared with epileptic seizures. Apart from seizures, the other major consideration in patients presenting with vigorous motor activity is obstructive sleep apnea with resulting arousals from sleep. Diagnosis is confirmed by video-EEG polysomnography (VPSG), demonstrating either a behavioral episode consistent with RBD or the persistence of muscle tone during REM sleep.

Sleep-related movement disorders

Movement disorders occurring during sleep that may resemble seizures include periodic limb movements, sleep-onset myoclonus, bruxism, and rhythmic movement disorder. Periodic limb movements in sleep (PLMS) may result in vigorous kicking or thrashing. A history of restless legs syndrome commonly is elicited [49]. In contrast to seizures, PLMS occur at periodic intervals (usually every 20 to 40 seconds) and involve a characteristic flexion of the leg, although the upper extremities occasionally may be involved. Sleep-onset myoclonus, also known as sleep starts, sleep jerks, or hypnic jerks, is a normal physiologic event occurring at the transition from wakefulness to sleep, often associated with sensory phenomena, including a sensation of falling. In contrast to myoclonic seizures, sleep-onset myoclonus is limited to sleep onset. Bruxism, manifested as stereotyped teeth grinding resembling rhythmic jaw movements of epilepsy, may lead to excessive tooth wear, which does not occur in epilepsy [50]. Rhythmic movement disorder, also known as head banging or body rocking, can occur during any sleep stage [51]. It is manifested in a variety of ways, including recurrent banging of the head while the patient is prone or rocking of the body back and forth while on hands and knees. Vocalizations may accompany the repetitive movements. Rhythmic movement disorder can occur at any age, although it is more common in children than adults and is associated with mental retardation. Although complex partial seizures, particularly those of frontal lobe origin, may include similar behaviors, bilateral body rocking is more characteristic of rhythmic movement disorder. Body rocking also may occur in psychogenic seizures.

Psychiatric disorders

Psychiatric disorders occurring during sleep that resemble seizures include panic attacks during sleep, post-traumatic stress disorder, and psychogenic seizures. Some patients who have panic disorder present exclusively or predominantly with panic episodes that cause multiple abrupt awakenings from sleep. Symptoms on awakening include apprehension and autonomic arousal, with palpitations, dizziness, and trembling [52]. In contrast to nightmare of REM sleep, dreams are not recalled. In contrast to night terrors, which arise out of deep NREM sleep, sleep panic usually occurs in the transition from NREM stages 2 to 3 [53]. Although a history of daytime panic attacks can be useful diagnostically, panic attacks may occur exclusively during sleep. An abrupt return to consciousness and autonomic arousal is more characteristic of panic disorder than seizures, although these features may occur in seizures. Simple partial seizures of parietal lobe origin may manifest occasionally as panic symptoms [54].

Post-traumatic stress disorder occurs after major psychologic trauma, such as combat situations and physical abuse. Repetitive rocking or head banging may occur, and the characteristic nightmares or flashbacks may arise from any stage of sleep [55]. In contrast to seizures, patients often experience the recall of true traumatic experiences.

Psychogenic seizures may occur during apparent sleep [56]. The diagnosis of these nonepileptic events is supported by the presence of a well-organized posterior alpha rhythm immediately before the onset of clinical changes despite the appearance of sleep and the lack of ictal or postictal EEG changes. Provocative testing with suggestion may be helpful in confirming the diagnosis of psychogenic seizures.

Video-electroencephalogram polysomnography

VPSG combines video-EEG monitoring with standard polysomnographic recordings and can be helpful in distinguishing epilepsy from other sleep disorders (Fig. 5) [57]. The video component is essential in characterizing spells; a stereotyped behavioral pattern, such as consistent head turning to one side, or a consistent automatism is highly suggestive of epilepsy. The stage of sleep from which the spells emerge can be useful in supporting the diagnosis of confusional arousals or RBD. Seizures, however, may emerge from any stage of sleep and may coexist with sleep disorders. The extensive EEG coverage provided by VPSG may detect interictal epileptiform activity or seizures; nonetheless, EEG studies may be completely normal in epilepsy. Finally, the coexisting standard PSG monitoring may detect coexisting sleep disorders, such as obstructive sleep apnea, which may exacerbate an underlying seizure disorder (discussed later) or mimic RBD.

An important limitation of VPSG is that the patient's habitual events, even if nightly, may not occur in the sleep laboratory; a similar phenomenon is observed in epilepsy monitoring units and may be related to the

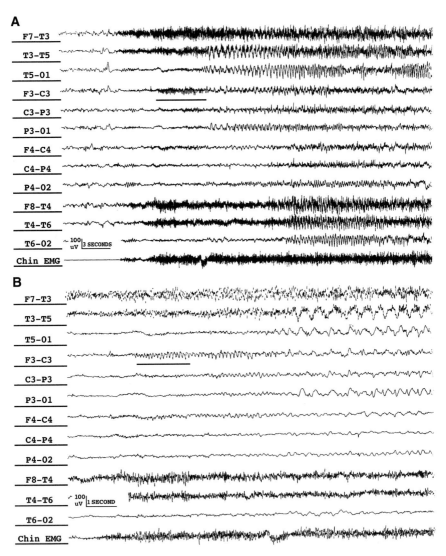

Fig. 5. EEG polysomnogram showing the onset of a partial seizure recroded at 10 mm/s paper speed. Clinically, the seizure began with an abrupt arousal, followed by turning of head and eyes to the left and movements of the arms beneath the bedclothes. On EEG, there is an initial electrodecremental event followed by a progressive increase in the amplitude of the ictal discharge over the left hemisphere and a spread to the right hemisphere derivations. The underlined activity (*A*) from the F3–C3 derivation seems to be muscle artifact; however, in (*B*), at 30 mm/s paper speed, the same underlined segment is the initial focal surface representation of the ictal discharge. Additional polysomnographic measurements recorded on channels 14 to 21 are not shown. (*From* Aldrich MS, Jahnke BA. Diagnostic value of video-EEG polysomnography. Neurology 1991;41:1060–6; with permission.)

unfamiliar surrounding or a change in the usual routine. Sleep deprivation may be useful in provoking events consistent with NREM arousal disorders. In patients who have suspected RBD, it is not necessary to capture a behavioral event; the persistence of chin EMG with increased phasic activity during REM sleep in the setting of compelling history is sufficient. In patients who have suspected epileptic seizures, subclinical ictal and interictal seizures in the absence of behavioral events support the diagnosis of epilepsy but are not diagnostic.

Sleep disorders and epilepsy

Sleep disorders are common, treatable conditions that frequently coexist with epilepsy. Epilepsy and its treatment, including antiepileptic drugs, may affect sleep organization and contribute to daytime sleepiness, insomnia, or sleep disorders, such as obstructive sleep apnea. Conversely, treatment of a coexisting sleep disorder may improve seizure control, daytime alertness, or both. Sleep disorders are covered in detail in articles elsewhere in this issue; the focus of this discussion is on the overlap of sleep disorders with epilepsy.

Antiepileptic medications may influence sleep. The barbiturates and benzodiazepines, which are sedating and suppress REM sleep [58], should be avoided if possible. In two independent studies of lamotrigine in patients who have epilepsy, this medication enhanced REM sleep [59] or did not suppress REM sleep [60]. Therefore, lamotrigine may be a useful antiepileptic drug in patients who have suppressed REM sleep at baseline. Gabapentin increases slow wave sleep in healthy adults [61] and may be useful in patients who have epilepsy and suppressed slow wave sleep at baseline. A provocative question is whether or not part of the beneficial effect of antiepileptic drugs on seizure control is related to consolidation of sleep.

Vagus nerve stimulation, a novel treatment option for refractory partial seizures, improved daytime sleepiness in 16 patients who had epilepsy [62]. This improvement may result from vagal afferents projecting to brainstem regions that promote alertness, such as the parabrachial nucleus. Alternatively, vagus nerve stimulation produces decreases in respiratory airflow and effort during sleep, and may exacerbate obstructive sleep apnea [63,64]. The etiology of these sleep-related respiratory effects might be either peripheral (vagal efferents to upper airway musculature) or central (vagal input to brainstem nuclei that regulates breathing).

Symptoms of drowsiness in a patient on antiepileptic drugs that do not seem dose-dependent or related to frequent seizures may be the result of a sleep disorder. In a study of predictors of sleepiness in patients who have epilepsy, symptoms of obstructive sleep apnea or restless legs syndrome were more significant predictors of elevated scores on the Epworth Sleepiness Scale than the number or type of antiepileptic medication, seizure frequency, epilepsy syndrome, or the presence of sleep-related seizures [65]. In a separate study, patients who had refractory epilepsy had a high prevalence of obstructive sleep apnea, one third with an apnea-hypopnea index of 5 or more episodes an hour on polysomnography. Increased age, male gender, and seizures during sleep were associated with obstructive sleep apnea [66]. Of note, treatment of obstructive sleep apnea in case series [67–69] and open-label trials [70] has led to improvements in seizure frequency and daytime sleepiness. The mechanism underlying the improvement in seizure frequency is not clear and may be related to amelioration of sleep deprivation or consolidation of sleep with reductions in sleep stage shifts, which tend to facilitate seizures [18].

Management considerations in patients who have sleep-related seizures

The treatment of nonepileptic sleep disorders mimicking epilepsy is described in this article and in detail elsewhere in this issue. The reader is referred to a standard textbook on epilepsy for treatment of epileptic seizures, including medications, epilepsy surgery, and other modalities [71]. In patients who have sleep-related seizures, it often is helpful for the largest dose to be taken before bedtime to maximize seizure control. Avoidance of sleep deprivation is recommended. Somnolence is a common adverse effect of antiepileptic medications; small initial doses of medication with gradual increases as needed minimize but do not eliminate somnolence.

In patients who have rare seizures limited to sleep, the decision to initiate medication therapy should be individualized. Some patients prefer to have an occasional seizure and avoid the side effects of daily antiepileptic medication. Patients who have seizures during sleep should be counseled about state driving restrictions; some licensing authorities may permit those who have seizures occurring only during sleep to drive, although requirements vary greatly among states [72].

The prognosis of seizures is influenced by the epilepsy syndrome and the underlying cause. For example, benign epilepsy of childhood with centrotemporal spikes has an excellent prognosis, and antiepileptic drugs can be discontinued in most cases by late adolescence. Patients who have complex partial seizures of temporal or frontal lobe origin have an intermediate and variable prognosis. Lennox-Gastaut syndrome is poorly responsive to medications in most cases.

Summary

This article examines the relationship between sleep and epilepsy, an association that has been recognized since antiquity. The mechanisms whereby sleep facilitates seizures are under investigation, although the synchronizing role of thalamocortic networks seems contributory. Recognition of the variety of generalized and partial epileptic syndromes associated with sleep, familiarity with the differential diagnosis of nocturnal spells, and awareness of the role that antiepileptic drugs and sleep disorders may play in epilepsy are helpful in evaluating patients presenting with behavioral and motor disturbances of sleep.

References

[1] Gowers WR. Epilepsy and other chronic convulsive diseases, vol. 1. London: Williams Wood; 1885.

[2] Langdon-Down M, Brain WR. Time of day in relation to convulsions in epilepsy. Lancet 1929;2:1029.

[3] Goldensohn ES. Historical perspectives and future directions. In: Wyllie E, editor. The treatment of epilepsy: principles and practice. Philadelphia: Lea & Febiger; 1993. p. 173.

[4] Gibbs E, Gibbs FA. Diagnostic and localizing value of electroencephalographic studies in sleep. Res Publ Assoc Res Nerv Ment Dis 1947;26:366.

[5] Janz D. The grand mal epilepsies and the sleeping-waking cycle. Epilepsia 1962;3:69.

[6] Niedermeyer E. Generalized seizure discharges and possible precipitating mechanisms. Epilepsia 1966;7:23.

[7] Lothman EW, Bertram EH III, Stringer JL. Functional anatomy of hippocampal seizures. Prog Neurobiol 1991;32:1.

[8] Gloor P, Fariello RG. Generalized epilepsy: some of its cellular mechanisms differ from those of focal epilepsy. Trends Neurosci 1988;11:63.

[9] Timofeev I, Bazhenov M, Sejnowski T, et al. Cortical hyperpolarization-activated depolarizing current takes part in the generation of focal paroxysmal activities. Proc Natl Acad Sci USA 2002;99:9533.

[10] Steriade M, McCormick DA, Sejnowski TJ. Thalamocortical oscillations in the sleeping and aroused brain. Science 1993;262:679.

[11] Steriade M, Contreras D, Amzica F. Synchronized sleep oscillations and their paroxysmal developments. Trends Neurosci 1994;17:199.

[12] Saper CB, Chou T, Scammell TE. The sleep switch: hypothalamic control of sleep and wakefulness. Trends Neurosci 2001;24:726.

[13] Janz D, Wolf P. Epilepsy with grand mal on awakening. In: Engel J Jr, Pedley T, editors. Epilepsy: a comprehensive textbook. Philadephia: Lippincott Raven; 1998. p. 2347.

[14] Young GB, Blume WT, Wells GA, et al. Differential aspects of sleep epilepsy. Can J Neurol Sci 1985;12:317.

[15] Commission on Classification and Terminology of the International League Against Epilepsy. Proposal for revised classification of epilepsies and epileptic syndromes. Epilepsia 1989;30:389.

[16] Crespel A, Baldy-Moulinier M, et al. The relationship between sleep and epilepsy in frontal and temporal lobe epilepsies: practical and physiopathologic considerations. Epilepsia 1998; 39:150.

[17] Herman ST, Walczak TS, Bazil CW. Distribution of partial seizures during the sleep wake cycle. Differences by seizure onset site. Neurology 2001;56:1453.

[18] Minecan DA, Natarajan A, Marzec M. Relationship of epileptic seizures to sleep stage and sleep depth. Sleep 2002;25:899.

[19] Williamson PD, Engel J Jr. Complex partial seizures. In: Engel J Jr, Pedley TA, editors. Epilepsy: a comprehensive textbook. Philadelphia: Lippincott-Raven Publishers; 1997. p. 557.

[20] Bernasconi A, Andermann F, et al. Nocturnal temporal lobe epilepsy. Neurology 1998;50: 1772.

[21] Sammaritano M, Gigli GL, Gotman J. Interictal spiking during wakefulness and sleep and localization of foci in temporal lobe epilepsy. Neurology 1991;41:290.

[22] Lieb J, Joseph JP, Engel J Jr, et al. Sleep state and seizure foci related to depth spike activity in patients with temporal lobe epilepsy. Electroencephalogr Clin Neurophysiol 1980;49:538.

[23] Rossi GF, Colicchio G, Pola P. Interictal epileptic activity during sleep: a stereo-EEG study in patients with partial epilepsy. Electroencephalogr Clin Neurophysiol 1984;58(2):97–106.

[24] Malow BA, Selwa LM, Ross D, et al. Lateralizing value of interictal spikes on overnight sleep-EEG studies in temporal lobe epilepsy. Epilepsia 1999;40:1587.

[25] Scheffer IE, Bhatia KP, Lopes-Cendes I. Autosomal dominant frontal epilepsy misdiagnosed as sleep disorder. Lancet 1994;343:515.

[26] di Corcia G, Blasetti A, De Simone M, et al. Recent advances in autosomal dominant nocturnal frontal lobe epilepsy: 'understanding the nicotinic acetylcholine receptor (nAChR)'. Eur J Paediatr Neurol 2005;9:59.

[27] Oldani A, Zucooni M, Asselta R, et al. Autosomal dominant nocturnal frontal lobe epilepsy. A video-polysomnographic and genetic appraisal of 40 patients and delineation of the epileptic syndrome. Brain 1998;121:205.

[28] Kellinghaus C, Lüders HO. Frontal lobe epilepsy. Epileptic Disord 2004;6:223.

[29] Kanner AM, Morris HH, Lüders H, et al. Supplementary motor seizures mimicking pseudoseizures: some clinical differences. Neurology 1990;40:1404.

[30] Goldstick L, Lesser RP, Lüders H, et al. The need for anticonvulsant drug withdrawal in the diagnosis of supplementary motor seizures. Epilepsia 1985;26:231.

[31] Pedley TA, Guilleminault C. Episodic nocturnal wanderings responsive to anticonvulsant drug therapy. Ann Neurol 1977;2:30.

[32] Montagna P, Sforza E, Tinuper P, et al. Paroxysmal arousals during sleep. Neurology 1990; 40:1063.

[33] Louseau P, Duche B. Benign childhood epilepsy with centrotemporal spikes. Clev Clin J Med 1989;56:17.

[34] Wirrel E. Benign epilepsy of childhood with centrotemporal spikes. Epilepsia 1998;39:S32.

[35] Grunewald R, Panayiotopoulos C. Juvenile myoclonic epilepsy: a review. Arch Neurol 1993; 50:594.

[36] Gomez MR, Westmoreland BF. Absence seizures. In: Lüders H, Lesser RP, editors. Epilepsy: electroclinical syndromes. New York: Springer-Verlag; 1987. p. 105.

[37] Theodore WH, Porter RJ, Penry JK. Complex partial seizures: clinical characteristics and differential diagnosis. Neurology 1983;33:1115.

[38] Sato S, Dreifuss F, Penry JK. The effect of sleep on spike-wave discharges in absence seizures. Neurology 1973;2:1335.

[39] Markand ON. Lennox-Gastaut syndrome (childhood epileptic encephalopathy). J Clin Neurophysiol 2003;20:426.

[40] Patry G, Lyagoub S, Tassinari CA. Subclinical electrical status epilepticus induced sleep in children. Arch Neurol 1971;24:242.

[41] Tassinari CA, Rubboli G, Volpi L. Encephalopathy with electrical status epilepticus during slow sleep or ESES syndrome including the aquired aphasia. Clin Neurophysiol 2000; 111(Suppl 2):S94.

[42] Lugaresi E, Cirignotta F, Montagna P. Nocturnal paroxysmal dystonia. Epilepsy Res Suppl 1991;2:137–40.

[43] Tinuper P, Cerullo A, Cirignotta F, et al. Nocturnal paroxysmal dystonia with short lasting attacks: three cases with evidence for an epileptic frontal lobe origin of seizures. Epilepsia 1990;31:549.

[44] Peled R, Lavie P. Paroxysmal awakenings from sleep associated with excessive daytime somnolence: a form of nocturnal epilepsy. Neurology 1986;36:95.

[45] Malow BA, Bowes R, Ross D. Relationship of temporal lobe seizures to sleep and arousal—a combined scalp-intracranial electrode study. Sleep 2000;23:231.

[46] Broughton RJ. Sleep disorders: disorders of arousal? Science 1968;159:1070.

[47] Mahowald MW, Ettinger MG. Things that go bump in the night: the parasomnias revisited. J Clin Neurophysiol 1990;7(1):119–43.

[48] Mahowald M, Schenck C. REM sleep parasomnias. In: Kryger M, Roth T, Dement W, editors. Principles and practice of sleep medicine. 4th edition. Philadelphia: Elsevier-Saunders; 2005. p. 897.

[49] Walters AS, Hening WA, Chokroverty S. Review and videotape recognition of idiopathic restless legs syndrome. Mov Disord 1991;6:105.

[50] Lavigne GJ, Manzini C, et al. Sleep bruxism. Principles and practice of sleep medicine. In: Kryger M, Roth T, Dement W, editors. Principles and practice of sleep medicine. 4th edition. Philadelphia: Elsevier-Saunders; 2005. p. 946.

[51] Hoban TF. Rhythmic movement disorder in children. CNS Spectr 2003;8:135.

[52] Mellman TA, Uhde TW. Patients with frequent sleep panic: clinical findings and response to medication treatment. J Clin Psychiatry 1990;51:513.

[53] Mellman TA, Uhde TW. Electroencephalographic sleep in panic disorder. Arch Gen Psychiatry 1989;46:178.

[54] Alemayehu S, Bergey GK, Barry E, et al. Panic attacks in ictal manifestations of parietal lobe seizures. Epilepsia 1995;36:824–30.

[55] Hefez A, Metz L, Lavie P. Long-term effects of extreme situational stress on sleep and dreaming. Am J Psychiatry 1987;144:344.

[56] Thacker K, Devinsky O, Perrine K, et al. Nonepileptic seizures during apparent sleep. Ann Neurol 1993;33:414.

[57] Aldrich MS, Jahnke B. Diagnostic value of video-EEG polysomnography. Neurology 1991; 41:1060.

[58] Placedi F, Marciani MG, Diomedi M, et al. Effects of lamotrigine on nocturnal sleep, daytime somnolence and cognitive functions in focal epilepsy. Acta Neurol Scand 2000;102:81.

[59] Placedi F, Scalise A, Marciani MG, et al. Effect of antiepileptic drugs on sleep. Clin Neurophys 2000;111(Suppl 2):S115.

[60] Foldvary N, Perry M, Lee J, et al. The effects of lamotrigine on sleep in patients with epilepsy. Epilepsia 2001;42:1569.

[61] Foldvary-Schaefer N, Sanchez ID, Karafa M, et al. Gabapentin increases slow-wave sleep in normal adults. Epilepsia 2002;43:1493.

[62] Malow BA, Edwards J, Marzec M, et al. Vagus nerve stimulation reduces daytime sleepiness in epilepsy patients. Neurology 2001;57:879.

[63] Malow BA, Edwards J, Marzec M, et al. Effects of vagus nerve stimulation on respiration during sleep: a pilot study. Neurology 2000;55:1450.

[64] Marzec M, Edwards J, Sagher O, et al. Effects of vagus nerve stimulation on sleep-related breathing in epilepsy patients. Epilepsia 2003;44:930.

[65] Malow BA, Bowes R, Lin X. Predictors of sleepiness in epilepsy patients. Sleep 1997;20:1105.

[66] Malow BA, Levy K, Maturen K, et al. Obstructive sleep apnea is common in medically refractory epilepsy patients. Neurology 2000;55:1002.

[67] Devinsky O, Ehrenberg B, Barthlen GM, et al. Epilepsy and sleep apnea syndrome. Neurology 1994;44:2060.

[68] Vaughn BV, Messenheimer JA, D'Cruz OF. Sleep apnea in patients with epilepsy. Epilepsia 1993;34:136.

[69] Malow BA, Fromes GA, Aldrich MS. Usefulness of polysomnography in epilepsy patients. Neurology 1997;48(5):1389–94.

[70] Malow BA, Weatherwax KJ, Chervin RD, et al. Identification and treatment of obstructive sleep apnea in adults and children with epilepsy: a prospective pilot study. Sleep Med 2003;4: 509.

[71] Engel J Jr, Pedley T, editors. Epilepsy: a comprehensive textbook. Philadephia: Lippincott Raven; 1998. p. 2347.

[72] Yale SH, Hansotia P, Knapp D, et al. Neurologic conditions: assessing medical fitness to drive. Clin Med Res 2003;1:177.

ELSEVIER
SAUNDERS

NEUROLOGIC
CLINICS

Neurol Clin 23 (2005) 1149–1163

Pharmacologic and Nonpharmacologic Treatments of Insomnia

Philip M. Becker, MD[a,b,c,*]

[a]Sleep Medicine Associates of Texas, Dallas, TX, USA
[b]Sleep Medicine Institute, Presbyterian Hospital of Dallas, Dallas, TX, USA
[c]Department of Psychiatry, UT Southwestern Medical Center at Dallas, Dallas, TX, USA

Insomnia is a symptom that arises from many environmental, medical, and psychologic and mental disorders [1]. Insomnia can be transient, short-term, or chronic in its presentation. When patients have difficulty falling asleep, staying asleep, or waking early, they begin to dread the night and the resultant daytime fatigue, mental clouding, and irritability. In a typical physician's practice, nearly 50% of adult patients experience a problem with falling or staying asleep during any year [2]. Research on sleep problems in the general population documents that between 10% and 18% of adults consider sleep to be a serious, chronic problem, with women and the elderly reporting more frequent problems [3]. The focus of this article is the practical management of chronic insomnia that is defined as poor sleep during 3 nights or more per week that has been present for at least 1 month (often much longer).

Definitions of insomnia

The diagnosis of insomnia requires that patients have a sleep disturbance that reduces daytime function. The disturbed sleep can present as delayed sleep onset, unwanted wakefulness later in the night, or nonrestorative sleep. A small percentage of adults are short sleepers who are capable of functioning normally without evidence of medical or psychiatric disturbance on 5 or fewer hours of nightly sleep [4].

Physicians should not be concerned with the specific number of minutes that persons report themselves to be awake. It is difficult for insomnia

---

* Sleep Medicine Institute, Presbyterian Hospital of Dallas, 8140 Walnut Hill Lane, Suite 100, Dallas, TX 75231.

   E-mail address: pbecker@sleepmed.com

0733-8619/05/$ - see front matter © 2005 Elsevier Inc. All rights reserved.
doi:10.1016/j.ncl.2005.05.002

sufferers to determine when they are asleep; therefore, physicians should focus on the impact of poor sleep on daytime functioning. For some, the minutes of lost sleep may be small, but the daytime impairments of fatigue, tiredness, mental slowing, reduced concentration, memory lapses, irritability, disinterest, decreased motivation, and reduced performance may be significant.

Insomnia often is characterized by the number of days it has been present. Transient insomnia lasts for 1 to 6 nights and most commonly is the result of a time zone change (jet lag) or stress from work, home, or other relationships. After the schedule or stress normalizes, sleep also returns to normal. Short-term insomnia involves 1 to 3 weeks of poor sleep. Life changes, such as job loss, separation, divorce, or health concerns, are the most common reasons for short-term insomnia. Sometimes substances, such as caffeine, decongestant or sinus medicines, or prescribed medications, can cause a significant disturbance in sleep. Chronic insomnia lasts for weeks, months, or years and proves distressing and sometimes disabling to sufferers. The causes of chronic insomnia arise from a variety of medical, psychiatric, and lifestyle problems. Chronic insomnia often waxes and wanes in its severity.

Factors causing chronic insomnia

The etiology of chronic insomnia most commonly is multifactorial. Table 1 shows the common causes of different types of chronic insomnia

Table 1
Causes of chronic insomnia based on time of presentation

Insomnia type	Causes
Sleep onset	Learned or conditioned activation (psychophysiologic)
	Anxiety, including situational, panic disorder, generalized anxiety disorder, and obsessive compulsive disorder
	Depressive disorders, including major depression, bipolar disorder I or II, and dysthymia
	Delayed sleep phase syndrome
	Restless legs syndrome
	Upper airway resistance (and less commonly OSAHS)
	Substances, such as caffeine, decongestants, and so forth
Sleep maintenance	Excessive time in bed
	Major depression, dysthymia, or bipolar disorder in association with anxiety
	Sleep disordered breathing, OSAHS, UARS
	Medical illness, particularly if associated with pain
	Periodic limb movements in sleep
Early awakening	Major depression
	Advance sleep phase syndrome
	Learned or conditioned activation (psychophysiologic)

Abbreviations: OSAHS, obstructive sleep apnea hypopnoea syndrome; UARS, upper airway resistance syndrome.

according to the time of presentation during the night. Often the specific factors that initiate insomnia no longer are operational. Spielman and colleagues propose organizing the multitude of factors into the behavioral medicine model of the "3 Ps"—predisposing, precipitating, and perpetuating [5]. Genetic, familial, and environmental factors predispose some individuals to poor sleep. Although not yet fully described, genetic factors determine the need for sleep and the length of the circadian rhythm, or "biologic clock." With good parenting, children learn how to settle themselves and manage the anxieties and stresses of life through good sleep habits, such as a regular bedtime. A chaotic environment predisposes a child to later sleep disturbance. A precipitating factor typically is a major loss or threat, resulting in heightened anxiety, mental activation, and inability to sleep. In predisposed individuals, precipitants grow into poor sleep habits and maladaptive behavior and then perpetuate a pattern of worsening sleep. To patients who have chronic insomnia, it is as if the mind and body conspire to activate individuals and push them further from sleep.

Strategies to improve sleep

To improve insomnia requires an understanding of what has changed in patients' lives. If patients have had poor sleep for a short time, the physician will find it easier to understand etiology and to recommend changes. If insomnia endures for months or years, the original reasons for poor sleep become less important. Behavior and lifestyle are more important. It is a physician's role to assess the causes for insomnia and to rank for patients those strategies that offer the highest likelihood of improved sleep and daytime function.

Better sleep should begin with a goal. It is important for patients to set a realistic goal rather than, for example, "8 hours of uninterrupted sleep." Physicians who evaluate insomnia complaints must gain some perspective through appropriate questioning, for example, "How did the patient sleep in the month or two before beginning to have trouble with sleep?" If it has been more than a year since patients have slept well consistently, physicians may have to set a goal for the patients, recognizing any changes in their sleep needs. Patients may find that 6 or 7 hours of better sleep are enough to feel good and function well during the day.

Box 1 offers some question that physicians might ask, with supplemental comments as to each question's relevance.

Treatment of insomnia focuses on three strategies—lifestyle changes, behavioral changes, and biologic treatments. Lifestyle changes involve good sleep habits. Box 2, written in language for patients, provides 10 steps, with explanations that can offer improvements to better sleep. Behavioral changes include stress management techniques, relaxation methods, interrupting sleep disruptive behaviors, management of negative thoughts, and working through negative emotional reactions. The biologic treatments

Box 1. Questions to explore with patients who report insomnia

1. "Have you experienced any medical problems in the month or 2 before your sleep changed?".

Comment: If medical illness or medical treatment is causing patients to sleep poorly, particularly in situations with pain, lost function, or neurocognitive dysfunction, physicians have to determine whether or not to alter treatment and whether or not to offer medication to assist sleep. Patients also should follow the *10 Steps to Better Sleep* (Box 2)

2. "What were or continue to be the stresses and other lifestyle changes that coincide with the problems of sleep?"

Comment: Disturbance of relationships is a common reason for developing sleep problems. Conflicts with family members or close friends, work supervisors, and other significant people in patients' lives increase activation. Some people are more sensitive to such problems. The poor sleeper must protect the 1 to 2 hours of time before bed. Wind down and relax, exercise midday, reduce or eliminate caffeine (or other xanthines), and avoid evening alcohol.

3. "Do you feel more sad, discouraged, irritable, or withdrawn? Have you felt a loss of interest and pleasure in work, home, normal activities, hobbies, and so forth? Have you become more anxious, worried, preoccupied, and generally tense?"

Comments: Disorders of significant depression and anxiety can be important reasons for chronic insomnia. Often insomnia is one of the earliest symptoms of depression. Poor sleep also can make people feel more discouraged and poorly focused. Patients who report loss of pleasure, easy tearfulness, guilt, hopelessness, easy anger and irritability, or thoughts of death require treatment for depression. Antidepressant medication with sedative properties, such as nefazodone, paroxetine, mirtrazapine, trazodone, amitriptyline, or doxepin, are helpful for sleep and mood. For those who have anxious thoughts that race through the mind, often the fears, worries, and concerns take over. Everything seems destined for disaster. Patients who have insomnia and who report tension, tightness, sweat, urinary frequency, shortness of breath, tachycardia, fatigue, poor focus, and tiredness should be treated for an anxiety disorder. Such patients often benefit from medication or referral to a mental health specialist. Selecting medications for depression or anxiety requires consideration of side effects and concurrent medications. Tables 2 and 3 list pharmacologic properties of various agents for anxiety and sleep.

4. "Does your body want to sleep when other people seem to be awake?" *Advanced sleep phase syndrome (ASPS)*. People who have advanced sleep phase experience sleepiness in the evening between 6:00 and 10:00 PM and then wake up at 3:00 or 4:00 AM. People who have ASPS often force themselves to stay awake at night but discover that they wake up at nearly the same early hour no matter when they go to bed. The elderly are affected more commonly with ASPS. Maximizing bright light from 6:00 to 9:00 PM can be helpful. The use of an artificial light box at 10,000 lux (phototherapy) for at least 30 to 60 minutes approximately 2 hours before desired bedtime may prove helpful.

Delayed sleep phase syndrome (DSPS). People who have DSPS prefer to go to sleep at 1:00 to 4:00 AM and arise between 10:00 AM and noon. Phototherapy of at least 10,000 lux (from a light box or the sun) for 30 to 60 minutes at the desired time of arising can be helpful. For 7 to 14 days, the circadian pattern resets to the new arising time. Patients who have DSPS also are wise to reduce exposure to light at night. Some advocate the use of the pineal hormone, melatonin (1 to 6 mg taken 1 hour before the desired bedtime), as a treatment of DSPS. Others are reluctant to recommend it. Melatonin is marketed as a health food supplement. Even if a person buys a synthesized form of melatonin, the controls on manufacture are not the same as for prescription medicines.

5. "Does your bed partner observe snoring, choking, or breathing pauses during sleep? Do your legs bother you when going to bed or are your legs creepy, crawly, jumpy, or restless when you lie down or are still around bedtime?"

Comments: People who snore are at risk of having obstructive sleep apnea (OSA) or upper airway resistance. A person who has sleep apnea or one of its variants may experience disturbed sleep. Although OSA is a less common reason to cause insomnia, it represents a potentially serious medical problem that deserves evaluation and treatment. Upper airway resistance may result in more problems of insomnia.

People who have creepy, crawly, jumpy legs may have problems of restless legs syndrome (RLS). RLS presents between 4:00 PM and 4:00 AM. Patients have to stretch, move, or walk to provide relief. RLS often is associated with periodic limb movements in sleep. This involuntary movement occurs in a regular pattern every 20 to 40 seconds and may cause disturbed sleep.

If patients fall asleep when still during the day, there is a higher likelihood of OSA, RLS, or periodic limb movement disorder in sleep. Other articles in this issue provide information about treatment of these medical disorders of sleep.

6. Is the etiology of insomnia still uncertain? None of these questions or answers seem to apply to patients. If the reasons for poor sleep continue to perplex physicians and patients, consider referral to a sleep specialist. Not all sleep specialists are expert on insomnia but they are able to give some direction.

include the use of medications, bright light therapy, and alternative therapies.

Managing chronic insomnia

Begin with concerns and worries

Often patients feel trapped by the vicious cycle of unwanted wakefulness that leaves mind and body fatigued, tired, and slowed. There is frustration and loneliness that comes with being awake at night. Worry and concern about anything connected with sleep begins to preoccupy the mind. Depression may increase and the ability to function in normal daily activities seems to be less.

People who have chronic insomnia want to know why they can not sleep. A better question is, What is keeping them awake? Many people who have insomnia can identify a life event or change that occurred at approximately the time they began to sleep poorly. After 2 or 3 months, the event or change becomes less relevant to why unwanted wakefulness continues to occupy the nighttime. Insomnia sufferers need to explore other possible causes that might be arising from medical illness or its treatment, psychiatric disorders, or abnormal behavioral patterns. If someone has slept poorly for years, it is common for many disorders to have been layered on top of the original reason for poor sleep.

If mental activation (eg, "my mind won't shut off") is a regular problem, patients need to set aside "thinking time" after supper. Hauri and Linde offer suggestions in their book, *No More Sleepless Nights* [6]. Patients should sit down with a pad of paper, draw a line down the page, and at the top of the left column, put the heading, "Thought, feeling, concern." At the top of the right column, they should write, "What I plan to do about it."

Box 2. Good sleep habits

There are 10 behavioral strategies and three mental strategies to improve the ability to sleep. Progress in sleeping can be enhanced by practicing these good sleep habits for at least 4 weeks in a row:

Ten behavioral strategies
1. **Maintain a regular sleep schedule.** It is helpful to maintain a regular bedtime and arise time on weekdays and weekends. Failure to do so, for example, by frequently staying up late, can reset the internal biologic clock to a later bedtime, leading to a biologic clock disorder called DSPS. Also, it is especially important to avoid sleeping in the morning after a night of poor sleep. Instead, arise at the same time every morning on weekdays and weekends, regardless of how poor the prior night's sleep has been. Although this can be difficult to initiate at first, it can, after a few weeks, help normalize the sleep-wake rhythm and increase sleep efficiency.
2. **Get enough daylight.** Lack of sufficient daily exposure to sunlight often is partially responsible for difficulty sleeping at night (daylight is a powerful regulator of the circadian cycle). It is beneficial to spend at least 30 minutes per day outside, in natural sunlight, preferably during the first hour or two in the morning. If unable to do so, try for a minimum of 30 minutes per day in strong artificial light.
3. **Avoid postlunch caffeine.** Most people know that that the intake of caffeine and similar stimulants in the evening can interfere with falling asleep and remaining asleep at night. Most doctors, therefore, advise avoiding caffeinated coffee, tea, and carbonated beverages beginning right after lunch and caffeine-like substances found in chocolate, cocoa, and some weight-control aids, pain relievers, diuretics, and cold and allergy remedies. Some individuals are highly sensitive to caffeine and should stop its use entirely.
4. **Avoid daytime napping.** With some exceptions (for example, in some cases of insomnia in the elderly), daytime napping solves only a short-term problem of fatigue, and it can contribute to the long-term development of insomnia at night by disrupting normal sleep-wake rhythms (discussed previously). In most cases, napping should be eliminated.
5. **Make the bedroom quiet and comfortable.** Insomniacs often overlook the fact that their bed and bedroom may not be as quiet or comfortable as they could be to promote restful sleep.

It is wise to assess for any disruptive lights, sounds, temperatures, or touch sensations and adopt whatever measures are necessary to reduce or eliminate these discomforts (for example, use eyeshades, earplugs, a low-volume background sound, or a new mattress or pillow). A bedroom temperature of 65 to 68°F is recommended for good sleep.

6. **Avoid alcohol within 3 hours of bedtime.** Aside from the risk of developing alcoholism, it is not productive to use alcohol as a sleeping aid, despite the popular notion that an evening nightcap promotes sleep. Research shows that although one to two drinks within 2 or 3 hours of bedtime may assist with falling asleep, they tend to disrupt subsequent sleep by increasing later wakefulness. Also, alcohol intake prior to bedtime tends to relax the muscles of the throat and to suppress awakening mechanisms, making snoring and sleep apnea episodes more likely.

7. **Avoid smoking nicotine products within 2 hours of bedtime.** Aside from the health risks associated with smoking, it is not productive to smoke up until bedtime. Like caffeine, nicotine is a central nervous system stimulant, and evening smoking tends to increase heart rate and blood pressure and stimulate brain activity in ways that are incompatible with sleep. Also, nicotine withdrawal symptoms during the night can contribute to wakefulness. People who stop smoking are likely to sleep better after 10 days of abstinence.

8. **Avoid large meals within 2 hours of bedtime.** Although a light snack before bed can be beneficial, consuming large meals in the late evening is not recommended. It can be sleep incompatible to assign the gastrointestinal tract the task of digesting a large meal at night, and it can increase the risk of heartburn during the night.

9. **Avoid exercise within 2 hours of bedtime.** As part of the circadian cycle, core body temperature begins to decrease in the late evening, and this assists with falling asleep and remaining asleep later. Engaging in vigorous exercise within 2 hours of bedtime can be counterproductive because it tends to raise core body temperature and activate the nervous system. In the interest of improving sleep, the best time to exercise is in the late afternoon.

10. **Wind down before bedtime.** Insomniacs commonly complain of physical tension and mental alertness when they should be sleeping. In the interest of physical relaxation and

mental calm, it is wise to wind down for 1 to 2 hours before bed by engaging in an enjoyable, relaxing activity. During this wind-down period, avoid working, studying, talking on the telephone, arguing, watching exciting television shows, reading exciting books, and so forth.

Three mental strategies

1. **Avoid worrying, clockwatching, trying.** Clinicians routinely prescribe only 2 activities for the bedroom: sleep and romance. Virtually all other activities belong outside the bedroom, by night and by day. It is not useful for to associate sleep-incompatible activities with the bedroom. This holds true particularly for insomniacs, who are prone to associating the bedroom with sleep-preventing activities, such as worrying, watching the clock, and trying to force the onset of sleep—all of which generally serve only to increase body tension and mental alertness. It is better to conceal clocks from view and simply wake up when they ring.

2. **Leave the bedroom when unable to sleep.** One method to stop associating the bedroom with non–sleep-inducing activities is to
   - Leave the bedroom, after approximately 10 minutes (20 minutes for people ages 60 and over) of sleeplessness, in order to worry or, for example, watch television or read in another room for as long as it takes to feel sleepy, and then
   - Return to the bedroom with positive expectations of sleeping.

This sequence should be repeated in a given night as many times as necessary to achieve sleep. Although this so-called "stimulus control" technique can be difficult to initiate, it can be helpful after at least 4 weeks of practice.

3. **Associate the bedroom with relaxing.** Good sleepers cultivate strong mental associations of physical relaxation, mental calm, and good sleep with their bedtime, bed, bedroom, and bedtime rituals (such as tooth brushing and setting the alarm clock). Insomniacs can learn to become better sleepers by establishing and strengthening these associations. Practicing muscle relaxation and deep breathing and focusing on relaxing mental imagery while in bed can help—particularly in conjunction with listening to relaxing, recorded guided imagery programs.

Unless the problem is an emergency, a plan of action should begin, at the earliest, in 24 hours. A plan for improvement might best begin next week, or next month, or next year. When patients arrive in bed and their mind creeps toward any of the thoughts, feelings, or concerns, patients must talk to themselves: "Hold it! I've taken care of that. I have considered the problem and decided on my plan of action. It's written down over there on that piece of paper. I have done what I can for now. I know what I'm going to do." Patients then should begin a distracting method of relaxation.

Specific treatments for chronic insomnia

Nonpharmacologic therapies
Stimulus control or "the 10-minute rule". Bootzin demonstrates that 70% of patients who have sleep-onset insomnia show improvement when they follow the practice of having only 10 minutes to fall asleep (20 minutes is allowed for the elderly) consistently [7]. If patients are not asleep in 10 minutes, they are to get up, go into another room, and come back to bed only when feeling sleepy. They should repeat the process as many times as needed to fall asleep quickly. After 5 to 15 days of ups and downs, patients experience rapid sleep onset. If insomnia returns, they should start again to get out of bed after 10 minutes of being awake.

Sleep restriction therapy. Spielman and colleagues demonstrate that almost any type of insomnia improves with sleep restriction therapy. It follows a simple principle. Restrict the time in bed to only the number of hours that are slept [8]. Many insomniacs stay in bed when awake in hopes of capturing any potential moment of sleep. But lying awake in bed only makes insomnia worse. Patients begin sleep restriction therapy by recording 7 nights in a sleep diary. They total up all the hours that are slept each night and then divide by the number of recorded nights. If patients average only 6 (or 6.5, 7, and so forth) hours of sleep during the hours that are spent in bed, then for the next week they should restrict the number of hours in bed to that number of hours actually slept according to the tally. If patients can sleep for 85% or more of the time in bed during the week, they should add another 15 minutes to the time in bed (eg, stay in bed for 6.25 hours during the next week). If wake time increases, causing sleep to occupy less than 85% of time in bed during the next week, they should decrease time in bed by 15 minutes. For the first week or two, patients may feel sleepy during the day but most people report that their nighttime sleep becomes deeper and more consistent.

Cognitive-behavioral therapy. Various researchers have written extensively about how beliefs, attitudes, and maladaptive behaviors worsen the sleep of chronic insomniacs [9–11]. Cognitive-behavioral therapy (CBT) helps people recognize that (1) they can function adequately on reduced sleep, (2) they sleep more than they realize, (3) they can manage the stresses of the day, and (4) they must become more responsibe for their thoughts during the day so that sleep improves. A study by Jacobs and coworkers of patients selected as typical of a primary care population demonstrates that CBT produces more durable improvements in sleep than the use of medications alone [12]. Research shows that insomnia sufferers of any age, including patients ages 75 and older, can improve sleep with CBT [10].

Relaxation therapy and imagery. Methods that help relax the mind and body can help sleep onset. The key to success is practice [13]. Most insomniacs want immediate relief. But relaxation takes practice. Relaxation requires the same type of daytime practice applied to learning to drive a car. Practice helps quiet the mind and body. Relaxation methods must be practiced twice a day for 10 afternoons or more before bringing the technique to the bedroom. It often is helpful to combine it with pleasant imagery. Imagery also is a talent that can be strengthened to improve sleep.

Pharmacologic therapies

Alternative and over-the-counter agents. Medicines for sleep include over-the-counter agents (OTCs) and prescribed medications. Common OTCs for sleep contain an antihistamine that causes drowsiness and dry mouth. Antihistamines should be avoided if patients take cardiovascular medicines, have cognitive impairment, or have urinary hesitancy or retention [14]. Alternative therapies that can be found in health food stores include melatonin, 5-hydroxytryptophan, St. John's Wort, valerian root, and others. OTCs and alternative therapies are studied inadequately, so effectiveness is uncertain, particularly for long-term use [4].

Antidepressants. Antidepressants can cause insomnia and anxiety in some patients who have depression. The percentages of adverse events that are derived from the *Physician's Desk Reference* are listed in Table 4 and show how often patients who are treated for depression demonstrate worsened sleep or anxiety during the first 2 months of treatment on the most commonly prescribed antidepressants.

Sedating antidepressants, particularly trazodone, have increased in use as treatments for chronic insomnia [15]. Although information is available about supplemental trazodone (25 to 150 mg by mouth at bedtime) in the management of insomnia secondary to depression, there is little data to determine the effectiveness of trazodone for chronic insomnia that is not related to depression. The dosages, such as 50 mg of trazodone or 10 mg, of a tricyclic antidepressant that are used are much lower than the dosages required to treat major depression. The tricyclic antidepressants, such as amitriptyline, doxepin, imipramine and others, have sedating properties that often improve sleep but also have significant anticholinergic side effects [16]. The newer antidepressants may have fewer side effects but often are available in dosages that do not allow easy adjustment of the sedative property of medicines (mirtrazapine is an example).

Sedative and hypnotic agents. Progress has been made during the past 50 years in the pharmacologic management of insomnia. Barbiturates and similar compounds offered improvements in sleep for only 10 to 14 days, yet carried risk for dependency and overdosage. The negative public image of sleeping pills began with the deaths of Marilyn Monroe and Elvis Presley, who had excessive levels of barbiturates at autopsy. The deaths of these stars may have been prevented if they had been prescribed the then-available benzodiazepine hypnotics, such as flurazepam.

Benzodiazepines represented an advance but also demonstrated problems of occasional dependence, particularly in addiction-prone individuals; withdrawal symptoms on abrupt discontinuation; wandering behavior; memory disturbance; and next-day residual side effects, including carryover sedation, reduced coordination, and psychomotor performance (falls, accidents, and work-related errors) [17].

Availability of more selective benzodiazepine receptor agonists, such as zolpidem, zaleplon, eszopiclone (and future agents, such as short and long-acting indiplon and zolpidem modified-release), are effective hypnotic agents with reduced side effects, less withdrawal reaction, and lessened risks for addiction [18]. For the first time, with the release of eszopiclone, the United States Food and Drug Administration (FDA) permitted labeling for long-term use of a hypnotic agent based on demonstrated effectiveness over 6 months of therapy in patients who had primary insomnia [19].

Benzodiazepines produce varying levels of therapeutic benefit for anxiety, convulsions, myalgia, and neuralgia based on pharmacologic targets. Although not labeled as hypnotics, any benzodiazepine may be used outside of FDA-approved designation as a sedative to assist insomnia. Table 2 lists the benzodiazepines that are labeled for anxiety, seizure disorder, or muscle relaxant rather than as a hypnotic. The primary concern in the use of these

Table 2
Pharmacologic properties of nonhypnotic benzodiazepines

Medication	Brand name	Daily dose	Speed of action	Length of action	Carry-over sedation	Daytime problems
Alprazolam	Xanax	0.25–3 mg	Rapid	10–14 hours	Mild-moderate	Moderate
Chlordiazepoxide	Librium	5–80 mg	Fairly rapid	30–50 hours	Significant	Moderate
Clonazepam	Klonopin	0.5–4 mg	Rapid	30–60 hours	Significant	Moderate
Clorazepate	Tranxene	7.5–37.5 mg	Fairly rapid	30–50 hours	Significant	Moderate
Diazepam	Valium	2–40 mg	Rapid	30–50 hours	Significant	Moderate
Lorazepam	Ativan	0.5–4 mg	Rapid	12–14 hours	Moderate	Moderate
Oxazepam	Serax	5–40 mg	Slow	6–8 hours	Mild	Mild

Table 3

Hypnotic agents that are active at the benzodiazepine receptor

Medication	Brand name	Daily dosage	Speed of action	Length of action	Carry-over sedation	Daytime problems
Nonspecific						
Estazolam	ProSom	1–2 mg	Rapid	12–20 hours	Mild-moderate	Mild to moderate
Flurazepam	Dalmane	15–30 mg	Fairly rapid	40–120 hours	Significant	Moderate
Quazepam	Doral	7.5–15 mg	Fairly rapid	30–80 hours	Significant	Moderate
Temazepam	Restoril	7.5–30 mg	Slower	10–14 hours	Mild-moderate	Mild to moderate
Triazolam	Halcion	0.125–.25 mg	Rapid	2–5 hours	Minimal to mild	Moderate
Benzodiazepine receptor-1 selectivity						
Eszopiclone	Lunesta	1, 2, 3 mg	Rapid	6–7 hours	Mild	Minimal
Zaleplon	Sonata	5–10 mg	Rapid	1–4 hours	Minimal	Minimal
Zolpidem	Ambien	5–10 mg	Rapid	2.5–6 hours	Minimal to mild	Minimal

agents for sleep is the longer half-life and the increased risks of daytime impairment, particularly falls or accidents in the elderly. Such agents carry risks for wandering at night, poor coordination, increased automobile accidents, daytime memory disturbance, and paradoxic reactions. Short-acting agents, such as zaleplon, show reduced risks for such adverse events [20].

Table 3 lists the FDA-labeled hypnotic agents that are active at one or more of the benzodiazepine receptor sites at the γ-aminobutryric acid–benzodiazepine–chloride complex. Newer agents are more selective for the benzodiazepine receptor-1 site that is believed to be important to the initiation of sleep. Sleep laboratory studies provide evidence of benefit for hypnotic agents for 2 to 6 weeks of nightly use [17]. Studies of eszopiclone demonstrate efficacy compared with placebo for 6 months of therapy [19]; recent behavioral research suggests that in selected populations,

Table 4

Treatment-emergent side effects of common antidepressants

Antidepressant	Insomnia	Anxiety	Somnolence
Trazodone	6%	6%	41%
Mirtrazapine	6%	—	54%
Fluoxetine	16%–33%	12%–14%	13%–17%
Sertraline	16%–28%	6%	13%–15%
Paroxetine	13%	5%	23%
Venlafaxine	18%	6%–13%	23%
Buproprion	11%–16%	5%–6%	2%–3%
Nefazodone	11%	—	25%

Data from Physician's Desk Reference. Montvale (NJ): Thomson PDR; 2004.

cognitive-behavioral interventions demonstrate superiority over chronic hypnotic use [12]. The debate about nightly use of hypnotic agents continues. Various strategies are proposed to reduce the nightly use of hypnotics, including alternating nightly use of zolpidem and placebo for 3 months [21]. A meta-analysis comparing the efficacy of behavioral versus pharmacologic interventions demonstrates a similar degree of benefit in various therapeutic interventions [2]. Discontinuation of medication for chronic insomnia is difficult. In a study that intervened in the long-term use of benzodiazepines for the treatment of chronic insomnia, efforts to discontinue medication resulted in a high return rate to the hypnotic over the 2 years of follow-up, with better success seen in patients who underwent gradual taper of the hypnotic over months rather than days or a few weeks [22].

Summary

Insomnia in its chronic form is present in high numbers of patients presenting to physicians. As older women who have medical problems have the highest rates of chronic insomnia, physicians must have a high index of suspicion and be prepared to explore various etiologic factors that might be operative. Treatment should focus on setting specific goals, with patients using strategies that combine lifestyle changes, behavioral interventions, and appropriate medications. OTC agents, sedating antidepressants at low dosages (trazodone, doxepin, amitriptyline, and others), and nonhypnotic benzodiazepines are insufficiently studied to provide evidence-based support for their use to treat chronic insomnia. Particularly in the elderly, close monitoring is needed to prevent falls, accidents, and cognitive impairment from these agents. FDA-labeled hypnotic agents are efficacious, but long-term studies have not been available until the recent release of eszopiclone in the United States. Recent work encourages the use of CBT even in patients who have used sleeping pills for several years, although the success of CBT has been less encouraging when applied to chronic insomnia sufferers who have concurrent psychiatric disorders and who have taken hypnotics for years.

References

[1] Kupfer DJ, Reynolds CF. Management of insomnia. N Engl J Med 1997;336:341–6.
[2] Smith MT, Perlis ML, Park A, et al. Comparative meta-analysis of pharmacotherapy and behavior therapy for persistent insomnia. Am J Psychiatry 2002;150:5–11.
[3] Ohayon MM. Epidemiology of insomnia: what we know and what we still need to learn. Sleep Med Rev 2002;6:97–111.
[4] NHLBI Working Group on Insomnia. Bethesda (MD): NHLBI; September 1998. NIH publication no. 98–4088.
[5] Spielman AJ, Caruso LS, Glovinsky PB. A behavioral perspective on insomnia treatment. Psychiatric Clin North Am 1987;10:541–53.

[6] Hauri P, Linde S. No more sleepless nights: a proven program to conquer insomnia. New York: Wiley; 1996.

[7] Bootzin R. Stimulus control treatment for insomnia. Proceedings of the 80th annual convention of the American Psychological Association 1972;7:395–6.

[8] Spielman AJ, Saskin P, Thorpy MJ. Treatment of chronic insomnia by restriction of time in bed. Sleep 1987;10:45–56.

[9] Espie CA. Insomnia: conceptual issues in the development, persistence, and treatment of sleep disorder in adults. Annu Rev Psychol 2002;53:215–43.

[10] Lichstein KL, Morin CM, editors. Treatment of late-life insomnia. Thousand Oaks (CA): Sage Publications; 2000.

[11] Morin CM, Hauri PJ, Espie CA, et al. Nonpharmacologic treatment of chronic insomnia. An American Academy of Sleep Medicine review. Sleep 1999;22:1134–56.

[12] Jacobs GD, Pace-Schott EF, Stickgold R, et al. Cognitive behavior therapy and pharmacotherapy for insomnia: a randomized controlled trial and direct comparison. Arch Intern Med 2004;164(17):1888–96.

[13] Hauri PJ. Sleep hygiene, relaxation therapy, and cognitive interventions. In: Hauri PJ, editor. Case studies in insomnia. New York: Plenum Publishing; 1991. p. 65–84.

[14] Borbely AA, Youmbi-Balderer G. Effect of diphenhydramine on subjective sleep parameters and on motor activity during bedtime. Int J Clin Pharmacol Ther Toxicol 1988;26:392–6.

[15] Mendelson WB. A review of the evidence for the efficacy and safety of trazodone in insomnia. J Clin Psychiatry 2005;66:469–76.

[16] Ringdahl EN, Pereira SL, Delzell JE Jr. Treatment of primary insomnia. J Am Board Fam Pract 2004;17:212–9.

[17] Mendelson WB, Roth T, Cassella J, et al. The treatment of chronic insomnia: drug indications, chronic use and abuse liability. Summary of a 2001 New Clinical Drug Evaluation Unit meeting symposium. Sleep Med Rev 2004;8:7–17.

[18] Sateia MJ, Nowell PD. Insomnia. Lancet 2004;364:1959–73.

[19] Krystal AD, Walsh JK, Laska E, et al. Sustained efficacy of eszopiclone over 6 months of nightly treatment: results of a randomized, double-blind, placebo-controlled study in adults with chronic insomnia. Sleep 2003;26:793–9.

[20] Barbera J, Shaprio C. Benefit-risk assessment of zaleplon in the treatment of insomnia. Drug Saf 2005;28:301–18.

[21] Perlis ML. Long-term, non-nightly administration of zolpidem in the treatment of patients with primary insomnia. J Clin Psychiatry 2004;65:1128–37.

[22] Morin CM, Belanger L, Bastien C, et al. Long-term outcome after discontinuation of benzodiazepines for insomnia: a survival analysis of relapse. Behav Res Ther 2005;43:1–14.

ELSEVIER
SAUNDERS

NEUROLOGIC
CLINICS

Neurol Clin 23 (2005) 1165–1185

Restless Legs Syndrome

William G. Ondo, MD

Baylor College of Medicine, Houston, TX, USA

A National Institutes of Health (NIH) consensus panel recently characterized restless legs syndrome (RLS) as (1) an urge to move the limbs with or without sensations; (2) worsening at rest; (3) improving with activity; and (4) worsening in the evening or night [1]. The diagnosis of RLS is based exclusively on those criteria. A validated diagnostic phone interview [2], rating scale [3], and quality-of-life scale [4] have been developed based on these features.

Clinical restless legs syndrome

Patients, however, seldom quote the RLS inclusion criteria at presentation and often have difficulty describing their sensory component of their RLS. The descriptions are varied and tend to be suggestible and education dependent. The sensation always is unpleasant but not necessarily painful. It usually is deep within the legs. In a study of patients who have RLS, the most common terms used, in descending order of frequency, are: need to move, crawling, tingling, restless, cramping, creeping pulling, painful, electric, tension, discomfort, and itching [5]. Patients usually deny any burning or pins-and-needles sensations, commonly experienced in neuropathies or nerve entrapments, although neuropathic pain and RLS can coexist.

Essentially all patients report transient symptomatic improvement by walking, although some use stationary bike riding or kicking. Other therapeutic techniques reported by my patients include rubbing or pressure, stretching, and hot water. Symptom relief strategies increase sensory stimulation to the legs and generally are alerting. Other clinical features typical of RLS include the tendency for symptoms to worsen gradually with age, improvement with dopaminergic treatments, a positive family history of RLS, and periodic limb movements of sleep (PLMS).

E-mail address: wondo@bcm.tmc.edu

Periodic limb movements of sleep

PLMS are defined by the Association of Sleep Disorders as "periodic episodes of repetitive and highly stereotyped limb movements that occur during sleep." The incidence in the general population increases with age and is reported to occur in as many as 57% of elderly people [6–8]. Bixler and colleagues report that 29% of people over the age of 50 have PLMS, whereas only 5% of those aged 30 to 50 and almost none under 30 are affected [9]. The largest single study, using a cut-off of 5 PLMS per hour, reports that 81% of patients who have RLS show pathologic PLMS [10]. The prevalence increases to 87% if two nights are recorded. Although PLMS accompany most cases of RLS, the only data evaluating RLS prevalence in the setting of polysomnographically documented PLMS finds that only 9 of 53 (17.0%) patients who have PLMS complain of RLS symptoms [11]. The degree of diligence with which RLS symptoms were queried, however, is unclear. Most people who have RLS have PLMS, but many patients who have isolated PLMS do not have RLS. The exact relationship between the two phenotypes is unclear.

PLMS can occur simultaneously in both legs, alternate between legs, or occur unilaterally. The duration of movement typically is between 1.5 and 2.5 seconds and varies in intensity from slight extension of the great toe to a triple flexion response. Other tonic and myoclonic patterns are observed less frequently, and arms are involved in a minority of cases. Patients frequently demonstrate a movement periodicity of between 20 and 40 seconds, although wide ranges of frequencies are reported [12]. Movements are most pronounced in stage I and stage II of sleep, where they often are accompanied by K complexes and by increases in pulse and blood pressure [13]. The K complexes usually precede the PLMS and may persist even if PLMS are reduced with L-dopa [14]. PLMS intensity and frequency lessen as sleep deepens. They may persist during REM sleep but their amplitude and frequency are reduced significantly. When severe, PLMS may result in arousals, but they generally do not cause insomnia [9,15].

Restless legs syndrome in children

RLS in children can be difficult to diagnose. Although some children report classic RLS symptoms that meet inclusion criteria, others complain of "growing pains" [16,17], and some seem to present with an attention-deficit hyperactivity disorder (ADHD) phenotype. Kotagal and Silber report that children who have RLS have lower than expected serum ferritin levels and in most cases seem to inherit the disorder from their mother [18]. NIH diagnostic criteria for RLS in children is less well validated but emphasize supportive criteria, such as a family history of RLS, sleep disturbances, and the presence of PLMS, which is less common in pediatric controls [1]. The exact relationship between RLS and ADHD is not known.

Children diagnosed with ADHD, however, often have PLMS [19–22] and meet criteria for RLS [19]. Children who have ADHD also have a higher prevalence of a parent who has RLS [23] and children diagnosed with PLMS often have ADHD [24]. Dopaminergic treatment of RLS/PLMS in children also improves ADHD symptoms [25]. There is some association between RLS and ADHD.

Diagnostic evaluation of restless legs syndrome

In most cases, only a simple evaluation is justified for clinically typical RLS. Serum ferritin, and possibly iron binding saturation, for serum iron deficiency and electrolytes for renal failure should be obtained. Nerve conduction velocities (NCV) and electromyogram (EMG) should be performed in cases without a family history of RLS, of atypical presentations (ie, sensations beginning in the feet or superficial pain), that have a predisposition for neuropathy (ie, diabetes), or when physical symptoms and signs are consistent with a peripheral neuropathy. If EMG/NCV abnormalities are found, they should be evaluated further. Polysomnographic evaluation usually is reserved for patients in whom the diagnosis is in doubt, in cases where PLMS are suspected to be severe and result in arousals, or if other sleep disorders are suspected. A careful history and physical examination generally are sufficient to make a diagnosis of RLS; however, historically, diagnostic sensitivity has been low.

There are several potential diagnostic dilemmas. Akathisia represents an inner sense of restlessness accompanied by an intense desire to move. Subjects who have akathisia typically do not complain of limb paresthesia. The restlessness usually is generalized but may be most prominent in the legs. The condition usually is associated with the use of neuroleptic drugs. Patients who have akathisia generally have milder sleep complaints and less severe PLMS than are seen in RLS [26]. Akathisia tends to be associated with whole body rocking movements or marching in place and concurrently may show mild extrapyramidal features or tardive dyskinesias.

Painful legs and moving toes present with neuropathic leg pain associated with persistent, semirhythmic toe movements that cannot easily be reproduced volitionally and may be only partially suppressed [27]. The condition may be associated with peripheral nerve injury or minor leg trauma, but many patients have no identifiable etiology or pathology. This syndrome differs clinically from RLS in that the sensory symptoms are described as painful, are not worsened by immobility, are not necessarily worse at night, and are not improved with movement.

Nocturnal leg cramps are a common, multifactorial, disorder manifested by paroxysmal, disorganized spasms that usually involve the feet or calf muscles. The presentation is different from RLS, but patients initially may describe their RLS symptoms simply as "night cramps," which can lead to misdiagnosis if a more extensive history is not taken.

Epidemiology

Historically, epidemiologic studies of RLS were limited by the subjective nature of the disease, the lack of standardized diagnostic criteria, and the indolent onset of the condition (Table 1). Ekbom initially estimated a 5% prevalence of RLS in the general population [28]. Subsequent general population prevalence surveys vary from 1% to 29% [29–31].

The largest epidemiologic study of RLS involved more than 23,000 persons from five countries [32]. Similar to smaller reports, 9.6% met criteria for RLS. In general, northern European countries demonstrated a higher

Table 1
Epidemiology of restless legs syndrome in general population, since 1995

Author (year)	N	Restless legs syndrome diagnostic criteria	Population	Location	Restless legs syndrome (%)
Hening (2004) [32]	23,052	NIH written	Adults	Europe/United States	9.6
Garbarino (2002) [169]	2560	Written	Police shift	Genoa, Italy	8.5: shift workers 4.2: day workers
Ohayon (2002) [170]	18,980	ICSD phone interview	15–100	Europe	5.5
Berger (2004) [171]	4310	IRLSSG interview	20–79	Northeast Germany	10.6
Rothdach (2000) [172]	369	IRLSSG interview	65–83	Ausberg, Germany	9.8
Nichols (2003) [173]	2099	IRLSSG	Adult	Idaho, United States (single PCP)	24.0
Ulfberg (2001) [174]	200	IRLSSG written	Women 18–64	Sweden	11.4
Ulfberg (2001) [175]	4000	IRLSSG written	Men 18–64	Sweden	5.8
Phillips (2000) [31]	1803	Single phone question	n > 18	Kentucky, United States	10.0
Lavigne (1997) [176]	2019	2 written questions	Adults	Quebec, Canada	10–15
Sevim (2002) [177]	3234	IRLSSG interview	Adults, no secondary RLS	Turkey	3.2
Tan (2001) [33]	1000	IRLSSG interview	>21	Singapore	0.1
Kageyama (2000) [34]	3600 women 1012 men	Single written	Adults	Japan	1.5

Abbreviations: ICSD, International Classification of Sleep Disorders; IRLSSG, International Restless Legs Study Group diagnostic criteria; NIH, National Institutes of Health RLS diagnostic criteria; PCP, primary care physician.

prevalence compared with Mediterranean countries. The vast majority of these subjects were not diagnosed previously, despite frequently reporting symptoms to their physicians.

RLS can occur in all ethnic backgrounds; however, most investigators believe that Whites are affected most. Although most surveys of White populations demonstrate approximately a 10% prevalence, two surveys in Asian populations report much lower prevalences. Tan and colleagues, in a door-to-door survey of 1000 people over age 21 in Singapore, found only one person (0.1%) who met International Restless Legs Study Group diagnostic criteria for RLS [33]. Kageyama and coworkers distributed a written questionnaire asking "if you ever experience sleep disturbances due to creeping sensations or hot feeling in your legs" to 3600 women and 1012 men [34]. They report that approximately 5% responded affirmatively to that single question, but far fewer met all criteria for RLS. People from African descent never have been studied specifically but, anecdotally, African-Americans present only rarely with RLS. It is unclear if this represents a true lower prevalence or, rather, differences in medical sophistication and referral patterns.

Genetics of restless legs syndrome

In approximately 60% of cases, a family history of RLS can be found, although often this is not reported initially by patients [5]. Twin studies also show a high concordance rate [35]. Most pedigrees suggest an autosomal dominant pattern [36], although an autosomal recessive pattern with a high carrier rate is possible. A complex segregation analysis performed in German families revealed a single gene autosomal pattern in subjects with a young onset of RLS (<30 years) but no clear pattern in older-onset subjects [36]. To date, several gene linkages have been demonstrated, although specific causative proteins remain elusive. Given the wide distribution of RLS, however, it is likely that additional specific genetic etiologies will be discovered.

Desautels first reported a linkage using an autosomal recessive pattern with a high penetrance on chromosome 12q in a large French-Canadian family [37]. Multipoint linkage calculations yielded a LOD score of 3.59. Haplotype analysis refined the genetic interval, positioning the RLS-predisposing gene in a 14.71-cM region between D12S1044 and D12S78. This linkage site has been corroborated in Iceland (David Rye, personal communication, 2005).

Bonati and colleagues next identified an autosomal dominant linkage in a single Italian family on chromosome 14q13-21 region. The maximum two-point log of odds-ratio score value of 3.23 at theta = 0.0 was obtained for marker D14S288 [38].

Chen and coworkers [38a] characterized 15 large and extended multiplex pedigrees, consisting of 453 subjects (134 affected with RLS). Model-free linkage analysis identified one novel significant susceptibility locus for RLS on chromosomal 9p24.2-22.3 with a multipoint nonparametric linkage score 3.22. Model-based linkage analysis assuming an autosomal dominant mode of inheritance validated the 9p24.2-22.3 linkage to RLS in two families (two-point LOD score of 3.77; multipoint LOD score of 3.91). This site has been corroborated independently in a separate German family (Winkelmann, personal communication).

Specific protein mutations have not been identified. The Montreal group reports that a specific allele of monoamine oxidase A conferred a modest risk for RLS [39]. Many other candidate genes of dopaminergic and iron regulation, however, do not show any association [40,41].

Pathophysiology of restless legs syndrome

Recent pathologic research suggests that the pathophysiology of RLS involves central nervous system (CNS) iron homeostatic dysregulation. Cerebrospinal fluid ferritin is lower in RLS cases [42], and specially sequenced MRI studies show reduced iron stores in the striatum and red nucleus [43]. Recently, CNS ultrasonography also identified RLS based on reduced iron echogenicity in the substantia nigra [44]. Most importantly, pathologic data in RLS autopsied brains show reduced ferritin staining, iron staining, and increased transferrin stains but also reduced transferrin receptors. Research also demonstrates reduced Thy-1 expression, which is regulated by iron levels [45]. Substantia nigra dopaminergic cells are not reduced in number nor are there markers associated with neurodegenerative diseases, such as tau-or alpha-synuclein abnormalities [46,47]. The reduced transferrin receptor finding is important because globally reduced iron stores normally upregulate transferrin receptors. It seems, therefore, that primary RLS has reduced intracellular iron indices secondary to a perturbation of homeostatic mechanisms that regulate iron influx or efflux from the cell. Intracellular iron regulation is complex; however, subsequent staining of RLS brains shows reduced levels of iron regulatory protein-type 1 [48]. This potentiates or inhibits (depending on feedback mechanisms involving iron atoms themselves) the production of ferritin molecules, which are the main iron storage proteins in the CNS the periphery, and transferrin receptors, which facilitate intracellular iron transport.

CNS dopaminergic systems are implicated strongly in RLS. Most researchers agree that dopamine agonists (DA) treat RLS most robustly; dopaminergic functional brain imaging studies inconsistently show modest abnormalities [49–52]; and normal circadian dopaminergic variation also is augmented in patients who have RLS [53]. There are several potential interactions between iron and dopamine systems. First, iron is a cofactor for tyrosine-hydroxylase, which is the rate-limiting step in the production of dopamine. Iron chelation reduces dopamine transporter protein expression and activity in mice [54]. Human cerebrospinal fluid studies, however, fail to demonstrate reduced dopaminergic metabolites [55,56]. Second, iron is a component of the dopamine type-2 (DRD2) receptor. Iron deprivation in rats results in a 40% to 60% reduction of DRD2 postsynaptic receptors [57,58]. The effect is specific, as other neurotransmitter systems, including D1 receptors, are not affected. Third, iron is necessary for Thy-1 protein regulation. This cell adhesion molecule, which is expressed robustly on dopaminergic neurons and is reduced in brain homogenates in iron-deprived mice [59] and in brains of patients who have RLS [45]. Thy-1 regulates vesicular release of monoamines, including dopamine [60]. It also stabilizes synapses and suppresses dendritic growth [61].

Another puzzle that remains is identification of a specific anatomy culpable for RLS. There are many dopaminergic systems in the brain, but patients who have RLS do not have symptoms consistent with dysfunction seen in most known dopaminergic systems, such as parkinsonism or olfactory loss [62]. Involvement of the seldom-studied diencephalospinal dopaminergic tract, originating from the A11-A14 nuclei, might explain some RLS features. It is involved in antinoscioception, is near circadian control centers, and could explain why legs are involved more than arms. A preliminary animal model with A11 lesions demonstrates increased standing episodes, which improved after the administration of ropinirole, a DA [63]. Subsequent studies of this model in mice, with and without dietary iron deprivation, also demonstrate increased movement, as measured in laser marked cages, in the lesioned animals. This hyperkinesis is normalized by D2 agonists, such as ropinirole and pramipexole, but not by the D1 agonist, SKF.

Secondary restless legs syndrome

Despite the appropriate attention given to RLS genetics, between 2% and 6% of the population probably suffer from RLS without any identifiable highly penetrant genetic pattern. It is not known if some "genetic" forms of RLS could express low penetrance and mimic a sporadic pattern of onset. Currently, however, there is no evidence to support this pattern of penetrance [36]. Therefore, patients who do not have a positive family history are classified as either primary RLS, if no other explanation is found, or secondary RLS, if they concurrently posses a condition known to be associated with RLS.

The most common causes of secondary RLS include renal failure, iron deficiency, neuropathy, myelinopathy, pregnancy, and, possibly, Parkinson's disease (PD) and essential tremor. There is some evidence to support an association of RLS with some genetic ataxias [64–66], fibromyalgia [67,68], and rheumatologic diseases [69–71]. A variety of other associations are tenuous at best. Finally, several medications are known to exacerbate existing RLS or possibly precipitate RLS. The most notable of these include antihistamines, dopamine antagonists (including many antinausea medications, mirtazapine, and possibly tricyclic antidepressants), and serotonergic reuptake inhibitors.

Many forms of neuropathy, including diabetes, alcoholism, amyloid, motor neuron disease, poliomyelitis, and radiculopathy, are seen at higher than expected frequency in patients presenting with RLS [5,72–82]. In contrast, series evaluating RLS in populations presenting with neuropathy do not show a particularly high prevalence of RLS; the usual range is from 5% to 10%, similar to the general population [78,79].

For example, my series reports that 37 of 98 (36.6%) patients who had RLS demonstrated electrophysiologic evidence of neuropathy, using standard EMG/NCV techniques. The exact etiologies varied. Many of these patients demonstrated no evidence of neuropathy on clinical examination. The presence of neuropathy was much higher in patients who did not have a family history of RLS compared with those who did have a family history, 22 of 31 (71%) versus 15 of 67 (24%) ($P < 0.001$). Small fiber neuropathy, which is detectable only with biopsy, also is found in a large number of patients presenting with RLS [76].

Specific forms of neuropathy may incur different risks for the development of RLS. Gemignani and colleagues report that 10 of 27 (37%) patients who had Charcot-Marie-Tooth disease type II (CMT II), an axonal neuropathy, had RLS, whereas RLS was not seen in any of 17 patients who had CMT type I, a demyelinating neuropathy [72].

The phenotype of neuropathic RLS may be slightly different from idiopathic RLS [5,76]. In the population I studied, neuropathic RLS symptoms initially presented more acutely and at an older age and then progressed more rapidly. A large number of patients who had neuropathic RLS reached maximum symptom intensity within 1 year from initial symptom onset, which is unusual in idiopathic cases. Neuropathic RLS also may have accompanying neuropathic pain, which often is burning and more superficial. The painful component and the urge to move, however, are seldom differentiated by the patient.

The spinal cord is implicated in the pathogenesis of RLS [63,83] and cases of RLS and PLMS are seen after transient or permanent spinal cord lesions. Traumatic spinal cord lesions [84,85], neoplastic spinal lesions [86], demyelinating or postinfectious lesions [87–89], and syringomyelia [90] can precipitate RLS and PLMS. Spinal cord blocks used for anesthesia also frequently cause or exacerbate RLS [91,92]. Hogl and coworkers systematically evaluated RLS after spinal anesthesia [91]. Of 161 subjects who did not have any history of RLS, 8.7% developed RLS immediately after the procedure.

Uremia secondary to renal failure is associated strongly with RLS symptoms. Several series report a 20% to 57% prevalence of RLS in renal dialysis patients; however, only a minority of patients who have uremia volunteer RLS symptoms unless specifically queried (Table 2) [93–112]. The

Table 2
Studies evaluating restless legs syndrome in renal failure

Author (year)	Cohort	Restless legs syndrome diagnosis	Percentage and number with restless legs syndrome	Restless legs syndrome predictors
Unruh (2004) [178]	HD/United States	Single question for "severe" RLS	15% of 894	Associated with increased mortality
Mucsi (2004) [179]	HD/PD Hungary		15%	NR
Gigli (2004) [180]	HD/PD Italy	Written IRLSSG	21.5% of 601	Greater duration of dialysis
Bhowmik (2004) [181]	India	1.5% of 65		NR
Takaki (2003) [182]	HD Japan	IRLSSG (4/4)	60/490 (12.2%)	Hyperphosphatemia
		IRLSSG (≥2/4)	112/490 (22.9%)	Stress
Goffredo Filho (2003) [183]	HD Brazil	IRLSSG interview	/176 (14.8%)	Caucasion > noncaucasion
Bhatia (2003) [93]	HD India		6.6%	NR
Kutner (2002) [184]	HD United States	IRLSSG interview	308 68% Caucasion 48% African	Caucasion > African-American, no other significant predictors
Cirignotta (2002) [185]	HD Italy	Written questionnaire, IRLSSG interview	/127 (50%)	NR
Sabbatini (2002) [104]	HD Italy	RLS question	/127 (33.3%)	None
Miranda (2001) [186]	HD Chile	Interview	257/694 (37%)	None
Hui (2000) [98]	PD Hong Kong	Written question	43/166 (26%)	Insomnia
Virga (1998) [107]	HD	"RLS"	124/201 (62%)	None
Collado-Seidel (1998) [95]	HD Germany	IRLSSG (4/4)	(27.4%)	Increased parathyroid hormone
		IRLSSG (≥3/4)	32/138 (23%)	
			44/138 (32%)	
Winkelmann (1996) [109]	HD United States	IRLSSG (3/4)	/204 (20%)	None Decreased Hct, poor sleep
Walker (1995) [187]	HD Canada	ICSD	31/54 (57%)	Increased BUN, P = 0.04 Increased Cr, P = 0.08
Stepanski (1995) [105]	PD	"Leg twitching"	26/81 (32%)	NR
Holley (1992) [97]	HD/PD	"RLS"	30/70 (42%)	NR
Roger (1991) [103]	HD/PD United Kingdom	"RLS"	22/55 (40%)	Hct, P = 0.03 female
Bastani (1987) [188]	HD	"RLS"	6/42 (17%)	NR
Nielsen (1971) [112]	None	"RLS"	43/109 (39%)	NR

Abbreviations: BUN, blood urea nitrogen; Cr, creatinine; Hct, hematocrit; HD, hemodialysis; IRLSSG, International Restless Legs Study Group; NR, not reported; PD, peritoneal dialysis.

prevalence of RLS in mild to moderate renal failure that does not require dialysis is unknown.

The RLS seen in dialysis patients often is severe. Wetter and colleagues compared clinical and polysomnographic features of idiopathic RLS and uremic RLS in a large clinical series [108]. They report no differences in sensory symptoms but note increased wakeful leg movements (78% versus 51%) and significantly greater numbers of PLMS in uremic patients who have RLS. RLS and PLMS also are associated with increased mortality in the dialysis population [109,113].

Overall, dialysis does not improve RLS. One study suggests that RLS correlates with greater dialysis frequency [100]. Patients who receive a successful, but not those who received unsuccessful, kidney transplant usually experience dramatic improvement in RLS within days to weeks, however [114,115]. The degree of symptom alleviation seems to correlate with improved kidney function.

As discussed previously, reduced CNS iron is implicated in all cases of RLS. It is intuitive to suggest that reduced body stores of iron also could result in low CNS intracellular iron and cause RLS symptoms. A series of recent reports associate low serum ferritin levels with RLS [42,43,116–120]. Serum ferritin is the best indicator of low iron stores and the only serum measure to correlate consistently with RLS. Anemia is not associated independently with RLS; however, blood donors frequently develop RLS symptoms [118,121].

Low serum iron stores are associated only with certain demographics of patients who have RLS. I have reported that serum ferritin is lower in patients who have RLS and who lack a family history compared to those who have familial RLS [116,122]. Earley and colleagues make the same general observation but segregated the groups based on age of RLS onset [123]. The patients who had an older age of RLS onset had lower serum ferritin levels compared with patients who had a younger age of onset. These groups, however, generally represent the same dichotomy as genetic-based segregations, because there is a strong correlation between a younger age of onset of RLS and the presence of a family history of RLS.

The development of RLS during pregnancy has long been recognized [28,124,125]. Manconi and colleagues recently evaluated risk factors for RLS in 606 pregnancies [126]. They report that 26% of these women suffered from RLS, usually in the last trimester. The investigators could find no significant differences in age, pregnancy duration, mode of delivery, tobacco use, the women's body mass index, baby weight, or iron/folate supplementation in those who had RLS. Hemoglobin, however, was significantly lower in the RLS group, and plasmatic iron tended to be lower, compared with those who did not have RLS. Lee and colleagues report that 23% of 29 third-trimester women developed RLS during pregnancy [127]. The RLS resolved shortly post partum in all but one subject. Women who had RLS in their population demonstrated lower preconception levels of ferritin but were similar to women who did not have RLS during pregnancy.

RLS and PD respond to dopaminergic treatments, show dopaminergic abnormalities on functional imaging [51,128], and are associated with PLMS [129]. Now it is known, however, that the pathology of the two dopaminergically treated diseases are different and, in regard to iron accumulation, opposite [47].

In a survey of 303 consecutive patients who had PD, I found that 20.8% of all patients who had PD met the diagnostic criteria for RLS. Only lower serum ferritin was associated with RLS [116]. Similar epidemiologic findings recently have been found by other groups evaluating Caucasian populations [130] (Chaudhuri, personal communication) but not Asian populations [131,132]. Despite this high number of cases, there are several caveats that tend to lesson the clinical significance of RLS in PD. The RLS symptoms in patients who have PD often are ephemeral, usually not severe, and can be confused with other PD symptoms, such as wearing off dystonia, akathisia, or internal tremor. Furthermore, most patients in my group were not diagnosed previously with RLS and few recognized that this was separate from other PD symptoms.

Treatment of restless legs syndrome

The development of validated rating scales and standardized diagnostic criteria have improved the quality of RLS treatment trials vastly in the past 5 years. Although many medications demonstrate outstanding efficacy, all are believed to provide only symptomatic relief, rather than any curative effect. Therefore, treatment should be initiated only when the benefits are believed to justify potential adverse effects and costs. Treatment decisions also need to consider the chronicity and general progressive course of RLS. Over time, dosing and medication changes often are required to maximize benefit and minimize the risk of tolerance and adverse effects.

DA are the best-investigated and probably most effective treatments of RLS. The improvement is immediate and often dramatic. Although no evidence favors any particular DA, ropinirole currently is the best studied. Three similar large multicenter, placebo-controlled trials in Europe and North America [133–135] and a smaller polysomnogram-based study [136] evaluated ropinirole versus placebo in almost 1000 total subjects. These large studies titrated from 0.25 mg up to a maximum of 4 mg of ropinirole of placebo given as a single nightly dose over 8 weeks, but patients were allowed to stop titrating if necessary. The final dose was maintained for the final 4 weeks. The trials demonstrated consistently significant efficacy of ropinirole using the RLS rating scale and clinical global assessments. The polysomnogram study showed a marked reduction of PLMS and improved sleep architecture. Adverse events were similar but probably milder than those seen in PD, perhaps owing to the lower dose or differences in the disease state. Overall, 7% of subjects on drug and 4% of subjects on placebo withdrew for adverse events. A smaller crossover trial using two split doses showed even more robust efficacy [137].

Placebo-controlled trials also demonstrate similar robust efficacy of the DA pramipexole [138,139], pergolide [133,140–143], bromocriptine [144], apomorphine [145], cabergoline [146], and rotigotine [146] and of the dopamine precursor levodopa (L-dopa) [147–151]. L-dopa was inferior to pergolide in the only controlled comparative trial of dopaminergic medications [141]. It also is believed to have greater potential for augmentation [152]. There is no comparative trial of the DAs but all are believed to provide similar efficacy. Several of these are being petitioned for registration in North America and Europe.

Less data addresses the long-term use of DA for RLS. Although studies of up to 1 year show that most patients on DA continue to benefit from the medications [153,154], some reports raise specific concerns about the development of tolerance and dopaminergic-induced augmentation. Augmentation is defined by an earlier phase shift of symptom onset, an increased intensity of symptoms, increased anatomic involvement, or less relief with movement. This was noted first, and still is most problematic, with L-dopa, which has the shortest half-life of any dopaminergic medication [152]. The mechanisms behind augmentation, however, are not known, and it also is reported with pergolide [142,152,155], pramipexole [156–158], and ropinirole [159] but, to date, not with cabergoline [157,160,161]. Winkelman and Johnston [158] retrospectively assessed augmentation and tolerance in 59 patients treated for RLS with pramipexole for at least 6 months (mean duration, 21.2 ± 11.4 months). Augmentation developed in 32% (19/59) and tolerance occurred in 46% (27/59) of patients. These two complications were statistically related ($P < 0.05$). The only clinical predictors of these complications were previous augmentation or tolerance to L-dopa.

I evaluated for augmentation in 83 patients who had RLS and who were started initially on a DA. Patients who had at least 6 months' use of DA were followed for a mean of 39.2 ± 20.9 months. Efficacy was maintained over time but at the expense of moderate but significant increases in dose ($P < 0.01$). Adverse events were frequent but usually mild and seldom resulted in discontinuation. Augmentation was frequent (48%) but usually modest and predicted by a positive family history for RLS and especially the lack of any neuropathy on EMG/NCV.

Opioid medications, also known as narcotics, have been used to treat RLS successfully. Open-label trials consistently demonstrate good initial and long-term results without difficulty with tolerance, dependence, or addiction [162]. There are, however, only two controlled trials that demonstrate efficacy [150,163]. I use opioids as second-line therapy and recently collated my experience with methadone (a μ-specific opioid agonist) in patients who had RLS and who failed DAs because of lack of efficacy, adverse events, or severe augmentation [164]. Overall, methadone (5 to

20 mg/d) benefits most refractory patients markedly who have RLS without augmentation, tolerance, or evidence of dependency.

Gabapentin is an antiepileptic with several but still unclear mechanisms of action, which treats a variety of neurologic conditions. Garcia-Borreguero and colleagues [164a] conducted a 24-patient, 6-week per arm, crossover study of gabapentin (mean dose 1855 mg/d) and placebo. RLS Rating Scale, Clinical Global Impression, a pain analog scale, and the Pittsburgh Sleep Quality Index all improved on gabapentin. In addition, sleep studies showed significantly reduced PLMS and improved sleep architecture (increased total sleep time, sleep efficiency, slow wave sleep, and decreased stage 1 sleep). The PLMS did not improve as robustly as in DA studies.

Despite past widespread use, there is little data to support the use of benzodiazepines for RLS. In the opinion of most experts, benzodiazepines help facilitate sleep but seldom improve RLS cardinal features. These can be used successfully in mild cases of RLS and as adjunct therapy for residual insomnia.

Although open-label oral iron supplementation is reported to improve RLS [165], the only controlled study of oral iron supplementation failed to improve RLS symptoms [166]. Oral iron, however, has many limitations related to absorption and tolerance. In contrast, the administration of intravenous iron can increase serum ferritin levels dramatically and an open-label study of intravenous iron demonstrates robust efficacy [167]. Controlled trials of iron dextran with uremic RLS also show efficacy [168]. Additional studies are ongoing.

Many other agents, including other antiepileptic medications, clonidine, baclofen, tramadol, and magnesium, are reported to help RLS but suffer from limited data and cannot be recommended as either first- or second-line therapy.

References

[1] Allen RP, Picchietti D, Hening WA, et al. Restless legs syndrome: diagnostic criteria, special considerations, and epidemiology. A report from the restless legs syndrome diagnosis and epidemiology workshop at the National Institutes of Health. Sleep Med 2003;4:101–19.

[2] Hening WA, Allen RP, Thanner S, et al. The Johns Hopkins telephone diagnostic interview for the restless legs syndrome: preliminary investigation for validation in a multicenter patient and control population. Sleep Med 2003;4:137–41.

[3] Walters AS, LeBrocq C, Dhar A, et al. Validation of the International Restless Legs Syndrome Study Group rating scale for restless legs syndrome. Sleep Med 2003;4:121–32.

[4] Atkinson MJ, Allen RP, DuChane J, et al. Validation of the Restless Legs Syndrome Quality of Life Instrument (RLS-QLI): findings of a consortium of national experts and the RLS Foundation. Qual Life Res 2004;13:679–93.

[5] Ondo W, Jankovic J. Restless legs syndrome: clinicoetiologic correlates. Neurology 1996; 47:1435–41.

[6] Ancoli-Israel S, Kripke DF, Klauber MR, et al. Periodic limb movements in sleep in community-dwelling elderly. Sleep 1991;14:496–500.

[7] Mosko SS, Dickel MJ, Paul T, et al. Sleep apnea and sleep-related periodic leg movements in community resident seniors. J Am Geriatr Soc 1988;36:502–8.

[8] Roehrs T, Zorick F, Sicklesteel J, et al. Age-related sleep-wake disorders at a sleep disorder center. J Am Geriatr Soc 1983;31:364–70.

[9] Bixler EO, Kales A, Vela-Bueno A. Nocturnal myoclonus and nocturnal myoclonic activity in a normal population. Res Commun Chem Pathol Pharmacol 1982;36:129–40.

[10] Montplaisir J, Boucher S, Poirier G, et al. Clinical, polysomnographic, and genetic characteristics of restless legs syndrome: a study of 133 patients diagnosed with new standard criteria. Movement Disorders 1997;12:61–5.

[11] Coleman RM, Miles LE, Guilleminault CC, et al. Sleep-wake disorders in the elderly: polysomnographic analysis. J Am Geriatr Soc 1981;29:289–96.

[12] Smith RC. The Babinski response and periodic limb movement disorder. J Neuropsychiatry Clin Neurosci 1992;4:233–4.

[13] Lugaresi E, Coccagna G, Mantovani M, et al. Some periodic phenomena arising during drowsiness and sleep in man. Electroencephalogr Clin Neurophysiol 1972;32:701–5.

[14] Montplaisir J, Boucher S, Gosselin A, et al. Persistence of repetitive EEG arousals (K-alpha complexes) in RLS patients treated with L-DOPA. Sleep 1996;19:196–9.

[15] Wiegand M, Schacht-Muller W, Starke C. [Psychophysiologic insomnia and periodic leg movements in sleep syndrome]. Wien Med Wochenschr 1995;145:527–8.

[16] Ekbom KA. Growing pains and restless legs. Acta Paediatr Scand 1975;64:264–6.

[17] Rajaram SS, Walters AS, England SJ, et al. Some children with growing pains may actually have restless legs syndrome. Sleep 2004;27:767–73.

[18] Kotagal S, Silber MH. Childhood-onset restless legs syndrome. Ann Neurol 2004;56:803–7.

[19] Chervin RD, Archbold KH, Dillon JE, et al. Associations between symptoms of inattention, hyperactivity, restless legs, and periodic leg movements. Sleep 2002;25:213–8.

[20] Picchietti DL, England SJ, Walters AS, et al. Periodic limb movement disorder and restless legs syndrome in children with attention-deficit hyperactivity disorder. J Child Neurol 1998;13:588–94.

[21] Chervin RD, Dillon JE, Archbold KH, et al. Conduct problems and symptoms of sleep disorders in children. J Am Acad Child Adolesc Psychiatry 2003;42:201–8.

[22] Konofal E, Lecendreux M, Bouvard MP, et al. High levels of nocturnal activity in children with attention-deficit hyperactivity disorder: a video analysis. Psychiatry Clin Neurosci 2001;55:97–103.

[23] Picchietti DL, Underwood DJ, Farris WA, et al. Further studies on periodic limb movement disorder and restless legs syndrome in children with attention-deficit hyperactivity disorder. Mov Disord 1999;14:1000–7.

[24] Picchietti DL, Walters AS. Moderate to severe periodic limb movement disorder in childhood and adolescence. Sleep 1999;22:297–300.

[25] Walters AS, Mandelbaum DE, Lewin DS, et al. Dopaminergic therapy in children with restless legs/periodic limb movements in sleep and ADHD. Dopaminergic Therapy Study Group. Pediatr Neurol 2000;22:182–6.

[26] Sachdev P, Longragan C. The present status of akathisia [comments]. J Nerv Ment Dis 1991;179:381–91.

[27] Dressler D, Thompson PD, Gledhill RF, et al. The syndrome of painful legs and moving toes. Movement Disorders 1994;9:13–21.

[28] Ekbom KA. Restless legs syndrome 1960;10:868–73.

[29] Lavigne GJ, Montplaisir JY. Restless legs syndrome and sleep bruxism: prevalence and association among Canadians. Sleep 1994;17:739–43.

[30] Oboler SK, Prochazka AV, Meyer TJ. Leg symptoms in outpatient veterans. West J Med 1991;155:256–9.

[31] Phillips B, Young T, Finn L, et al. Epidemiology of restless legs symptoms in adults. Arch Intern Med 2000;160:2137–41.

[32] Hening W, Walters AS, Allen RP, et al. Impact, diagnosis and treatment of restless legs syndrome (RLS) in a primary care population: the REST (RLS epidemiology, symptoms, and treatment) primary care study. Sleep Med 2004;5:237–46.

[33] Tan EK, Seah A, See SJ, et al. Restless legs syndrome in an Asian population: a study in Singapore. Mov Disord 2001;16:577–9.

[34] Kageyama T, Kabuto M, Nitta H, et al. Prevalences of periodic limb movement-like and restless legs-like symptoms among Japanese adults. Psychiatry Clin Neurosci 2000;54: 296–8.

[35] Ondo WG, Vuong KD, Wang Q. Restless legs syndrome in monozygotic twins: clinical correlates. Neurology 2000;55:1404–6.

[36] Winkelmann J, Muller-Myhsok B, Wittchen HU, et al. Complex segregation analysis of restless legs syndrome provides evidence for an autosomal dominant mode of inheritance in early age at onset families. Ann Neurol 2002;52:297–302.

[37] Desautels A, Turecki G, Montplaisir J, et al. Identification of a major susceptibility locus for restless legs syndrome on chromosome 12q [comment]. Am J Hum Genet 2001;69: 1266–70.

[38] Bonati MT, Ferini-Strambi L, Aridon P, et al. Autosomal dominant restless legs syndrome maps on chromosome 14q. Brain 2003;126(Pt 6):1485–92.

[38a] Chen S, Ondo WG, Rao S, et al. Genome-wide linkage scan identifies a novel susceptibility locus for restless legs syndrome on chromosome 9p. Am J Hum Gen 2004;74:876–85.

[39] Desautels A, Turecki G, Montplaisir J, et al. Evidence for a genetic association between monoamine oxidase A and restless legs syndrome. Neurology 2002;59:215–9.

[40] Li J, Hu LD, Wang WJ, et al. Linkage analysis of the candidate genes of familial restless legs syndrome. I Chuan Hsueh Pao 2003;30:325–9.

[41] Desautels A, Turecki G, Montplaisir J, et al. Dopaminergic neurotransmission and restless legs syndrome: a genetic association analysis [comment]. Neurology 2001;57: 1304–6.

[42] Earley CJ, Connor JR, Beard JL, et al. Abnormalities in CSF concentrations of ferritin and transferrin in restless legs syndrome. Neurology 2000;54:1698–700.

[43] Allen RP, Barker PB, Wehrl F, et al. MRI measurement of brain iron in patients with restless legs syndrome. Neurology 2001;56:263–5.

[44] Schmidauer C, Sojer M, Stocckner H, et al. Brain parenchyma sonography differentiates RLS patients from normal controls and patients with Parkinson's disease. Mov Disord 2005;20(Suppl 10):S43.

[45] Wang X, Wiesinger J, Beard J, et al. Thy1 expression in the brain is affected by iron and is decreased in Restless Legs Syndrome. J Neurol Sci 2004;220:59–66.

[46] Pittock SJ, Parrett T, Adler CH, et al. Neuropathology of primary restless leg syndrome: absence of specific tau- and alpha-synuclein pathology. Mov Disord 2004;19:695–9.

[47] Connor JR, Boyer PJ, Menzies SL, et al. Neuropathological examination suggests impaired brain iron acquisition in restless legs syndrome. Neurology 2003;61:304–9.

[48] Connor JR, Wang XS, Patton SM, et al. Decreased transferrin receptor expression by neuromelanin cells in restless legs syndrome. Neurology 2004;62:1563–7.

[49] Staedt J, Stoppe G, Kogler A, et al. Nocturnal myoclonus syndrome (periodic movements in sleep) related to central dopamine D2-receptor alteration. Eur Arch Psychiatry Clin Neurosci 1995;245:8–10.

[50] Trenkwalder C, Walters AS, Hening WA, et al. Positron emission tomographic studies in restless legs syndrome. Mov Disord 1999;14:141–5.

[51] Turjanski N, Lees AJ, Brooks DJ. Striatal dopaminergic function in restless legs syndrome: 18F-dopa and 11C-raclopride PET studies. Neurology 1999;52:932–7.

[52] Tribl GG, Asenbaum S, Happe S, et al. Normal striatal D2 receptor binding in idiopathic restless legs syndrome with periodic leg movements in sleep. Nucl Med Commun 2004;25: 55–60.

[53] Garcia-Borreguero D, Larrosa O, Granizo JJ, et al. Circadian variation in neuroendocrine response to L-dopa in patients with restless legs syndrome. Sleep 2004;27:669–73.

[54] Nelson C, Erikson K, Pinero DJ, et al. In vivo dopamine metabolism is altered in iron-deficient anemic rats. J Nutr 1997;127:2282–8.

[55] Stiasny-Kolster K, Moller JC, Zschocke J, et al. Normal dopaminergic and serotonergic metabolites in cerebrospinal fluid and blood of restless legs syndrome patients. Mov Disord 2004;19:192–6.

[56] Earley CJ, Hyland K, Allen RP. CSF dopamine, serotonin, and biopterin metabolites in patients with restless legs syndrome. Mov Disord 2001;16:144–9.

[57] Ben-Shachar D, Finberg JP, Youdim MB. Effect of iron chelators on dopamine D2 receptors. J Neurochem 1985;45:999–1005.

[58] Ashkenazi R, Ben-Shachar D, Youdim MB. Nutritional iron and dopamine binding sites in the rat brain. Pharmacol Biochem Behav 1982;17(Suppl 1):43–7.

[59] Ye Z, Connor JR. Identification of iron responsive genes by screening cDNA libraries from suppression subtractive hybridization with antisense probes from three iron conditions. Nucleic Acids Res 2000;28:1802–7.

[60] Jeng CJ, McCarroll SA, Martin TF, et al. Thy-1 is a component common to multiple populations of synaptic vesicles. J Cell Biol 1998;140:685–98.

[61] Shults CW, Kimber TA. Thy-1 immunoreactivity distinguishes patches/striosomes from matrix in the early postnatal striatum of the rat. Brain Res Dev Brain Res 1993;75: 136–40.

[62] Adler CH, Gwinn KA, Newman S. Olfactory function in restless legs syndrome. Mov Disord 1998;13:563–5.

[63] Ondo WG, He Y, Rajasekaran S, et al. Clinical correlates of 6-hydroxydopamine injections into A11 dopaminergic neurons in rats: a possible model for restless legs syndrome. Mov Disord 2000;15:154–8.

[64] Abele M, Burk K, Laccone F, et al. Restless legs syndrome in spinocerebellar ataxia types 1, 2, and 3. J Neurol 2001;248:311–4.

[65] Schols L, Haan J, Riess O, et al. Sleep disturbance in spinocerebellar ataxias: is the SCA3 mutation a cause of restless legs syndrome? Neurology 1998;51:1603–7.

[66] van Alfen N, Sinke RJ, Zwarts MJ, et al. Intermediate CAG repeat lengths (53,54) for MJD/SCA3 are associated with an abnormal phenotype. Ann Neurol 2001;49: 805–7.

[67] Yunus MB, Aldag JC. Restless legs syndrome and leg cramps in fibromyalgia syndrome: a controlled study. BMJ 1996;312:1339.

[68] Moldofsky H. Management of sleep disorders in fibromyalgia. Rheum Dis Clin North Am 2002;28:353–65.

[69] Reynolds G, Blake DR, Pall HS, et al. Restless leg syndrome and rheumatoid arthritis. Br Med J 1986;292:659–60.

[70] Salih AM, Gray RE, Mills KR, et al. A clinical, serological and neurophysiological study of restless legs syndrome in rheumatoid arthritis. Br J Rheumatol 1994;33:60–3.

[71] Gudbjornsson B, Broman JE, Hetta J, et al. Sleep disturbances in patients with primary Sjogren's syndrome. Br J Rheumatol 1993;32:1072–6.

[72] Gemignani F, Marbini A, Di Giovanni G, et al. Charcot-Marie-Tooth disease type 2 with restless legs syndrome. Neurology 1999;52:1064–6.

[73] Gemignani F, Marbini A, Di Giovanni G, et al. Cryoglobulinaemic neuropathy manifesting with restless legs syndrome. J Neurol Sci 1997;152:218–23.

[74] Frankel BL, Patten BM, Gillin JC. Restless legs syndrome. Sleep-electroencephalographic and neurologic findings. JAMA 1974;230:1302–3.

[75] Iannaccone S, Zucconi M, Marchettini P, et al. Evidence of peripheral axonal neuropathy in primary restless legs syndrome. Mov Disord 1995;10:2–9.

[76] Polydefkis M, Allen RP, Hauer P, et al. Subclinical sensory neuropathy in late-onset restless legs syndrome. Neurology 2000;55:1115–21.

[77] Salvi F, Montagna P, Plasmati R, et al. Restless legs syndrome and nocturnal myoclonus: initial clinical manifestation of familial amyloid polyneuropathy. J Neurol Neurosurg Psychiatry 1990;53:522–5.

[78] O'Hare JA, Abuaisha F, Geoghegan M. Prevalence and forms of neuropathic morbidity in 800 diabetics. Ir J Med Sci 1994;163:132–5.

[79] Rutkove SB, Matheson JK, Logigian EL. Restless legs syndrome in patients with polyneuropathy. Muscle Nerve 1996;19:670–2.

[80] Harriman DG, Taverner D, Woolf AL. Ekbom's syndrome and burning paresthesiae: a biopsy study by vital staining and electron microscopy of the intramuscular innervation with a note on age changes in motor nerve endings. Brain 1970;93:393–406.

[81] Gorman CA, Dyck PJ, Pearson JS. Symptom of restless legs. Arch Int Med 1965;115: 155–60.

[82] Walters AS, Wagner M, Hening WA. Periodic limb movements as the initial manifestation of restless legs syndrome triggered by lumbosacral radiculopathy [letter]. Sleep 1996;19: 825–6.

[83] Bara-Jimenez W, Aksu M, Graham B, et al. Periodic limb movements in sleep: state-dependent excitability of the spinal flexor reflex. Neurology 2000;54:1609–16.

[84] de Mello MT, Lauro FA, Silva AC, et al. Incidence of periodic leg movements and of the restless legs syndrome during sleep following acute physical activity in spinal cord injury subjects. Spinal Cord 1996;34:294–6.

[85] Hartmann M, Pfister R, Pfadenhauer K. Restless legs syndrome associated with spinal cord lesions. J Neurol Neurosurg Psychiatry 1999;66:688–9.

[86] Lee MS, Choi YC, Lee SH, et al. Sleep-related periodic leg movements associated with spinal cord lesions. Mov Disord 1996;11:719–22.

[87] Brown LK, Heffner JE, Obbens EA. Transverse myelitis associated with restless legs syndrome and periodic movements of sleep responsive to an oral dopaminergic agent but not to intrathecal baclofen. Sleep 2000;23:591–4.

[88] Bruno RL. Abnormal movements in sleep as a post-polio sequelae. Am J Phys Med Rehabil 1998;77:339–43.

[89] Hemmer B, Riemann D, Glocker FX, et al. Restless legs syndrome after a borrelia-induced myelitis. Mov Disord 1995;10:521–2.

[90] Winkelmann J, Wetter TC, Trenkwalder C, et al. Periodic limb movements in syringomyelia and syringobulbia. Mov Disord 2000;15:752–3.

[91] Hogl B, Frauscher B, Seppi K, et al. Transient restless legs syndrome after spinal anesthesia: a prospective study. Neurology 2002;59:1705–7.

[92] Moorthy SS, Dierdorf SF. Restless legs during recovery from spinal anesthesia. Anesth Analg 1990;70:337.

[93] Bhatia M, Bhowmik D. Restless legs syndrome in maintenance haemodialysis patients. Nephrol Dial Transplant 2003;18:217.

[94] Callaghan N. Restless legs syndrome in uremic neuropathy. Neurology 1966;16:359–61.

[95] Collado-Seidel V, Kohnen R, Samtleben W, et al. Clinical and biochemical findings in uremic patients with and without restless legs syndrome. Am J Kidney Dis 1998;31:324–8.

[96] Fukunishi I, Kitaoka T, Shirai T, et al. Facial paresthesias resembling restless legs syndrome in a patient on hemodialysis [letter]. Nephron 1998;79:485.

[97] Holley JL, Nespor S, Rault R. Characterizing sleep disorders in chronic hemodialysis patients. ASAIO Trans 1991;37:M456–7.

[98] Hui DS, Wong TY, Ko FW, et al. Prevalence of sleep disturbances in chinese patients with end-stage renal failure on continuous ambulatory peritoneal dialysis. Am J Kidney Dis 2000;36:783–8.

[99] Hui DS, Wong TY, Li TS, et al. Prevalence of sleep disturbances in Chinese patients with end stage renal failure on maintenance hemodialysis. Med Sci Monit 2002;8:CR331–6.

[100] Huiqi Q, Shan L, Mingcai Q. Restless legs syndrome (RLS) in uremic patients is related to the frequency of hemodialysis sessions. Nephron 2000;86:540.

[101] Parker KP. Sleep disturbances in dialysis patients. Sleep Med Rev 2003;7:131–43.

[102] Pieta J, Millar T, Zacharias J, et al. Effect of pergolide on restless legs and leg movements in sleep in uremic patients. Sleep 1998;21:617–22.

[103] Roger SD, Harris DC, Stewart JH. Possible relation between restless legs and anaemia in renal dialysis patients [letter]. Lancet 1991;337:1551.

[104] Sabbatini M, Minale B, Crispo A, et al. Insomnia in maintenance haemodialysis patients. Nephrol Dial Transplant 2002;17:852–6.

[105] Stepanski E, Faber M, Zorick F, et al. Sleep disorders in patients on continuous ambulatory peritoneal dialysis. J Am Soc Nephrol 1995;6:192–7.

[106] Walker SL, Fine A, Kryger MH. L-DOPA/carbidopa for nocturnal movement disorders in uremia. Sleep 1996;19:214–8.

[107] Virga G, Mastrosimone S, Amici G, et al. Symptoms in hemodialysis patients and their relationship with biochemical and demographic parameters. Int J Artif Organs 1998;21:788–93.

[108] Wetter TC, Stiasny K, Kohnen R, et al. Polysomnographic sleep measures in patients with uremic and idiopathic restless legs syndrome. Mov Disord 1998;13:820–4.

[109] Winkelman JW, Chertow GM, Lazarus JM. Restless legs syndrome in end-stage renal disease. Am J Kidney Dis 1996;28:372–8.

[110] Read DJ, Feest TG, Nassim MA. Clonazepam: effective treatment for restless legs syndrome in uraemia. Br Med J (Clin Res Ed) 1981;283:885–6.

[111] Tanaka K, Morimoto N, Tashiro N, et al. The features of psychological problems and their significance in patients on hemodialysis—with reference to social and somatic factors. Clin Nephrol 1999;51:161–76.

[112] Nielsen V. The peripheral nerve function in chronic renal failure. Acta Med Scan 1971;190:105–11.

[113] Benz RL, Pressman MR, Peterson DD. Periodic limb movements of sleep index (PLMSI): a sensitive predictor of mortality in dialysis patients. J Am Soc Nephrology 1994;5:433.

[114] Yasuda T, Nishimura A, Katsuki Y, et al. Restless legs syndrome treated successfully by kidney transplantation–a case report. Clin Transpl 1986;1:138.

[115] Winkelmann J, Stautner A, Samtleben W, et al. Long-term course of restless legs syndrome in dialysis patients after kidney transplantation. Mov Disord 2002;17:1072–6.

[116] Ondo WG, Vuong KD, Jankovic J. Exploring the relationship between Parkinson disease and restless legs syndrome. Arch Neurol 2002;59:421–4.

[117] O'Keeffe ST, Gavin K, Lavan JN. Iron status and restless legs syndrome in the elderly. Age Ageing 1994;23:200–3.

[118] Silber MH, Richardson JW. Multiple blood donations associated with iron deficiency in patients with restless legs syndrome. Mayo Clin Proc 2003;78:52–4.

[119] Sun ER, Chen CA, Ho G, et al. Iron and the restless legs syndrome. Sleep 1998;21:371–7.

[120] Aul EA, Davis BJ, Rodnitzky RL. The importance of formal serum iron studies in the assessment of restless legs syndrome. Neurology 1998;51:912.

[121] Ulfberg J, Nystrom B. Restless legs syndrome in blood donors. Sleep Med 2004;5:115–8.

[122] Ondo W, Tan EK, Mansoor J. Rheumatologic serologies in secondary restless legs syndrome. Movement Disorders 2000;15:321–3.

[123] Earley CJ, Allen RP, Beard JL, et al. Insight into the pathophysiology of restless legs syndrome. J Neurosci Res 2000;62:623–8.

[124] Goodman JD, Brodie C, Ayida GA. Restless leg syndrome in pregnancy. BMJ 1988;297:1101–2.

[125] Botez MI, Lambert B. Folate deficiency and restless-legs syndrome in pregnancy [letter]. N Engl J Med 1977;297:670.

[126] Manconi M, Govoni V, Cesnik E, et al. Epidemiology of restless legs syndrome in a population of 606 pregnant women. Sleep 2003;26(Suppl):A300–1.

[127] Lee KA, Zaffke ME, Baratte-Beebe K. Restless legs syndrome and sleep disturbance during pregnancy: the role of folate and iron. J Womens Health Gend Based Med 2001; 10:335–41.

[128] Ruottinen HM, Partinen M, Hublin C, et al. An FDOPA PET study in patients with periodic limb movement disorder and restless legs syndrome. Neurology 2000;54:502–4.

[129] Wetter TC, Collado-Seidel V, Pollmacher T, et al. Sleep and periodic leg movement patterns in drug-free patients with Parkinson's disease and multiple system atrophy. Sleep 2000;23:361–7.

[130] Braga-Neto P, da Silva FP Jr, Sueli Monte F, et al. Snoring and excessive daytime sleepiness in Parkinson's disease. J Neurol Sci 2004;217:41–5.

[131] Krishnan PR, Bhatia M, Behari M. Restless legs syndrome in Parkinson's disease: a case-controlled study. Mov Disord 2003;18:181–5.

[132] Tan EK, Lum SY, Wong MC. Restless legs syndrome in Parkinson's disease. J Neurol Sci 2002;196:33–6.

[133] Trenkwalder C, Garcia-Borreguero D, Montagna P, et al. Ropinirole in the treatment of restless legs syndrome: results from the TREAT RLS 1 study, a 12 week, randomised, placebo controlled study in 10 European countries. J Neurol Neurosurg Psychiatry 2004; 75:92–7.

[134] Walters AS, Ondo WG, Dreykluft T, et al. Ropinirole is effective in the treatment of restless legs syndrome. TREAT RLS 2: a 12-week, double-blind, randomized, parallel-group, placebo-controlled study. Mov Disord 2004;19:1414–23.

[135] Bogan R, Connolly G, Rederich G. Ropinirole is effective, well tolerated treatment for moderate-to-severe RLS: results of a US study. Mov Disord 2005;20(Suppl 10):S61.

[136] Allen R, Becker PM, Bogan R, et al. Ropinirole decreases periodic leg movements and improves sleep parameters in patients with restless legs syndrome [comment]. Sleep 2004; 27:907–14.

[137] Adler CH, Hauser RA, Sethi K, et al. Ropinirole for restless legs syndrome: a placebo-controlled crossover trial. Neurology 2004;62:1405–7.

[138] Montplaisir J, Nicolas A, Denesle R, et al. Restless legs syndrome improved by pramipexole: a double-blind randomized trial. Neurology 1999;52:938–43.

[139] Oertel W, Stiasney-Kolster K. Pramipexole is effective in the treatment of restless legs syndrome (RLS): results of a 6 week, multi-centre, double, and placebo controlled study. Movement Disorders 2005;20(Suppl 10):S58.

[140] Earley CJ, Yaffee JB, Allen RP. Randomized, double-blind, placebo-controlled trial of pergolide in restless legs syndrome. Neurology 1998;51:1599–602.

[141] Staedt J, Wassmuth F, Ziemann U, et al. Pergolide: treatment of choice in restless legs syndrome (RLS) and nocturnal myoclonus syndrome (NMS). A double-blind randomized crossover trial of pergolide versus L-Dopa. J Neural Transm (Budapest) 1997;104:461–8.

[142] Trenkwalder C, Brandenburg U, Hundemer H, et al. A randomized long-term placebo controlled multicenter trial of pergolide in the treatment of restless legs syndrome with central evaluation of polysomnographic data. Neurology 2001;56(Suppl 3):A5.

[143] Wetter TC, Stiasny K, Winkelmann J, et al. A randomized controlled study of pergolide in patients with restless legs syndrome. Neurology 1999;52:944–50.

[144] Walters AS, Hening WA, Kavey N, et al. A double-blind randomized crossover trial of bromocriptine and placebo in restless legs syndrome. Ann Neurol 1988;24:455–8.

[145] Reuter I, Ellis CM, Ray Chaudhuri K. Nocturnal subcutaneous apomorphine infusion in Parkinson's disease and restless legs syndrome. Acta Neurol Scand 1999;100:163–7.

[146] Happe S, Trenkwalder C. Role of dopamine receptor agonists in the treatment of restless legs syndrome. CNS Drugs 2004;18:27–36.

[147] Benes H, Kurella B, Kummer J, et al. Rapid onset of action of levodopa in restless legs syndrome: a double-blind, multicenter, crossover trial. Sleep 1999;22: 1073–81.

[148] Brodeur C, Montplaisir J, Godbout R, et al. Treatment of restless legs syndrome and periodic movements during sleep with L-dopa: a double-blind, controlled study. Neurology 1988;38:1845–8.

[149] Collado-Seidel V, Kazenwadel J, Wetter TC, et al. A controlled study of additional sr-L-dopa in L-dopa-responsive restless legs syndrome with late-night symptoms. Neurology 1999;52:285–90.

[150] Kaplan PW, Allen RP, Buchholz DW, et al. A double-blind, placebo-controlled study of the treatment of periodic limb movements in sleep using carbidopa/levodopa and propoxyphene. Sleep 1993;16:717–23.

[151] Saletu M, Anderer P, Hogl B, et al. Acute double-blind, placebo-controlled sleep laboratory and clinical follow-up studies with a combination treatment of rr-L-dopa and sr-L-dopa in restless legs syndrome. J Neural Transm 2003;110:611–26.

[152] Allen RP, Earley CJ. Augmentation of the restless legs syndrome with carbidopa/levodopa. Sleep 1996;19:205–13.

[153] Stiasny K, Wetter TC, Winkelmann J, et al. Long-term effects of pergolide in the treatment of restless legs syndrome. Neurology 2001;56:1399–402.

[154] Montplaisir J, Denesle R, Petit D. Pramipexole in the treatment of restless legs syndrome: a follow-up study. Eur J Neurol 2000;7(Suppl 1):27–31.

[155] Silber MH, Shepard JW Jr, Wisbey JA. Pergolide in the management of restless legs syndrome: an extended study. Sleep 1997;20:878–82.

[156] Silber M, Girish M, Izurieta R. Pramipexole in the management of restless legs syndrome: an extended study. Sleep 2001;24(Suppl):A18.

[157] Ferini-Strambi L, Oldani A, Castronovo C, et al. Augmentation of restless legs syndrome after long term treatment with pramipexole and cabergoline. Neurology 2002;58(Suppl 3):A515.

[158] Winkelman JW, Johnston L. Augmentation and tolerance with long-term pramipexole treatment of restless legs syndrome (RLS). Sleep Med 2004;5:9–14.

[159] Ondo W, Romanyshyn J, Vuong KD, et al. Long-term treatment of restless legs syndrome with dopamine agonists. Arch Neurol 2004;61:1393–7.

[160] Stiasny K, Robbecke J, Schuler P, et al. Treatment of idiopathic restless legs syndrome (RLS) with the D2-agonist cabergoline—an open clinical trial. Sleep 2000;23:349–54.

[161] Porter MC, Appiah-Kubf LS, Chaudhuri KR. Treatment of Parkinson's disease and restless legs syndrome with cabergoline, a long-acting dopamine agonist. Int J Clin Pract 2002;56:468–74.

[162] Walters AS, Winkelmann J, Trenkwalder C, et al. Long-term follow-up on restless legs syndrome patients treated with opioids. Mov Disord 2001;16:1105–9.

[163] Walters AS, Wagner ML, Hening WA, et al. Successful treatment of the idiopathic restless legs syndrome in a randomized double-blind trial of oxycodone versus placebo. Sleep 1993;16:327–32.

[164] Ondo W. Methadone for refractory restless legs syndrome. Mov Disord 2005;20:345–8.

[164a] Garcia-Borreguero D, Larrosa O, de la Llave Y, et al. Treatment of restless legs syndrome with gabapentin: a double-blind, cross-over study. Neurology 2002;59(10):1573–9.

[165] O'Keeffe ST, Noel J, Lavan JN. Restless legs syndrome in the elderly. Postgrad Med J 1993;69:701–3.

[166] Davis BJ, Rajput A, Rajput ML, et al. A randomized, double-blind placebo-controlled trial of iron in restless legs syndrome. Eur Neurol 2000;43:70–5.

[167] Earley CJ, Heckler D, Allen RP. The treatment of restless legs syndrome with intravenous iron dextran. Sleep Med 2004;5:231–5.

[168] Sloand JA, Shelly MA, Feigin A, et al. A double-blind, placebo-controlled trial of intravenous iron dextran therapy in patients with ESRD and restless legs syndrome. Am J Kidney Dis 2004;43:663–70.

[169] Garbarino S, De Carli F, Nobili L, et al. Sleepiness and sleep disorders in shift workers: a study on a group of italian police officers. Sleep 2002;25:648–53.

[170] Ohayon MM, Roth T. Prevalence of restless legs syndrome and periodic limb movement disorder in the general population. J Psychosom Res 2002;53:547–54.

[171] Berger K, Luedemann J, Trenkwalder C, et al. Sex and the risk of restless legs syndrome in the general population. Arch Intern Med 2004;164:196–202.

[172] Rothdach AJ, Trenkwalder C, Haberstock J, et al. Prevalence and risk factors of RLS in an elderly population: the MEMO study. Memory and morbidity in Augsburg elderly. Neurology 2000;54:1064–8.

[173] Nichols DA, Allen RP, Grauke JH, et al. Restless legs syndrome symptoms in primary care: a prevalence study. Arch Intern Med 2003;163:2323–9.

[174] Ulfberg J, Nystrom B, Carter N, et al. Restless Legs Syndrome among working-aged women. Eur Neurol 2001;46:17–9.

[175] Ulfberg J, Nystrom B, Carter N, et al. Prevalence of restless legs syndrome among men aged 18 to 64 years: an association with somatic disease and neuropsychiatric symptoms. Mov Disord 2001;16:1159–63.

[176] Lavigne GL, Lobbezoo F, Rompre PH, et al. Cigarette smoking as a risk factor or an exacerbating factor for restless legs syndrome and sleep bruxism. Sleep 1997;20:290–3.

[177] Sevim S, Dogu O, Camdeviren H, et al. Unexpectedly low prevalence and unusual characteristics of RLS in Mersin, Turkey. Neurology 2003;61:1562–9.

[178] Unruh ML, Levey AS, D'Ambrosio C, et al. Restless legs symptoms among incident dialysis patients: association with lower quality of life and shorter survival. Am J Kidney Dis 2004;43:900–9.

[179] Mucsi I, Molnar MZ, Rethelyi J, et al. Sleep disorders and illness intrusiveness in patients on chronic dialysis. Nephrol Dial Transplant 2004;19:1815–22.

[180] Gigli GL, Adorati M, Dolso P, et al. Restless legs syndrome in end-stage renal disease. Sleep Med 2004;5:309–15.

[181] Bhowmik D, Bhatia M, Tiwari S, et al. Low prevalence of restless legs syndrome in patients with advanced chronic renal failure in the Indian population: a case controlled study. Ren Fail 2004;26:69–72.

[182] Takaki J, Nishi T, Nangaku M, et al. Clinical and psychological aspects of restless legs syndrome in uremic patients on hemodialysis. Am J Kidney Dis 2003;41:833–9.

[183] Goffredo Filho GS, Gorini CC, Purysko AS, et al. Restless legs syndrome in patients on chronic hemodialysis in a Brazilian city: frequency, biochemical findings and comorbidities. Arq Neuropsiquiatr 2003;61(3B):723–7.

[184] Kutner NG, Bliwise DL. Restless legs complaint in African-American and Caucasian hemodialysis patients. Sleep Med 2002;3:497–500.

[185] Cirignotta F, Mondini S, Santoro A, et al. Reliability of a questionnaire screening restless legs syndrome in patients on chronic dialysis. Am J Kidney Dis 2002;40:302–6.

[186] Miranda M, Araya F, Castillo JL, et al. Restless legs syndrome: a clinical study in adult general population and in uremic patients. Rev Med Chil 2001;129:179–86.

[187] Walker S, Fine A, Kryger MH. Sleep complaints are common in a dialysis unit. Am J Kidney Dis 1995;26:751–6.

[188] Bastani B, Westervelt FB. Effectiveness of clonidine in alleviating the symptoms of "restless legs" [letter]. Am J Kidney Dis 1987;10:326.

ELSEVIER
SAUNDERS

NEUROLOGIC
CLINICS

Neurol Clin 23 (2005) 1187–1208

Parkinson's Disease and Sleep

Michael J. Thorpy, MD[a],*,
Charles H. Adler, MD, PhD[b]

[a]*Sleep-Wake Disorders Center, Montefiore Medical Center, Bronx, NY, USA*
[b]*Parkinson's Disease and Movement Disorders Center, Mayo Clinic Scottsdale,
Scottsdale, AZ, USA*

Patients with Parkinson's disease have sleep difficulties that include not only difficulty falling or remaining asleep, but also excessive daytime sleepiness (EDS) and abnormal events during sleep. Often the clinical features of the Parkinson's disease (PD) tend to overshadow the sleep difficulties, but they can be as disrupting to patients as the motor symptoms. As patients age, their likelihood of sleep disturbance increases; so, in the elderly patients who have PD, not only are sleep disturbance associated with the primary disorder but also they can be made worse by underlying sleep problems associated with aging. Recognition and management of sleep issues in PD require an in-depth assessment because of the myriad of sleep disorders that can occur; however, it is important to assess these sleep problems, as treating them can improve the patient's overall health, quality of life, and psychologic well-being.

Normal sleep and sleep in the elderly

Normal sleep

The major sleep episode of the day in young, healthy adults typically is a single episode that occurs at night for an average of $7\frac{1}{2}$ to 8 hours. After a sleep latency of approximately 10 minutes, normal sleep begins with non–rapid eye movement (NREM) sleep. Ninety minutes later, REM sleep episodes begin and account for approximately 25% of the night. NREM sleep constitutes approximately 75% of total sleep. NREM and REM sleep

---

* Corresponding author. Sleep-Wake Disorders Center, Montefiore Medical Center, 111 East 210th Street, Bronx, NY 10467-2490.
E-mail address: thorpy@aecom.yu.edu (M.J. Thorpy).

doi:10.1016/j.ncl.2005.05.001   *neurologic.theclinics.com*

alternate cyclically approximately 5 times through the night, with slow wave sleep predominating in the first third of sleep and REM sleep in the last third. Normal, healthy people are awake less than 5% of the night.

Sleep in the elderly

There is greater variability in sleep quality in the elderly compared with that of the young. Nocturnal sleep length decreases as does the amount of slow wave sleep, which may be absent after age 60 [1]. The latency to the first REM sleep episode decreases, although the percentage of REM sleep does not change. Arousals and awakenings are common. Daytime naps become more frequent and older people tend to go to sleep earlier and arise earlier, leading to a phase advance of sleep.

With increasing age, the prevalence of sleep disorders increases [2]. This is explained partly by the increase in sleep pathologies that occur in the elderly, such as sleep apnea, periodic limb movements (PLMs), and REM sleep behavior disorder (RBD); however, other factors play a part, such as deteriorating general health, medication use, and psychologic problems, including the development of anxiety and depression. It is unclear if the elderly have a natural breakdown of the processes involved in sleep, although it seems likely that the ability to maintain good sleep does decrease as one gets older. Not infrequently, elderly people sleep normally and sleep as well as young adults.

The increase in the number of awakenings with increasing age may reflect an inability to maintain a consolidated nocturnal sleep episode, as daytime sleepiness and napping increase in the elderly. The ability to sleep well for the amount of time spent in bed reduces as one gets older. The ratio of sleep to time in bed, known as the sleep efficiency, gradually reduces with age. There is little difference between the sexes with regard to sleep efficiency. A major difference between the young and the elderly is in the tendency for daytime napping. The number of naps increases with age. This reflects a breakdown in the ability to maintain a single consolidated period of nocturnal sleep, and sleep becomes dispersed over the 24-hour period.

Objective measures of sleepiness, such as the Multiple Sleep Latency Test, show that the ability to fall asleep increases with age [3]. Adolescents who sleep well at night are well rested during the day and have little tendency to fall asleep at inappropriate times. With increasing age, the tendency to fall asleep in the daytime increases, and some otherwise healthy elderly are nearly as sleepy in the daytime as younger persons who have sleep apnea or even narcolepsy.

Sleep pathologies are common in the elderly but, when recognized, often can be treated effectively, especially sleep apnea, periodic limb movement disorder (PLMD), and restless legs syndrome (RLS) [4]. Too often, sleep disruption in the elderly is considered a normal part of aging and the underlying causes are not investigated or treated.

The effect of sleep disturbance in the elderly can manifest itself as difficulty sustaining attention, poor response time, decreased performance, and difficulty with memory. Accidents within the home and motor vehicle accidents are common because of these effects. Some elderly are believed demented because of the inability to sustain daytime alertness.

Sleep disorders

Sleep apnea

Sleep-related breathing disorders increase in prevalence with age. The most common disorder is obstructive sleep apnea, although central sleep apnea occurs as a result of cerebrovascular or cardiovascular disease. Breathing disturbances in sleep have an association with increased mortality in the elderly [5]. The elderly are less likely to complain of respiratory disturbance during sleep, despite having symptoms of snoring, gasping, choking, and shortness of breath at night. Episodes of cessation of breathing may be overlooked by elderly spouses.

Restless legs syndrome and periodic limb movement disorder

RLS is discomfort or pain in the legs associated with the uncontrollable desire to move the legs [6]. The symptoms occur typically at night when patients are lying in bed, although they can occur whenever patients are at rest. Sleep-onset insomnia can result and patients may have difficulty returning to sleep if the symptoms reoccur during the night. The criteria for the diagnosis of RLS includes the desire to move the limbs with or without paresthesias or dysesthesias, motor restlessness, symptom exacerbation during the evening or night, and symptom worsening at rest with some relief by activity. The disorder increases in prevalence with age and is believed to affect approximately 15% of elderly patients. Most patients who have RLS have PLMs that occur at 20- to 40-second intervals and last 0.5 to 5 seconds. The movements, which can cause awakenings and arousals, affect one or both of the lower limbs, although usually both limbs are affected.

Rapid eye movement sleep behavior disorder

RBD consists of vigorous and injurious behavior in REM sleep that usually represents attempted enactment of vivid, action-filled, and violent dreams [7]. The activity often involves violent behavior, such as fighting or fleeing from an enemy. Patients often report a prodromal phase, including sleep talking or limb movements in sleep, that often precedes onset of RBD by months or years. The prevalence of RBD is unknown but presents mostly in older males. Overall sleep architecture is normal and the REM/NREM cycle is intact. There is persistence of electromyographic tone during REM sleep, however, which can be seen without the complex RBD behaviors.

The pathophysiology involves functional depression or destruction of brainstem structures responsible for the atonia of REM sleep. There is reduced activity or destruction of brainstem serotonergic or noradrenergic structures responsible for inhibiting phasic activity. The diagnosis of RBD requires polysomnographic monitoring, which shows loss of the generalized muscle atonia of REM sleep or prominent phasic muscle twitching in REM.

Clonazepam is an effective treatment in approximately 90% of patients; 0.5 to 1.0 mg at bedtime usually is sufficient. Tolerance generally does not develop and on discontinuation there usually is immediate relapse. The mechanism of action of clonazepam is unknown. Desipramine may reduce RBD, although some tricyclics can exacerbate RBD. Unpredictable episodes may occur even with pharmacologic management; therefore, it is important to remove dangerous objects from the environment. If medications are ineffective, spouses should move to another bed.

Circadian rhythm sleep disorders

Circadian rhythm sleep disorders are sleep disorders associated with misalignment between patients' sleep pattern and the desired or societal norm [8]. The elderly have a natural tendency for an advancement of the sleep phase. Some elderly people may start to fall asleep as early as 6:00 PM and after 7 or 8 hours of sleep awaken and have difficulty returning to sleep. They may complain of insomnia, but the problem is an advancement of the sleep pattern, not a deterioration of the ability to sleep. The unhealthy elderly also can lose the ability to maintain a regular sleep-wake cycle so that sleep becomes disrupted, an irregular sleep-wake pattern develops, and the likelihood of being asleep at any particular time of day becomes unpredictable.

The sleep-wake cycle in the elderly, as in younger people, is influenced by bright light [9]. Light, via the retina and retinohypothalamic tract, influences the suprachiasmatic nucleus, thereby altering circadian rhythms. As light is an important synchronizer of the sleep-wake cycle, and in many cases elderly patients have a deficiency of bright light exposure, circadian rhythm disorders are not uncommon. In the elderly, advanced sleep phase syndrome often is seen and can be treated by exposure to bright light [10].

Insomnia

Insomnia increases in prevalence with age [4]. The ability to maintain a single episode of unbroken sleep is lost. Psychiatric disorders, such as depression or general anxiety disorder, are common causes, as are conditioned and learned sleep-preventing associations that develop with the breakdown of good sleep hygiene behaviors. Lack of regular exercise, reduced exposure to bright light, and the use of caffeinated beverages or alcohol can be exacerbating factors.

Depression

Depression is a common cause of sleep disturbance in the elderly [11]. Difficulty falling asleep and difficulty remaining asleep are typical features.

Early morning awakening is a cardinal feature of this type of sleep disturbance. Insomnia often is an early sign of mood change and often occurs before clinical depression is evident.

Anti–Parkinson's disease medication effects on sleep

Selegiline

Selegiline, which is metabolized to amphetamine, can disturb sleep and is associated with an increase in arousals at night. Electroencephalographic studies of sleep show increased wakefulness after selegiline [12]. Selegiline is used to treat narcolepsy.

Anticholinergic agents

Anticholinergic agents can have alerting effects on sleep at night and sedative effects in the daytime [13]. The regulation of the sleep-wake cycle is controlled partially by the M1 muscarinic receptor. Benztropine can counteract the sedative properties of chlorpromazine and haloperidol [13]. Sleep studies show that trihexyphenidyl increases wakefulness and decreases REM sleep [14].

Dopaminergic agonists

Dopaminergic agonists (DAs) increase stage 1 sleep and awakenings in healthy controls [15]. It is believed that low-dose dopaminergic medications are more likely to produce insomnia, whereas high-dose dopaminergic medications may produce daytime sleepiness. DAs can produce increased activity at night [16].

Catechol-O-methyltransferase inhibitors

Catechol-O-methyltransferase inhibitors cause an enhancement of dopaminergic activity and may cause an initial worsening of levodopa (L-dopa)–induced adverse effects, such as sleep disorders and hallucinations [17].

Sleep and sleepiness in Parkinson's disease

Fatigue and sleepiness

Disturbed nocturnal sleep, fatigue, and sleepiness are common symptoms in patients who have PD. Although sleepiness and fatigue often are seen as overlapping symptoms, fatigue is distinguished by a sense of tiredness or lack of energy but not necessarily the desire to sleep. Fatigue is difficult to assess accurately as it is a subjective symptom that may not be assessed easily by patients [18]. The relationship between fatigue, physical activity, physical function, and functional capacity has been explored in patients who have PD [19]. The Up and Go Test, leisure activity score, long compliance use, Vo_{2max}, and diastolic blood pressure are the best predictor variables of fatigue. Patients who have severe fatigue are more sedentary and have poorer functional capacity and physical function than those who have less severe fatigue.

Fatigue is reported in patients who have PD to have a prevalence ranging from 42% to 56% of patients [20–22]. Fatigue should not be regarded as part of the normal aging process, and the new onset of fatigue in elderly individuals should be considered a warning sign of psychiatric or somatic disease, including PD. Because patients who report fatigue may have sleep disorders, clinicians should conduct a thorough sleep history.

Fatigue does not correlate with PD disease severity, duration, or depression in patients who have PD but does correlate with depression in normal controls [23]. Fatigue, however, often fails to respond to antidepressants. If depression, dementia, or sleep disturbances are excluded from analysis in patients who have PD, fatigue still is highly prevalent in PD patients.

Amantadine commonly is used to treat fatigue in multiple sclerosis; however, there is no evidence that it is effective in PD, although no controlled studies assessing its efficacy have been performed. Modafinil is shown to treat sleepiness in patients who have PD effectively, but no significant improvement is seen with the fatigue assessment inventory, which includes the fatigue severity scale [24].

Sleep attacks can be considered one end of the sleepiness spectrum, although some patients who have sleep attacks say they are not aware of their sleepiness. Most patients report prodromal signs of tiredness, sometimes described as waves of sleep, followed by a slow and irresistible dozing off. These patients typically sleep for approximately 1 hour and can be awakened but do not remain awake during this time. Infrequently, patients describe irresistible attacks of sleep without warning signs. After 2 to 5 minutes, patients recover abruptly to full wakefulness but cannot give any account of the preceding event. These sudden events are documented with electroencephalograms that show sleep latencies of less than 1 minute. In one case, polysomnography showed abrupt slowing of electroencephalographic background activity and occurrence of slow eye movements and K complexes within 10 seconds after stable wakefulness. Within 60 seconds, the pattern proceeded to stable sleep stage 2 [25].

Consequences

EDS places a significant burden on patients who have PD by interfering with social interactions and work performance. Sleepiness results in feelings of insecurity, anxiety, and depression and can interfere with patients' independence and economic situation. Fatigue severity correlates with poor functional capacity and physical function [19]. Patients who are excessively sleepy may be unable to tolerate increases in the dosages of dopaminergic medications necessary for improved motor control, because these increases may add to their sleepiness.

An important issue to patients who have PD is whether or not they should be allowed to drive. Hobson finds that half of all patients who have PD who drove met criteria for EDS [26]. Many reports in the media and anecdotal word-of-mouth reports describe accidents involving patients who have PD, especially those receiving dopaminergic therapy [27,28]. Because patients who have PD and drive, generally are younger than those who do not and frequently are employed or required to drive for other reasons, the decision to treat these patients with agonists is a clinical dilemma [29]. The results of a recent literature review, however, find only 17 cases where a sleep event occurred during driving, leading to road crashes in 10 [30]. The investigators conclude that sleep attacks are too infrequent to recommend that all patients who have PD, and who take DAs, stop driving.

Risk factors

The evidence of risk factors for developing EDS in patients who have PD supports the influence of disease duration and severity and dopaminergic load and male gender, although some results are somewhat contradictory. Gjerstad and coworkers followed 142 patients who had PD for 4 years and find that the prevalence of EDS went from 7.7% to 29% as disease severity and duration increased [31]. Nocturnal sleeping problems were not considered major risk factors for EDS [31,32].

Pal and collegues propose that "EDS in PD is likely to be multifactorial, most probably arising secondarily to a complex interaction between advancing disease process, increased age, and dopaminergic therapies such as levodopa and dopamine agonists" [33]. These investigators find that the highest Epworth Sleepiness Scale (ESS) scores are seen in treated patients who have more advanced disease and older age.

Central nervous system pathophysiology

The pathophysiology of PD affects areas of the central nervous system that are involved in the control of sleep and wakefulness, particularly the pedunculotegmental nucleus. The pedunculotegmental nucleus is implicated in the control of REM sleep and the akinesia of PD. The caudally directed pathway from the pedunculotegmental nucleus mediates locomotion, whereas the cholinergic ascending thalamic pathways mediate the events of REM sleep [34]. In PD, there seems to be a dysregulation of REM sleep, possibly related to the loss of cholinergic neurons, that influences the balance in the monoaminergic and cholinergic control of sleep [35]. Circadian sleep-wake dysrhythmia in PD may reflect underlying central nervous system pathophysiology affecting the circadian system.

PD motor symptoms can affect sleep. Although tremor usually is reduced during sleep, it may continue and disturb sleep in some patients [36]. Nocturnal dystonia, and nocturnal akinesia that is associated with increased rigidity and stiffness, can affect sleep quality adversely [37,38]. The severity of motor symptoms is reported to be associated with sleep-related events, such as sleepwalking, heavy sweating, and nightmares [36].

Sleep disorders in Parkinson's disease

Nocturnal sleep disturbance

Sleep disorders are common and often severe in PD [11,39,40]. Nocturnal sleep disturbance occurs in 60% to 98% of patients [37,41]. The sleep disturbance correlates with disease severity, Schwab and England score, Unified Parkinsons Disease Rating Scale (UPDRS) part III, L-dopa score, rigidity, and bradykinesia [42].

Deficiencies are found in slow wave sleep, REM/sleep proportions, NREM stages 3 and 4, total sleep time, sleep latency, and sleep efficiency. Sleep fragmentation occurs approximately three times more frequently in patients who have PD than in healthy controls (38.9% versus 12%) [41]. Comparison of polysomnographic sleep measures in 10 drug-free patients who had PD and 10 age-matched healthy controls showed that patients who had PD had significantly less total sleep time, sleep period time, and sleep efficiency. Patients who had PD had more frequent awakenings and greater overall wake time than controls. The groups did not differ in the relative amount of stage 1 and stage 2 sleep, slow wave sleep, or REM sleep. Five patients who had PD, but no control subjects, showed abnormal REM sleep features [43].

Sleep disruptions were not observed in newly diagnosed patients who had PD compared with healthy controls [44]. Also, no significant differences in sleep parameters were observed between patients who had either mild or severe PD with mild and severe disease [44]. Mild and severe groups slept poorly compared with historic controls, with decreased sleep efficiency, increased sleep latency, and decreased REM sleep [44]. Treatment with dopaminergic medications, however, is shown to produce sleep-disruptive effects, with an increase in the number of awakenings and longer duration of stage 1 sleep [15]. The effects are more likely with higher doses of medication. Approximately 40% of patients who have PD take sleeping pills, significantly more than that taken by their healthy elderly contemporaries [41].

Poor nocturnal sleep does not always correlate with EDS. Tandberg and colleagues find the occurrence of nocturnal sleep disorders similar in patients who had PD and EDS compared with those who did not have EDS [41]. Arnulf and coworkers find that in 54 sleepy patients who had PD, shorter Multiple Sleep Latency Test latencies did not correlate with total sleep time or sleep efficiency [45]. In a study of 27 patients who had PD, Rye and colleagues report that sleepiness, defined as short mean sleep latency on the Multiple Sleep Latency Test, correlated with greater total sleep time, better sleep efficiency, shorter sleep latency, and greater stage 1 sleep [46]. One explanation for these findings is that fewer and briefer arousals and shorter awakenings occur as the sleepiness increases in severity.

Treatment of disturbed nocturnal sleep begins with determining the factors involved. Sleep hygiene; sleep disorders, such as sleep apnea, PLMs, RBD, and depression; anxiety disorders; dementia; circadian rhythm disorders; and the effects of medications all need to be assessed in any patients who have PD and disturbed sleep or daytime sleepiness.

Treatment always must include recommendations for good sleep hygiene. Maintaining a regular time for going to bed and a regular wake time with an appropriate amount of time in bed, usually no more than 8 hours, is the mainstay of sleep hygiene. Exposure to bright light, especially on awakening in the morning, and exercise and activity during the daytime are essential to maintaining a strong circadian pattern of sleep and wakefulness. Avoiding caffeinated products during the day and evening prevents excessive daytime stimulation that can affect nocturnal sleep adversely. Avoiding alcohol at night and hunger at sleep time is useful.

Excessive sleepiness

In patients who have PD, 15% to 51% complain of daytime sleepiness [11,26,32,47]. EDS is more frequent in patients who have PD than in healthy controls [32]. The sleepiness can cause cognitive impairment that can range from mild to severe, with deficits in attention, memory, and judgment.

In a review of the literature from July 1999 to May 2001, Homann and coworkers find descriptions of 124 out of 1787 patients (6.6%) who had "sleep events" ranging from "sudden and irresistible sleep confirmed by reliable sources" to "not sudden but irresistible onset of daytime sleep" [30]. In 17 cases, the sleep event happened during driving, leading to motor vehicle crashes in 10.

Factors contributing to daytime sleepiness include, insomnia, mood and anxiety disorders, dementia, motor disorders associated with PD, the effects of PD and other medications, specific sleep disorders, and concurrent medical illness. Severe daytime sleepiness is common in PD and can be related to poor sleep quality, with daytime alertness, as measured by the maintenance of wakefulness test, is impaired as the medication burden increases [48].

Clinicians often underestimate the severity of EDS if they do not get corroborating information from spouses or caretakers. In light of the burden EDS places on patients and caregivers, physicians can play a pivotal role in improving the lives of PD patients who have PD by understanding the causes of EDS and initiating treatment.

Sleep apnea

Airway obstruction or restrictive pulmonary dysfunction is highly prevalent in patients who have PD [49]. The spectrum of respiratory dysfunction includes the primary effects of PD on ventilation and medication-induced pulmonary effects, including L-dopa–induced respiratory dyskinesia [50,51].

Studies show the prevalence of sleep apnea to be 20% to 31% [45,52]. Whether or not sleep apnea is more common in patients who have PD than in healthy elderly subjects and whether or not it plays a major role in EDS is not clear. Several studies report that apnea is not more common in patients who have PD than in controls [11,43,52,53]. Arnulf and colleagues find that 20% of patients who had PD had significant sleep apnea with an apnea-hypopnea index greater than 15 per hour (range, 12–20/h), a prevalence greater than the 2.5% to 4.4% found in elderly Americans [45]. No correlation is found, however, between the apnea-hypopnea index and mean sleep latency, and the investigators conclude that obstructive sleep apnea is not a major factor contributing to the severity of sleepiness in patients who have PD. Snoring is shown to correlate with EDS [54].

Treatment of sleep apnea in the elderly begins with determining the severity of the apnea by polysomnography to determine the baseline respiratory status during sleep, followed by polysomnography with continuous positive airway pressure (CPAP) to determine CPAP's effectiveness. Treatment with CPAP not always is as easy as it is in younger age groups. The elderly tolerate CPAP masks on their face less often and may need frequent instruction on correct use of the CPAP. A bed partner may need to be involved in assisting and encouraging patients to use the device. Other treatments are indicated less often, such as the use of oral appliances or upper airway surgery, unless multiple system atrophy is present with laryngeal stridor, in which case tracheostomy may be indicated.

Restless legs syndrome and periodic limb movements

Ondo and colleagues find that 20.8% of patients who have PD have RLS, twice that of the control population [47]. This can be compared with approximately 10% to 30% of the general population over the age of 65 years. PD preceded the development of RLS in 68% of patients [47]. Tan and colleagues, however, find that none of the 125 patients who had PD they studied met criteria for RLS [55]. The evidence does not support RLS as a major factor in the EDS of patients who have PD. Ondo and colleagues report that RLS is not associated with higher ESS scores [47].

Patients who have PD show increased PLMs during REM and NREM sleep, compared with patients who have multiple system atrophy and healthy controls [43]. Arnulf and coworkers find PLMs in 15% (PLMI range, 16–43/h) of patients who have PD, but no correlation between PLMs and MSL, and conclude that PLMs did not seem to be a significant cause of sleepiness in the 54 patients who had PD [45]. Happe and colleagues find no differences in the occurrence of PLM between 56 patients who had PD and 59 age-matched controls [11].

Whether or not any etiologic relationship exists between PD and RLS/PLMs is not clear. Clinically, both disorders respond to dopaminergic medication and often coexist in patients. Ondo and colleagues report that the presence of RLS did not correlate with factors, such as duration of PD, age, Hoehn and Yahr stage, gender, dementia, use of L-dopa or DAs, history of pallidotomy, or history of deep brain stimulation [47]. Functional imaging data by single photon emission computed tomography suggests impaired central dopaminergic transmission in RLS [56]. It is proposed that striatal dopaminergic nerve cell loss is involved in the increased number of PLMS in patients who have PD. Other evidence, however, suggests pathophysiologic differences between PD and RLS, including no reports of motor fluctuations in patients who have RLS on long-term dopaminergic treatment, lack of increasing RLS severity with progression of PD, and different locations of dopaminergic pathophysiology. It is suggested that RLS may result from reduced dopamine cellular function secondary to local iron deficiency, rather than dopamine cell depletion.

Clinicians should be aware that patients who have PD usually do not reveal RLS symptoms unless specifically asked. Many patients who have PD and RLS believe that RLS symptoms are part of their PD symptom complex.

RLS usually responds well to L-dopa or DAs [57]. Adjustment or initiation of a nighttime dose of L-dopa or dopaminergic medications is helpful. Treatment also is effective in reducing the number of PLMs. Gabapentin (300 mg to 1200 mg dose) also is an effective agent for RLS and may help prevent adverse effects from increasing doses of dopaminergic medications [58].

Rapid eye movement sleep behavior disorder

The occurrence of RBD in PD is reported as varying from 15% to 47% [35,59]. In 45 patients who had PD, 40% had abnormal REM sleep features, defined as REM sleep without atonia and RBD. Those patients who had abnormal REM sleep had lower sleep period times than patients who did not have PD [35].

In a group of 33 patients who had PD, one third met the diagnostic criteria of RBD based on polysomnography recordings, but only one half of these cases would have been detected by history [60]. RBD may be the sole heralding manifestation of eventual PD in older men. In a group of 29 male patients 50 years and older, PD comprised 85% (11/13) of all neurologic disorders emerging after RBD was diagnosed [61]. Compared with patients who had idiopathic RBD, patients who had RBD and who eventually developed PD had significantly longer REM sleep percentages of total sleep time ($P = .007$) and significantly greater limb movements per hour of NREM sleep ($P = .003$). Excessive daytime somnolence was not detected in either group.

Increased muscle activity in REM sleep, an early sign of RBD, is reported in asymptomatic patients who have PD [62]. The prevalence of RBD also seems greater in patients who have PD and who are taking dopaminergic medications [43,45]. Other medications, such as mirtazapine, are reported to cause RBD in patients who have PD [63].

Clonazepam (.5 mg to 3 mg) is shown effective in the treatment of RBD [7]. This medication, however, is long acting and sedative and, therefore, may add to daytime sedation. Other alternatives include the use of melatonin, which also may be helpful as a mild hypnotic agent [64].

Circadian rhythm sleep disorders

PD with severe sleep disruption and daytime sleepiness can lead to an irregular sleep-wake pattern. Patients who have EDS may fall into a cycle of frequent dozing during the daytime and nocturnal wakefulness, a problem for patients and caregivers. In PD, autonomic dysfunction reveals many alterations in circadian regulations, including loss of circadian rhythm of blood pressure, increased diurnal blood pressure variability, and postprandial hypotension [65].

Treatment of day/night reversal relies on restoring normal sleep patterns, and patients should be encouraged to follow the rules of good sleep hygiene to promote daytime activity and wakefulness [41]. Exposure to bight light during the daytime, quiet and rest at night, and physical activity during the daytime all help to reestablish a good sleep-wake pattern.

Insomnia

Insomnia occurs in 32% of patients who have PD [42]. The most common types of insomnia reported by patients who have PD are sleep fragmentation and early awakenings, which are seen more frequently than in age-matched controls. No differences are found between groups in sleep initiation, however [41].

Treatment includes sleep hygiene and consideration of whether or not to use a hypnotic medication, such as zolpidem or zaleplon, or a sedating antidepressant medication, such as a tricyclic medication, such as amitriptyline or doxepin. Melatonin (3 mg 1 to 2 hours before bedtime) can be helpful for some patients, not only to treat insomnia but also to treat RBD effectively [64]. If depression is a factor, then a sedating antidepressant may be indicated or, alternatively, a daytime antidepressant medication, such as a selective serotonin reuptake inhibitor (SSRI), in conjunction with a hypnotic at night.

Other conditions affecting sleep

Depression

Depression occurs in almost 40% of patients who have PD [20,66,67]. Causes of depression in PD range from neurochemical imbalances associated with PD to the consequences of living with a chronic, progressive, degenerative illness. Depression in PD is not correlated with age, disease duration or severity, or cognitive impairment. Depression scores in PD, however, are associated with sleep-onset difficulties and sleep interruptions [35]. It is believed that depressive symptoms and increasing L-dopa doses in patients who had PD caused mainly sleep-onset difficulties and sleep interruptions. Fatigue is not correlated with depression in patients who have PD, although it is correlated in depressed control subjects [23]. SSRIs can be effective, although they can cause excessive agitation, disturb sleep, and worsen Parkinsonian symptoms.

Psychosis

Psychosis can affect almost one fifth of patients who have PD and can add to sleep problems [68]. Hallucinations can develop at any stage of PD and may occur spontaneously or secondary to medications [69]. Psychosis may become more frequent with increasing age and greater cognitive impairment.

The treatment of psychosis involves the reduction of antiparkinsonian medications, by tapering and stopping, if necessary. An antipsychotic drug may need to be added. Clozapine is an effective agent for psychosis in PD and does not producing worsening of parkinsonism [70]. Quetiapine, another atypical neuroleptic drug that does not have the risk of blood dyscrasia, may be as effective as clozapine. Olanzapine and risperidone can aggravate parkinsonism and should be used only as a last resort.

Pain

Pain, associated most commonly with foot dyskinesia, is noted in approximately 50% of all patients who have PD. Because the pain often is linked to "off" states or insufficient doses of dopaminergic therapy, adjustment of antiparkinsonian medications may provide relief. Treatment of pain in PD may require the use of pain medications, such as acetaminophen or an opiate derivative. Acupuncture therapy is reported as helpful [71].

Cognitive impairment

Cognitive impairment is becoming a common and troublesome issue now that patients are living longer. The prevalence of dementia has risen to almost 70% in those over 80 years old [40]. Patients who have dementia generally are older, have developed PD at an older age, have longer disease durations, and have a history of hallucinations. More than three quarters of a representative PD cohort developed dementia during an 8-year study period [72]. Early hallucinations and akinetic-dominant PD are associated with an increased risk of dementia.

Cholinesterase inhibitors may help in the amelioration of some symptoms in patients who have dementia of the Alzheimer's type with PD. The three most widely used cholinesterase inhibitors are donepezil, rivastigmine, and galantamine [73]. Olanzapine may affect the progression of PD adversely. As well as providing cognitive benefits, there also is evidence that cholinesterase inhibitors can produce beneficial effects on the neuropsychiatric and behavioral disturbances and activities of daily living. Donepezil (5 mg daily), in addition to an ongoing treatment with perphenazine, was shown to be helpful in improving delusions or psychotic symptoms [74].

Autonomic disorders

Autonomic disorders affect most patients who have PD [39,75]. Some are related to the normal aging process (nocturia, daytime urge incontinence, impotence, and hypothermia), but other symptoms, such as dysphagia and paroxysmal sweating, are associated more specifically with PD. Still other problems, such as orthostatic hypotension, constipation, and bladder retention, may be secondary to antiparkinsonian medications.

Pharmacotherapy may be useful to treat orthostasis, gastrointestinal, urinary, and sexual dysfunction. Treatment with the salt-retaining steroid fludrocortisone may help reduce orthostasis.

Nocturia

Frequent urination can disrupt sleep [76]. There is an increased prevalence of nocturia in PD, and overflow incontinence and spastic bladder also can occur [37]. In patients who have PD, 80% have two or more episodes of nocturia per night and 33% urinate at least three times per night [37]. The frequency of nocturia increases with PD severity [44]. In a group of 41 idiopathic patients who had Parkinson' disease, 32 (78%) had urinary symptoms with frequency in 27 cases (65%), urgency in 9 cases (21%), urge incontinence in one case and dysuria in one case [77].

A urologic evaluation is useful in assessing the exact cause of the nocturia. Treatment of an underlying sleep disorder, such as sleep apnea, often can reduce nocturia. Urinary frequency also may occur as the dose of dopaminergic medication wears off and, therefore, a change to a longer-acting form of medication at night may be required. Anticholinergic medications can produce urinary dysfunction and the dose of such medications may need to be reduced. Intranasal desmopressin can be helpful [78]. Specific bladder medications may be required for some patients. If prostatic enlargement is a factor, a long-acting $\alpha(1)$-adrenergic receptor blocking agent, such as terazosin, may be helpful. The antimuscarinic anticholinergic drugs, tolterodine and extended-release oxybutynin, may be useful if an overactive bladder is a factor.

Nightmares

Kumar reports that 32% of patients who have PD had nightmares [42]. He finds that nightmares correlate with the Hoehn and Yahr stage, high UPDRS, and L-dopa dose. Some patients who have PD also manifest other parasomnias associated with dreams, such as vivid dreams, altered dream content, night terrors, RBD, and hallucinations.

Nightmares may be helped by reducing medications that could contribute to disrupted REM sleep, including anticholinergic medications, antidepressants, L-dopa, and DAs.

Hallucinations

Up to 40% of patients who have PD are reported to have hallucinations [79]. In patients who have PD and who have hallucinations, the hallucinations seem to be related temporally with either REM sleep at night or daytime NREM sleep [80]. Hallucinations often are associated with RBD [59,81]. RBD was detected in 10 patients who had PD without dementia who had hallucinations [59]. Hallucinators tended to be sleepier during the day. Delusions following nighttime REM periods and daytime REM onsets were observed in some of the hallucinators. Daytime hallucinations, coincident with REM sleep intrusions during periods of wakefulness, were reported only by hallucinators. Hallucinations also can be induced by PD medications [79]. Other investigators find that hallucinations increase with duration of disease and can be independent of the degree of sleep disturbance. Vivid dreams or nightmares in nonhallucinators do not predict future development of hallucinations [73].

The treatment of hallucinations includes treating underlying sleep disorders, such as RBD, and assessing the effects of dopaminergic medications. Clozapine or quetiapine may be required [73].

Medications

Effects on nocturnal sleep

Medications that can disrupt nocturnal sleep include PD medications, antidepressants, anticholinergics, and stimulants. Of the PD medications, selegiline, which is metabolized to amphetamine, is one of the most likely to cause sleep-onset insomnia. DAs, stimulating antidepressants, and amantadine also may disrupt nighttime sleep. Withdrawal from benzodiazepines and other sedatives can cause rebound insomnia [82].

Sleep disturbance is more common in those taking DAs [11]. There is little difference in sleep prevalence of sleep disturbances between those who take ergoline medications (11.9%) compared with nonergoline medications (9.1%). Those taking DAs continuously, however, had less sleep disturbance than those newly taking DAs. Sleep problems increase in those who discontinue DAs.

Nausieda and colleagues report that chronic L-dopa therapy was associated with disturbed nocturnal sleep in 74% of patients who had PD [83]. In addition, L-dopa is shown to reduce REM sleep latency and cause inhibition of REM sleep [84,85]. With prolonged treatment, REM returns to normal levels [86]. The sudden stopping of L-dopa can give a REM rebound that can last as long as 10 days [85]. Others find that chronic therapy with L-dopa can lead to increased REM sleep [87]. Garcia-Borreguero and coworkers did not find a difference in the sleep of patients who had PD treated with L-dopa as compared with controls [58]. In patients newly diagnosed with PD, Brunner and colleagues find an increase in stage 1 sleep and the number of awakenings after administration of PD medications [15]. There also is an increase in nocturnal activity and dyskinesias in patients taking PD medications [16].

It seems that low-dose DAs can improve sleep by preventing PD symptoms from interfering with sleep, but high doses can suppress REM sleep and be disruptive to sleep by causing awakenings and increasing nocturnal activity.

Excessive daytime sleepiness

Frucht and coworkers were the first to bring attention to the role of dopaminergic medications in producing EDS in patients who have PD [27].

He described eight patients who had PD who were taking pramipexole and one taking ropinirole who fell asleep when driving, causing accidents. Five experienced no warning before falling asleep, but the attacks ceased when the drugs were stopped. In an open-label trial of pramipexole, 57% of patients who had PD reported somnolence as an adverse event [88]. Since then, studies of patients who have PD report that up to 30% of patients who have PD and who take DAs have sleep attacks [89]. EDS was reported more prevalent in patients who had PD and were taking DAs than in those not taking DAs [90]. There seems no greater prevalence of EDS in those taking ergoline DAs (11.9%) than those taking nonegoline DAs (9.1%), whereas those taking no medications had a prevalence of 4.5% [90]. Patients who commenced taking DAs have a higher prevalence of EDS than those taking DAs continuously [90]. Other large population studies show that, independent of medication taken, patients who have PD have a high prevalence (51%) of EDS [26]. Patients who have sleepiness report relatively continuous drowsiness that may lead to falling asleep without acute warning during periods of inactivity [88].

Sleepiness may be a common side effect of L-dopa and DAs. In a 10-week safety and efficacy study of pramipexole for PD, somnolence was the most frequently noted adverse event and was reported in approximately 30% of patients receiving pramipexole (3–6 mg/d) [91]. In controlled, randomized, double-blind clinical trials, somnolence occurred as an adverse event in 32.4% of patients treated with pramipexole compared with 17.3% of those treated with L-dopa ($P < .01$) and in 27.4% of patients treated with ropinirole versus 19.1% of L-dopa–treated patients (not significant) [92,93]. No differences were found in the level of EDS between patients treated with a nonergot DA plus L-dopa, an ergot DA plus L-dopa, and L-dopa monotherapy, suggesting it is a class effect of all dopaminergic drugs [33].

Sleepiness in PD is reported to be associated with the total dopaminergic dose of medication rather than whether or not the medication is an ergot or nonergot DA or the specific type of DA [94]. Reducing the dose or discontinuing the medication usually resolves dopaminergic medication-induced sleepiness. The risk of somnolence is of particular concern for the elderly, those who have preexisting sleep disorders, and those receiving multiple medications. This can be problematic particularly for patients who drive [27]. Patients taking dopaminergic medications should be warned about this potential effect.

Many other types of medications can contribute to EDS in patients who have PD. Comella proposes that the high frequency of nocturnal sleep disorders with consequent sleep deprivation in patients who have PD may increase their susceptibility to the sedative adverse effects of many centrally active drugs [82]. Strategies to control medication-induced EDS are to reduce or discontinue the sedative medication if possible and, if necessary, substitute with one that has less sedative properties [95].

Deep brain stimulation and sleep

Deep brain stimulation is effective for the treatment of patients who have advanced PD whose condition can no longer be improved by adjustment of medical therapy. Deep brain stimulation of the subthalamic nucleus reduces motor disability and total medication intake; therefore, sleep disturbance often is improved. Chronic deep brain stimulation of the subthalamic nucleus may improve sleep quality through increased nocturnal mobility and reduction of sleep fragmentation [96].

Treatment of excessive sleepiness

Amphetamines and methylphenidate have been used for many years to treat sleepiness, especially that associated with narcolepsy. These medications are used to treat sleepiness in PD but there is little information available about their use. Concerns are expressed about the cardiovascular consequences of stimulants; they also can cause rebound hypersomnolence as they wear off.

More recently, modafinil has become available for the treatment of sleepiness in narcolepsy. Two double-blind studies show that modafinil (100 to 200 mg per day) can be useful in treating sleepiness in PD [24,97]. Modafinil has the advantage of having fewer side effects and less evidence of cardiovascular consequences than the stimulants.

Other medications used to treat sleepiness include buproprion, which not only helps depression but also has stimulant effects and may improve alertness in some patients [98]. Caffeine can be used to improve alertness but may be limited because of its general stimulant slide effects that can cause nervousness and cardiovascular side effects.

Summary

Sleep disorders are common in PD and many factors can contribute to disturbed nocturnal sleep and daytime sleepiness. Factors contributing to sleep disturbance include the presence of insomnia, mood or anxiety disorders, dementia, specific sleep disorders, PD motor disorders, and the effects of PD or medications. Patients who have PD should be interrogated about sleep disturbance and daytime sleepiness and preferably, because of underestimation of the severity of sleepiness or lack of awareness, patients should be interviewed in the presence of a close friend or relative. The ability to drive, if sleepiness is present, should be assessed and appropriate recommendations made. Treatment of sleepiness involves treating any underlying sleep disturbance and may involve the use of stimulant or alerting medications in the daytime.

References

[1] Williams R, Karacan I, Hursch C. Electroencephalography (EEG) of human sleep: cinical applications. New York: John Wiley & Sons; 1974.

[2] Karacan I, Thornby JI, Anch M, et al. Prevalence of sleep disturbance in a primarily urban Florida County. Soc Sci Med 1976;10:239–44.

[3] Carskadon MA, van den Hoed J, Dement WC. Sleep and daytime sleepiness in the elderly. J Geriatr Psychiatry 1980;13:135–51.

[4] Ancoli-Israel S. Epidemiology of sleep disorders. Clin Geriatr Med 1989;5:347–62.

[5] Ancoli-Israel S, Kripke DF, Klauber MR, et al. Morbidity, mortality and sleep-disordered breathing in community dwelling elderly. Sleep 1996;19:277–82.

[6] Stacy M. Sleep disorders in Parkinson's disease: epidemiology and management. Drugs Aging 2002;19:733–9.

[7] Schenck CH, Bundlie SR, Mahowald MW. Delayed emergence of a parkinsonian disorder in 38% of 29 older men initially diagnosed with idiopathic rapid eye movement sleep behaviour disorder. Neurology 1996;46:388–93 [published erratum appears in Neurology 1996; 46:1787].

[8] Dagan Y. Circadian rhythm sleep disorders (CRSD). Sleep Med Rev 2002;6:45–54.

[9] Youngstedt SD, Kripke DF, Elliott JA, et al. Circadian abnormalities in older adults. J Pineal Res 2001;31:264–72.

[10] Fukuda N, Kobayashi R, Kohsaka M, et al. Related Articles, links effects of bright light at lunchtime on sleep in patients in a geriatric hospital II. Psychiatry Clin Neurosci 2001;55: 291–3.

[11] Happe S, Pirker W, Sauter C, et al. Sleep disorders and depression in patients with Parkinson's disease. Acta Neurol Scand 2001;104:275–80.

[12] Thornton C, Dore CJ, Elsworth JD, et al. The effect of deprenyl, a selective monoamine oxidase B inhibitor, on sleep and mood in man. Psychopharmacology (Berl) 1980;70:163–6.

[13] Singh MM, Kay SR. A comparative study of haloperidol and chlorpromazine in terms of clinical effects and therapeutic reversal with benztropine in schizophrenia. Theoretical implications for potency differences among neuroleptics. Psychopharmacologia 1975;43: 103–13.

[14] Zoltoski RK, Velazquez-Moctezuma J, Shiromani PJ, et al. The relative effects of selective M1 muscarinic antagonists on rapid eye movement sleep. Brain Res 1993;608:186–90.

[15] Brunner H, Wetter TC, Hoegl B, et al. Microstructure of the non-Rapid Eye Movement Sleep Electroencephalogram in patients with newly diagnosed Parkinson's disease: Effects of dopaminergic treatment. Mov Disord 2002;17:928–33.

[16] van Hilten B, Hoff JI, Middelkoop HA, et al. Sleep disruption in Parkinson's disease. Assessment by continuous activity monitoring. Arch Neurol 1994;51:922–8.

[17] Kaakkola S. Clinical pharmacology, therapeutic use and potential of COMT inhibitors in Parkinson's disease. Drugs 2000;59:1233–50.

[18] Schwid SR. Are studies of fatigue worth the effort? Neurology 2003;60:1057.

[19] Gerber CE, Friedman JH. Effects of fatigue on physical activity and function in patients with Parkinson's Disease. Neurology 2003;60:1119–24.

[20] Friedman JH, Friedman H. Fatigue in Parkinson's disease: a nine-year follow-up. Mov Disord 2001;16:1120–2.

[21] Herlofson K, Larsen JP. The influence of fatigue on health-related quality of life in patients with Parkinson's disease. Acta Neurol Scand 2003;107:1–6.

[22] Karlsen K, Larsen JP, Tandberg E, et al. Fatigue in patients with Parkinson's disease. Mov Disord 1999;14:237–41.

[23] Abe K, Takanashi M, Yanagihara T. Fatigue in patients with Parkinson's disease. Behav Neurol 2000;12:103–6.

[24] Adler CH, Caviness JN, Hentz JG, et al. Randomized trial of modafinil for treating subjective daytime sleepiness in patients with Parkinson's disease. Mov Disord 2003;18:287–93.

[25] Tracik F, Ebersbach G. Sudden daytime sleep onset in Parkinson's disease: polysomnographic recordings. Mov Disord 2001;16:500–6.

[26] Hobson DE, Lang AE, Martin WR, et al. Excessive daytime sleepiness and sudden-onset sleep in Parkinson disease: a survey by the Canadian Movement Disorders Group. JAMA 2002;287:455–63.

[27] Frucht S, Rogers JD, Greene PE, et al. Falling asleep at the wheel: motor vehicle mishaps in persons taking pramipexole and ropinirole. Neurology 1999;52:1908–10.

[28] Schlesinger I, Ravin PD. Dopamine agonists induce episodes of irresistible daytime sleepiness. Eur Neurol 2003;49:30–3.

[29] Comella CL. Daytime sleepiness, agonist therapy, and driving in Parkinson's disease. JAMA 2002;287:509–11.

[30] Homann CN, Wenzel K, Suppan K, et al. Sleep attacks in patients taking dopamine agonists: review. BMJ 2002;324:1483–7.

[31] Gjerstad MD, Aarsland D, Larsen JP. Development of daytime somnolence over time in Parkinson's disease. Neurology 2002;58:1544–6.

[32] Tandberg E, Larsen JP, Karlsen K. Excessive daytime sleepiness and sleep benefit in Parkinson's disease: a community based study. Mov Disord 1999;14:922–7.

[33] Pal S, Bhattacharya R, Agapito C, et al. A study of excessive daytime sleepiness and its clinical significance in three groups of Parkinson's disease patients taking pramipexole, cabergoline and levodopa mono and combination therapy. J Neural Trans 2001;108:71–7.

[34] Lee MS, Rinne JO, Marsden CD. The pedunculopontine nucleus: its role in the genesis of movement disorders. Yonsei Med J 2000;41:167–84.

[35] Wetter TC, Trenkwalker C, Gershanik O, et al. Polysomnographic measures in Parkinson's disease: A comparison between patients with and without REM sleep disturbances. Wien Klin Wochenschr 2001;113:249–53.

[36] Stern M, Roffwarg H, Duvoisin R. The parkinsonian tremor in sleep. J Nerv Ment Dis 1968;147:202–10.

[37] Lees AJ, Blackburn NA, Campbell VL. The nighttime problems of Parkinson's disease. Clin Neuropharmacol 1988;11:512–9.

[38] Happe S, Ludemann P, Berger K. The association between disease severity and sleep-related problems in patients with Parkinson's disease. Neuropsychobiology 2002;46:90–6.

[39] Hiner BC. Autonomic complications of Parkinson's disease. In: Adler CH, Ahlskog JE, editors. Parkinson's disease and movement disorders: diagnosis and treatment guidelines for the practicing physician. Rochester (MN): Mayo Foundation for Medical Education and Research; 2002.

[40] Mayeux R, Denaro J, Hemenegildo N, et al. A population-based investigation of Parkinson's disease. J Neurol Neurosurg Psychiatry 1992;55:566–71.

[41] Tandberg E, Larsen JP, Karlsen K. A community-based study of sleep disorders patients with Parkinson's disease. Mov Disord 1998;13:895–9.

[42] Kumar S, Bhatia M, Behari M. Sleep disorders in Parkinson's disease. Mov Disord 2002;17: 775–81.

[43] Wetter TC, Collado-Seidel V, Pollmacher T, et al. Sleep and periodic leg movement patterns in drug-free patients with Parkinson's disease and multiple system atrophy. Sleep 2000;23: 361–7.

[44] Young A, Horne M, Churchward T, et al. Comparison of sleep disturbance in mild versus severe Parkinson's disease. Sleep 2002;25:573–7.

[45] Arnulf I, Konofal E, Merino-Andreu M, et al. Parkinson's disease and sleepiness: an integal part of PD. Neurology 2002;58:1019–24.

[46] Rye DB, Bliwise DL, Dihenia B, et al. Daytime sleepiness in Parkinson's disease. J Sleep Res 2000;9:63–9.

[47] Ondo WG, Vuong KD, Khan H, et al. Daytime sleepiness and other sleep disorders in Parkinson's disease. Neurology 2001;57:1392–6.

[48] Stevens S, Cormella CL, Stepanski EJ. Daytime sleepiness and alertness in patients with Parkinson disease. Sleep 2004;27:967–72.

[49] Sabate M, Rodriguez M, Mendez E, et al. Obstructive and restrictive pulmonary dysfunction increases disability in Parkinson's disease. Arch Phys Med Rehabil 1996;77:29–34.

[50] Shill H, Stacy M. Respiratory function in Parkinson's disease. Clin Neurosci 1998;5: 131–5.

[51] Rice JE, Antic R, Thompson PD. Disordered respiration as a levodopa-induced dyskinesia in Parkinson's disease. Mov Disord 2002;17:524–7.

[52] Ferini-Strambi L, Franceschi M, Pinto P, et al. Respiration and heart rate variability during sleep in untreated Parkinson patients. Gerontology 1992;38:92–8.

[53] Apps MC, Sheaff PC, Ingram DA, et al. Respiration and sleep in Parkinson's disease. J Neurol Neurosurg Psychiatry 1985;48:1240–5.

[54] Hogl B, Seppi K, Brandauer E, et al. Increased daytime sleepiness in Parkinson's disease: a questionnaire survey. Mov Disord 2003;18:319–23.

[55] Tan EK, Lum SY, Wong MC. Restless legs syndrome in Parkinson's disease. J Neurol Sci 2002;196:33–6.

[56] Happe S, Pirker W, Klosch G, et al. Periodic leg movements in patients with Parkinson's disease are associated with reduced striatal dopamine transporter binding. J Neurol 2003; 250:83–6.

[57] Happe S, Trenkwalder C. Movement disorders in sleep: Parkinson's disease and restless legs syndrome. Biomed Tech (Berl) 2003;48:62–7.

[58] Garcia-Borreguero D, Larrosa O, de la Llave Y, et al. Treatment of restless legs syndrome with gabapentin: a double-blind, cross-over study. Neurology 2002;59:1573–9.

[59] Arnulf I, Bonnet AM, Damier P, et al. Hallucinations, REM sleep, and Parkinson's disease: a medical hypothesis. Neurology 2000;55:281–8.

[60] Eisensehr I, v Lindeiner H, Jager M, et al. REM sleep behavior disorder in sleep-disordered patients with versus without Parkinson's disease: is there a need for polysomnography? J Neurol Sci 2001;186:7–11.

[61] Gagnon JF, Bedard MA, Fantini ML, et al. REM sleep behavior disorder and REM sleep without atonia in Parkinson's disease. Neurology 2002;59:585–9.

[62] Sonka K, Juklickova M, Hnidkova P. [Manifestations of abnormal behavior during REM sleep in all-night polysomnography in patients with Parkinson disease]. Sb Lek 2000;101: 353–6.

[63] Onofrj M, Luciano AL, Thomas A, et al. Mirtazapine induces REM sleep behavior disorder (RBD) in parkinsonism. Neurology 2003;60:113–5.

[64] Kunz D, Bes F. Melatonin as a therapy in REM sleep behavior disorder patients: an open-labeled pilot study on the possible influence of melatonin on REM-sleep regulation. Mov Disord 1999;14:507–11.

[65] Bruguerolle B, Simon N. Biologic rhythms and Parkinson's disease: a chronopharmaco-logic approach to considering fluctuations in function. Clin Neuropharmacol 2002;25: 194–201.

[66] Cummings JL. Depression and Parkinson's disease: a review. Am J Psychiatry 1992;149: 443–54.

[67] Schrag A, Jahanshahi M, Quinn NP. What contributes to depression in Parkinson's disease? Psychol Med 2001;31:65–73.

[68] Cummings JL. Managing psychosis in patients with Parkinson's disease. N Engl J Med 1999; 340:801–3.

[69] Chacon JR, Duran E, Duran JA, et al. [Usefulness of olanzapine in the levodopa-induced psychosis in patients with Parkinson's disease.] Neurologia 2002;17:7–11.

[70] Pollak P. Rev Neurol (Paris) 2002;158(Spec no 1):S125–31.

[71] Shulman LM, Wen X, Weiner WJ, et al. Acupuncture therapy for the symptoms of Parkinson's disease. Mov Disord 2002;17:799–802.

[72] Aarsland D, Andersen K, Larsen JP, et al. Prevalence and characteristics of dementia in Parkinson disease: an 8-year prospective study. Arch Neurol 2003;60:387–92.

[73] Goetz CG, Wuu J, Curgian LM, et al. Hallucinations and sleep disorders in PD: six-year prospective longitudinal study. Neurology 2005;64:81–6.

[74] Bergman J, Brettholz I, Shneidman M, et al. Donepezil as add-on treatment of psychotic symptoms in patients with dementia of the Alzheimer's type. Clin Neuropharmacol 2003;26: 88–92.

[75] Zesiewicz TA, Baker MJ, Wahba M, et al. Autonomic nervous system dysfunction in Parkinson's disease. Curr Treat Options Neurol 2003;5:149–60.

[76] Araki I, Kitahara M, Oida T, et al. Voiding dysfunction and Parkinson's disease: urodynamic abnormalities and urinary symptoms. J Urol 2000;164:1640–3.

[77] Krygowska-Wajs A, Weglarz W, Szczudlik ZD. [Micturition disturbances in Parkinson's disease. Clinical and urodynamic evaluation.] Neurol Neurochir Pol 2002;36:25–32.

[78] Rembratt A, Norgaard JP, Andersson KE. Desmopressin in elderly patients with nocturia: short-term safety and effects on urine output, sleep and voiding patterns. BJU Int 2003;91: 642–6.

[79] Fenelon G, Mahieux F, Huon R, et al. Hallucinations in Parkinson's disease: prevalence, phenomenology and risk factors. Brain 2000;123(Pt 4):733–45.

[80] Manni R, Pacchetti C, Terzaghi M, et al. Hallucinations and sleep-wake cycle in PD. Neurology 2002;59:1979–81.

[81] Comella CL, Tanner CM, Ristanovic RK. Polysomnographic sleep measures in Parkinson's disease patients with treatment-induced hallucinations. Ann Neurol 1993;34:710–4.

[82] Comella CL. Sleep and Parkinson's disease. In: Adler CH, Ahlskog JE, editors. Parkinson's disease and movement disorders: diagnosis and treatment guidelines for the practicing physician. Totawa (NJ): Humana Press; 2000.

[83] Nausieda PA, Weiner WJ, Kaplan LR, et al. Sleep disruption in the course of chronic levodopa therapy: an early feature of the levodopa psychosis. Clin Neuropharmacol 1982;5: 183–94.

[84] Gillin JC, Post RM, Wyatt R, et al. REM inhibitory effect of L-Dopa infusion during human sleep. Electroenceph Clin Neurophys 1973;35:181–6.

[85] Wyatt RJ, Chase TN, Scott J, et al. Effect of L-Dopa on the sleep of man. Nature 1970;228: 999–1001.

[86] Kales A, Ansel RD, Markham CH, et al. Sleep in patients with Parkinson's Disease and in normal subjects prior to and following levodopa administration. Clin Pharmacol Ther 1971; 12:397–406.

[87] Schmidt HS, Knopp W. Sleep in Parkinson's Disease: the effect of L-dopa. Psychophys-iology 1972;9:88–9.

[88] Hauser RA, Gauger L, Anderson WM, et al. Pramipexole-induced somnolence and episodes of daytime sleep. Mov Disord 2000;15:658–63.

[89] Montastruc JL, Brefel-Courbon C, Senard JM, et al. Sudden sleep attacks and antiparkinsonism drugs: a pilot prospective pharmacoepidemiological study. Clin Neuropharmacol 2001;24:181–3.

[90] Happe S, Berger K. The association of dopamine agonists with daytime sleepiness, sleep problems and quality of life in patients with Parkinson's disease—a prospective study. J Neurol 2001;248:1062–7.

[91] Parkinson Study Group. Safety and efficacy of pramipexole in early Parkinson's disease. JAMA 1997;273:125–30.

[92] Parkinson Study Group. Pramipexole vs. levodopa as initial treatment for Parkinson disease. JAMA 2000;284:1931–8.

[93] Rascol O, Brooks DJ, Korczyn AD, et al. A five-year study of the incidence of dyskinesia in patients with early Parkinson's disease who were treated with ropinirole or levodopa. N Engl J Med 2000;342:1484–91.

[94] Razmy A, Lang AE, Shapiro CM. Predictors of impaired daytime sleep and wakefulness in patients with Parkinson disease treated with older (ergot) vs newer (nonergot) dopamine agonists. Arch Neurol 2004;61:97–102.

[95] Olanow CW, Watts RL, Koller WC. An algorithm (decision tree) for the management of Parkinson's disease (2001): treatment guidelines. Neurology 2001;56(Suppl 5):S1–88.

[96] Antonini A, Landi A, Mariani C, et al. Deep brain stimulation and its effect on sleep in Parkinson's disease. Sleep Med 2004;5:211–4.

[97] Hogl B, Saletu M, Brandauer E, et al. Modafinil for the treatment of daytime sleepiness in Parkinson's disease: a double-blind, randomized, crossover, placebo-controlled polygraphic trial. Sleep 2002;25:905–9.

[98] Goetz CG, Tanner CM, Klawans HL. Bupropion in Parkinson's disease. Neurology 1984;34:1092–4.

ELSEVIER
SAUNDERS

Neurol Clin 23 (2005) 1209–1223

NEUROLOGIC
CLINICS

Sleep and Neuromuscular Disorders

Antonio Culebras, MD[a,b,*]

[a]Department of Neurology, Upstate Medical University, Syracuse, New York, USA
[b]The Sleep Center Community General Hospital, Syracuse, New York, USA

The unique physiologic conditions that concur in sleep may reveal or aggravate respiratory dysfunction when ventilatory mechanisms are compromised as a result of neuromuscular disease. This includes lower motor neuron disease, alterations of the neuromuscular junction, and disorders of muscle. Reduction of muscle tone in non–rapid eye movement (NREM) sleep and frank loss of muscle tone and activity of intercostal muscles with preservation or enhancement of diaphragmatic drive in REM sleep determine a unique series of circumstances in patients who have muscular disorders. The pattern of ventilatory deficit may be diverse as a result of the various clinical forms of muscular weakness. Focal deficit of diaphragm function, as in acid maltase deficiency [1], is characterized by REM sleep-related nocturnal breathlessness and respiratory failure before limb weakness becomes symptomatic. The generalized myopathies, such as Duchenne's muscular dystrophy, present sleep-related ventilatory deficiency only in terminal stages of the disease. These alterations potentially are correctable so that their recognition and characterization become part of the work-up of patients who have a neuromuscular disorder.

Conditions that are associated with central neurologic disease may show other patterns of involvement. Although ventilatory dysfunction is the prime sleep-related abnormality in most patients who have neuromuscular disorders, some sleep alterations cannot be explained solely on the basis of a mechanical respiratory disorder. Patients who have myotonic dystrophy may have excessive daytime somnolence that is not corrected with ventilatory assistance or that appears in excess of, or in the absence of, a ventilatory impediment. These patients may have an intrinsic form of excessive daytime somnolence of central origin that remains poorly understood. In some forms of congenital myopathy, there is impairment of respiratory chemosensitivity

---

* Department of Neurology, Upstate Medical University, 750 East Adams Street, Syracuse, New York 13210.
 E-mail address: aculebras@aol.com

0733-8619/05/$ - see front matter © 2005 Elsevier Inc. All rights reserved.
doi:10.1016/j.ncl.2005.08.004
neurologic.theclinics.com

with reduced sleep-related ventilatory drive independent of hypoxemia and hypercapnia, suggesting a central dysfunction and not a mere blunting of chemosensitivity.

Overview of neuromuscular factors associated with sleep-related respiratory dysfunction

In patients who have neuromuscular disease, weakness of the diaphragm is a major determinant factor of the pattern of respiratory compromise. The diaphragm may be weak in isolation, as in phrenic nerve paralysis, or as part of a generalized muscle involvement, as in amyotrophic lateral sclerosis (ALS). Diaphragm muscle weakness becomes specifically manifest during REM sleep, when the diaphragm is, under normal circumstances, the only effective muscle pump. Patients who have diaphragm paralysis cannot breathe while supine, even in the awake state. Lesser forms of diaphragm muscle weakness become apparent during REM sleep, particularly if patients lie supine. Individuals who have neuromuscular disease and diaphragm involvement exhibit the greatest oxygen desaturations in REM sleep, so that this stage becomes a test of diaphragm muscle function.

Patients who have neuromuscular disease may have restrictive lung disorder as a consequence of chest wall muscle weakness, scoliosis, and pulmonary microatelectases that result from chronic hypoventilation, repeated episodes of aspiration, and retained secretions. These changes may lead to perfusion of nonventilated lung, a phenomenon that contributes to hypoxemia.

Inspiratory upper airway resistance and obstructive apnea are alterations of the respiratory function that may affect patients who have neuromuscular disorders, causing an additional burden on sleep-related ventilation. These conditions may appear as a result of weakness of pharyngeal muscle dilators causing collapse of the pharyngeal wall along with increased upper airway resistance. The alteration is aggravated further by tonsillar hypertrophy, obesity, or craniofacial dysmorphias and micrognathia that reduce the oropharyngeal lumen. Patients who have congenital myopathies and muscular dystrophies commonly have poor development of facial bones and mandible [2].

Scoliosis is of common observance in patients who have neuromuscular disease. Mechanical alteration of the spine causes a disadvantage of intercostal muscles and diaphragm function that is translated in a less efficient inspiratory mechanism.

Sedentarism in patients who have altered muscular function promotes obesity, another factor that burdens ventilatory efficiency during sleep. Obese patients suffer mechanical reduction of intercostal muscle function, and subjects who have abdominal obesity exhibit marked diaphragm dysfunction that is particularly evident during REM sleep. Accumulation of fat in oropharyngeal soft tissues may contribute to restriction of the oropharyngeal lumen.

Sleep-related ventilatory deficit in patients who have neuromuscular disease may cause nocturnal hypoxemia and many episodes of desaturation that precipitate restlessness, partial arousals, and sleep fragmentation. Depending on the severity of the ventilatory deficit, patients may have continuous alveolar hypoventilation, even in the awake state, which in the most advanced circumstances becomes complicated with carbon dioxide retention. These patients exhibit secondary daytime excessive somnolence, a development that should prompt a thorough investigation of sleep-related ventilatory function, including polysomnography. Development of excessive daytime somnolence in very weak subjects could constitute a marker of preterminal muscular disease and herald major vulnerability in the event of respiratory illness [3]. Sitting positions in sleep, nocturnal cyanosis, morning drowsiness, headaches, vomiting, and even cor pulmonale attributed to nocturnal hypoventilation are reported in patients who have advanced neuromuscular disease whose condition was reversed with appropriate ventilatory therapy [4].

Nocturnal hypoventilation with hypoxemia and hypercapnia, when not corrected, may lead to blunting of peripheral and central respiratory chemoreceptor responses that determine a state of chronic alveolar hypoventilation. In some forms of congenital myopathy, however, there is evidence of impairment of respiratory chemosensitivity that may be familial in nature [5,6]. The combination of ventilatory muscle dysfunction and reduced central ventilatory drive is a particularly dangerous situation.

Neuromuscular conditions with sleep disorder

Sleep and the postpolio syndrome

The acute episode of poliomyelitis may affect brainstem neuronal centers that control respiration, as described in patients coming to autopsy during the epidemics of the 1950s [7]. Some survivors of an acute attack developed, 20 to 30 years later, a condition characterized by progressive fatigue, joint pains, and weakness in muscles not affected before that has been termed, appropriately, the postpolio syndrome. In this condition, central respiratory control and peripheral respiratory function may be affected. Some patients present progressive deterioration of nocturnal sleep, whereas sleep apnea episodes with oxygen desaturation events become increasingly frequent. Sleep disturbances are common, appearing in 31% of patients, even in those who have no prior bulbar involvement [8]. Sleep studies show central sleep apnea episodes in patients weaned from respiratory support as a result of bulbar involvement [9]. Most apneas, however, are of the obstructive or mixed varieties with favorable response to noninvasive positive airway ventilation [10]. Some of the complaints typically attributed to the postpolio syndrome, such as increasing fatigue, may be the result of nocturnal respiratory dysfunction and, thus, potentially correctable. Sleep studies should be performed in all postpolio patients complaining of sleep disturbance and respiratory manifestations [10]. Patients who have kyphoscoliosis secondary to poliomyelitis often develop restrictive respiratory dysfunction, particularly if there is associated weakness of thoracoabdominal and respiratory accessory muscles.

Amyotrophic lateral sclerosis

The pattern of neuromuscular involvement in ALS is determined by progressive degeneration of corticobulbar, corticospinal, and anterior horn cells. The combination of central neurogenic dysfunction and peripheral muscle atrophy in ALS, particularly in patients who have bulbar involvement, sets the stage for sleep-related ventilatory abnormalities; however, severe sleep disruption is not observed in all patients. In a prospective study of 21 patients who had ALS to determine the relationship of pulmonary function test abnormalities with quality of sleep and survival [11], disordered breathing events mostly were obstructive or mixed apneas. Although commonplace, obstructive events were not accountable for nocturnal oxygen desaturation, whereas hypoventilation was found as the primary explanation for the decline in oxygen saturation. Bulbar involvement or phrenic nerve dysfunction were not prime factors determining severity of sleep-related respiratory disorder. Fasciculations were not reported to interfere with sleep and affective depression was not evident. The group as a whole was not excessively somnolent, as shown by the results of the multiple latency test, and the overall quality of sleep was surprisingly normal.

In patients who have ALS and diaphragm dysfunction, REM sleep is reduced and median survival time is shorter [12]. Investigators found remarkable phasic inspiratory sternomastoid activation during REM sleep in some patients who had diaphragm dysfunction. There is a case report [13] of a patient presenting with exertional dyspnea and hypersomnia followed several months later by respiratory failure that necessitated intubation. Neurologic examination, electromyographic testing, and histologic examination of the central nervous system confirmed a diagnosis of ALS with specific involvement of anterior horn cells from C3 to C7, corresponding to the phrenic nuclei, where recognizable nerve cells could not be found.

Noninvasive respiratory support with positive airway pressure machines may be indicated in patients who have motor neuron disease developing sleep-related respiratory disturbance as a result of diaphragm paralysis or bulbar involvement. In some patients who have ALS, nocturnal sleep-related ventilatory alterations may occur in disproportion to the severity of the neuromuscular disorder. Daytime tiredness and incapacitating fatigue may be the result of a potentially correctable sleep-related abnormality and not the result of relentless progression of the neuromuscular condition. Weakness of the diaphragm is critical particularly in REM sleep, a time when the only functional respiratory muscle is the diaphragm. Patients develop severe REM sleep deprivation along with orthopnea, daytime

sleepiness, nocturnal restlessness, unrefreshing sleep, nocturnal oxygen desaturations, and hypercapnia that affect the quality of life and may decrease
survival. Application of noninvasive positive airway pressure ventilation is
a simple, ambulatory therapeutic maneuver that may correct sleep-related
ventilatory alterations in patients who have ALS. Lechtzin and coworkers
[14] showed that nocturnal application of noninvasive positive airway pressure ventilation to patients who have ALS and a predicted baseline forced
vital capacity of less than 50% without tracheostomy increases survival
and decreases the risk of death by 34%. Noninvasive positive airway pressure ventilation also improves the quality of life in patients who have
ALS. Using various instruments to measure quality of life, Bourke and coworkers [15] showed that noninvasive positive airway pressure ventilation is
associated with improved quality of life. Quality-of-life benefit and survival
were related strongly to noninvasive positive airway pressure ventilation
compliance. In Bourke and coworker' study, patients who had orthpnea
showed the most compliance and benefit, whereas those who had bulbar
weakness had the least benefit.

Polysomnographic evaluation in the sleep laboratory is recommended for
patients who have ALS and who develop signs and symptoms of sleep-wake
abnormality or nocturnal respiratory failure [16]. In the author's laboratory,
criteria for noninvasive positive airway pressure ventilation are an apnea/
hypopnea index of more than 10 per hour, desaturations of oxygen below
89%, and an arousal index of more than 10 per hour.

Myasthenia gravis

Myasthenia gravis is an autoimmune disease in which autoantibodies
against muscle acetylcholine receptor attack the receptor at the neuromuscular junction. As a result, patients develop excessive muscular fatigability
that may involve the diaphragm and accessory respiratory muscles with resulting respiratory failure in unmedicated, uncontrolled patients. Sleep-
related complaints in some patients who have myasthenia gravis include
waking up with sensation of breathlessness, morning headaches, and daytime somnolence. Respiratory function may be altered during sleep, with
carbon dioxide retention and respiratory failure serious enough to require
ventilatory assistance [17]. Risk factors for development of sleep apnea in
patients who have myasthenia gravis are age, restrictive pulmonary syndrome, diaphragm weakness, and daytime alveolar hypoventilation [18].
Apneas and hypopneas mainly are nonobstructive [18]. The breathing alteration is evident particularly during REM stage when the diaphragm is the
only muscle that remains active in the exchange of air. Respiratory muscles
may be affected focally in patients who have myasthenia gravis [19]. Sleep
apneas are not related to a central cholinergic effect caused by
anticholinesterase used to treat myasthenia gravis or by antibodies to muscle acethylcholine receptores, because receptors in brain are antigenically

distinct from acethylcholine receptors in skeletal muscle [18]. Daytime somnolence in patients who have myasthenia gravis should suggest abnormal
breathing during sleep, even in the absence of abnormal daytime muscle
dysfunction. Adequate respiratory muscle strength during sleep is an often-
overlooked peripheral influence on mental functioning and general well being of patients who have myasthenia gravis [20]. Nocturnal manifestations
usually respond to the administration of slow release pyridostigmine at bedtime, although patients receiving appropriate treatment and who have satisfactory daytime functional capacity may have abnormal breathing during
sleep requiring noninvasive assisted ventilation [21]. There is one report of
improvement of sleep apnea disorder after thymectomy in a small series
of patients who had myasthenia gravis [22].

In the myasthenic syndrome, dysfunction of respiratory muscles may
cause sleep hypoventilation and sleep apnea to the point of requiring assisted ventilation.

Myotonic dystrophy

Myotonic dystrophy is an autosomal dominant, multisystem disease affecting skeletal and cardiac muscle, central nervous system structures, and
endocrine function. Cataracts, frontal balding, skin atrophy, skeletal
changes, and hypogonadism are common abnormalities. Excessive daytime
sleepiness and respiratory failure during wakefulness and in sleep are observed commonly in these patients.

Excessive somnolence in patients who have myotonic dystrophy is characterized by daytime sleepiness [23], with occasional features suggestive of
narcolepsy, including sleep-onset REM periods [24,25]. Broughton and colleagues [26] found, in their group of patients who had myotonic dystrophy,
disrupted sleep structure characterized by sleep fragmentation, short REM
sleep latencies and reduced REM sleep amounts. In a sleep questionnaire
with assessment of wakefulness of 157 patients who had myotonic dystrophy type I (DMI), Laberge and coworkers [27] found excessive daytime
somnolence in 33.1% of patients, with severity of daytime sleepiness corre-
lating with the degree of muscular impairment. Patients reported a longer
sleep period, less restorative sleep, and more difficulty falling asleep. Patients
who had DM1 exhibited characteristics reminiscent of those found in patients who have idiopathic hypersomnia. In Meché and colleagues' series
[28] patients exhibited some episodes of central sleep apnea with minor fluctuations in oxygen saturation that, in the investigators' estimation, were insufficient to cause daytime somnolence. Hypersomnia may be aggravated by
alveolar hypoventilation [29] and the sleep apnea syndrome but is not reversed entirely by continuous positive airway pressure applications [25], suggesting that hypersomnia is an intrinsic disorder related to central nervous
system disease. In a study of six patients who had DM1 and excessive daytime sleepiness, Martínez-Rodríguez and colleagues [30] found that multiple

sleep latency tests were abnormal in all patients (<8 minutes sleep latency) and two patients had REM sleep periods. Hypocretin-1 levels in cerebrospinal fluid were significantly lower in patients who had myotonic dystrophy, suggesting dysfunction of the hypothalamic hypocretin system. Hypersomnia in myotonic dystrophy may respond successfully to the administration of methylphenidate [31] and modafinil [32].

In patients who have myotonic dystrophy, clinical manifestations of nervous system degeneration occur in parallel with progressive skeletal muscle changes. Hypersomnia, apathy, mental decline, and "slow alpha rhythms" in subjects who have moderately advanced disease are linked to morphologic changes and dysfunction of the dorsomedial nuclei of the thalamus [33]. In myotonic dystrophy, 10% to 30% of nerve cells of the dorsomedial nuclei contain eosinophilic cytoplasmic inclusion bodies that manifest neuronal damage. Eosinophilic bodies [34] are round, oval, or elongated with smooth, sharply defined contours and an occasional peripheral halo ranging in size from 4 to 8 microns in diameter. Staining histologic methods indicate that the bodies are acidophilic, composed of protein but not amyloid. Ultrastructural studies show a fibrillar material within ribosome-bearing membranes, suggestive of a proteic nature. Inclusion bodies probably develop as the contents of expanding cisternae coalesce and become enclosed by condensing membranes. It is proposed that they represent the morphologic expression of a block in the excretion or transport of a protein formed by the thalamic nerve cells and a sign of neuronal degeneration. Structures adjacent to the thalamus also may be affected by neuronal degenerative changes; however, further histologic studies are required to verify hypothalamic involvement.

Cognitive, sleep, EEG, and morphologic brain changes worsen as the disease advances. It is likely that progressive enlargement of the third ventricle observed in some patients who have this disorder [35] results from progressive degeneration of the medial thalamus. Mental decline, psychosocial deterioration, apathy, inattention, and memory defect suggest a medial thalamic syndrome [36], whereas EEG changes characterized by "slow alpha rhythms" also suggest a diencephalic disorder [37]. Neuropsychologic testing in patients who have myotonic dystrophy shows that the neuropsychologic deficit cannot be attributed to the effect of sleep apnea or sleep disruption [38].

The breathing sleep-related disorder in myotonic dystrophy may be another manifestation of central alteration. Nonobstructive sleep apneas and sleep-related alveolar hypoventilation are common [29] and may contribute to increased somnolence. Sleep-related breathing abnormalities probably are the result of central neuronal lesions and declining muscular function. In myotonic dystrophy, weakness of inspiratory effort during REM sleep and increased upper airway resistance during NREM sleep are the main mechanisms for the development of sleep-related respiratory disturbance. In one study, obesity correlated with levels of sleep hypoxemia, and body mass index was associated significantly with the nadir of oxygen saturation, time spent at saturations below 85%, and number of 4% drops in oxygen saturation [39]. In another study comparing patients who had myotonic dystrophy with those who had nonmyotonic respiratory muscle weakness [40], myotonic patients showed more frequent apnea and hypopnea events and more severe desaturation than the nonmyotonic group who had muscle weakness. The study reveals that abnormal breathing during sleep is common in myotonic dystrophy and suggests that sleep-related respiratory disturbance is not solely the result of the direct effects of muscle weakness. Furthermore, somnolence was not attributable clearly to the sleep apnea/hypopnea syndrome or the abnormal structure of nocturnal sleep.

Early muscular weakness in patients who have myotonic dystrophy affects craniofacial and mandibular growth, contributing to the development of obstructive sleep apnea by increasing airway resistance in a stenotic oropharynx.

Sleep-related neuroendocrine studies in myotonic dystrophy

The largest bursts of growth hormone (GH) secretion occur in normal individuals at night in association with slow wave sleep (SWS; stages 3 and 4) [41]. If sleep onset is delayed, the nocturnal rise of GH also is delayed. Not all episodes of SWS are accompanied by GH secretion, and dissociations may occur, suggesting that both events are related temporally but are not strictly interdependent. The evidence indicates that SWS-related GH secretion is regulated by neural pathways that are different from those intervening in the wake state release. The investigation of nocturnal sleep patterns and associated GH plasma concentrations in five patients who had myotonic dystrophy revealed no GH elevations related to SWS in the three individuals most affected [42]. It is proposed that a subcortical center is responsible for integrating SWS, a cortical event, with the hypothalamic-pituitary function of GH release [43]. Patients who have myotonic dystrophy and thalamic damage presumably have failure of integration of SWS with the hypothalamic-pituitary function of GH secretion. The early loss of GH as a consequence of thalamic damage may be responsible for manifestations of premature aging that include reduced muscle mass, increased abdominal adiposity, skin atrophy, and reduced bone density. In patients who have fatal familial insomnia with progressive degeneration of the dorsomedial nuclei of the thalamus and loss of sleep-related GH secretion, a dramatic acceleration of the aging process is reported. Rancurel and colleagues' 62-year-old patient "looked 20 years older than her age" [44] when she died 18 months after developing fatal familial insomnia.

Congenital and metabolic myopathies

Severe nocturnal respiratory failure is described in two siblings who had nemaline myopathy [45]. This is a congenital myopathy with a benign prognosis that affects all skeletal muscles, including the diaphragm. Both patients developed marked sleep inertia in the morning with headaches, vomiting, and daytime lethargy. Subsequent medical evaluation disclosed marked hypoxia, hypercapnia, and cor pulmonale. Breathing at night was irregular with progressive hypercapnia as soon as they fell asleep. Nocturnal respiratory failure was not the result of muscular weakness or obstructive sleep apnea but attributed to a disturbance of central respiratory control with poor sensitivity to carbon dioxide inhalation, also detected in relatives. Nocturnal mechanical ventilation reversed respiratory failure in both siblings and permitted a return to daytime activities, including school attendance.

In patients who have Duchenne's muscular dystrophy, restrictive lung disease develops as muscle weakness progresses and rib cage deformities take hold. Patients who have moderately advanced disorder develop nocturnal hypoventilation with profound desaturation during REM sleep despite normal awake minute ventilation [46]. Patients who have advanced muscular weakness and skeletal deformities [47] also may show abundant fragmentation of nocturnal sleep, many sleep stage changes, and reduced REM sleep without evidence of nocturnal hypoxia. Daytime predictors of sleep hypoventilation in patients who have Duchenne's muscular dystrophy are a forced expiratory volume of less than 40% and a base excess of greater than 4 mmol per liter [48]. The investigators recommend that polysomnography be considered when the $Paco_2$ is greater than 45 mm Hg, particularly if the base excess is high.

Various combinations of nocturnal respiratory dysfunction are described in isolated cases or short series of patients who have neuromuscular disorders, including congenital fiber-type disproportion syndrome [49], mitochondrial myopathy [50], and acid maltase deficiency [51].

As expected, obstructive sleep apnea syndrome with snoring and excessive daytime somnolence was found in a 75-year-old patient who had oculopharyngeal muscular dystrophy [52].

The impact of long-term noninvasive ventilation was investigated in 30 children and adolescents who had neuromuscular disorders [53]. The investigators found a favorable overall long-term effect. Noninvasive ventilation improved respiratory disturbance index, nocturnal heart rate, sleep architecture, and reduced nocturnal arousals. Gas exchanges also improved. The investigators conclude that noninvasive ventilation is indicated in children and adolescents who have symptomatic sleep-disordered breathing or ventilatory insufficiency resulting from neuromuscular disorders.

Neuropathy and phrenic nerve paralysis

Phrenic nerve damage causing diaphragm paralysis may be part of the spectrum of involvement in some polyneuropathies and motor neuron disease. Unilateral paralysis is asymptomatic but bilateral paralysis invariably is symptomatic and may be life threatening; paresis or weakness with partial diaphragm dysfunction may cause manifestations of ventilatory insufficiency that, despite their typical characteristics, may remain undiagnosed. Bilateral paralysis causes inspiratory orthopnea that is striking because of its severity out of proportion to the cardiopulmonary status. In the supine posture, patients complain of profound difficulty when breathing that is the result of a reduction in lung volume and increased inspiratory effort as the abdominal contents rise into the thorax. In severe or acute cases, patients present with nocturnal orthopnea, cyanosis, and fragmented sleep followed by morning headaches, vomiting, and daytime lethargy.

Polysomnography reveals hypoventilation that is particularly profound during REM sleep. As the desaturation event frequency increases in REM sleep, arousals and secondary daytime somnolence increasingly become prominent so that the condition resembles the sleep apnea syndrome. The severity of hypoventilation and the depth of oxygen desaturation in NREM sleep is determined by the degree of involvement of chest wall and accessory respiratory muscles. Undiagnosed bilateral diaphragm paralysis of any cause may lead to acute cardiopulmonary failure and death. Some reports describe unexplained failure to wean from respirator as the presenting manifestation of diaphragm paralysis in patients who have undiagnosed motor neuron disease [54] or myopathies. A recent polysomnographic study of patients who had bilateral diaphragm paralysis showed normal proportion of REM sleep achieved by inspiratory recruitment of extradiaphragmatic muscles in tonic and phasic REM sleep, suggesting brainstem reorganization of stimuli [55].

Phrenic nerve paralysis is reported in patients who have Charcot-Marie-Tooth disease (hereditary motor and sensory neuropathy) complicated by diabetes mellitus [56]. Other conditions in which diaphragm paralysis is observed include spinal cord injury, poliomyelitis, Guillain-Barré syndrome, diabetes, diphtheric neuropathy, beriberi, alcoholic neuropathy, brachial plexus neuropathy, lead neuropathy, trauma, ALS, myotonic dystrophy, Duchenne's muscular dystrophy, paraneoplastic syndrome, and idiopathic conditions [54,56].

The diagnosis of diaphragm paralysis is suspected when paradoxic respirations are observed in the supine posture and major discrepancies in vital capacity between the erect and supine postures are detected. Phrenic nerve stimulation studies, nerve conduction measurements, and EMG of selected muscles may aid in the diagnosis along with fluoroscopy and computerized imaging studies of the chest. Nocturnal polysomnography is of critical importance for evaluating the presence and degree of sleep-related respiratory dysfunction in patients who have suspected paralysis of the diaphragm.

Treatment of phrenic nerve paralysis with diaphragm insufficiency includes noninvasive positive airway ventilation, implantation of phrenic pacemakers [57], and plication of the diaphragm [58].

General approach and suggested management

Patients who have neuromuscular disorders are at high risk for the development of sleep-related respiratory disorders and respiratory failure. A variety of concurring abnormalities converge in patients who have neuromuscular disorder that explain their vulnerable status. Diaphragm weakness and failure is the most important determinant of sleep-related respiratory insufficiency. Chest wall weakness and restrictive lung diseases, such as those caused by chest-wall deformities and kyphoscoliosis, contribute to hypoventilation in REM and NREM sleep. Weakness of the pharyngeal wall compounded with obesity of sedentary origin and craniofacial maldevelopment may facilitate the appearance of obstructive sleep apneas. Some patients who have neuromuscular disorder exhibit nocturnal hypoventilation in excess of muscular weakness or of diaphragm failure, suggesting an alteration of central respiratory drive.

Patients who have neuromuscular disorder and develop a sleep-related respiratory alteration present a variety of symptoms and signs that should alert clinicians. Nocturnal restlessness, frequent unexplained awakenings, and loud snoring may be punctuated by occasional awakenings and gasping for breath. Patients and relatives report difficulty waking up in the morning and prolonged sleep inertia that may interfere with morning activities. During the day, these patients may present somnolence, fatigue, and inappropriate napping that underlie failure to thrive in the very young and declining school grades or poor work performance at later ages. More ominously, some patients develop nocturnal cyanosis, severe insomnia, morning lethargy, headaches, vomiting, and leg edema that indicate the insidious but relentless occurrence of acute respiratory failure and cor pulmonale.

Polysomnographic evaluation is necessary to distinguish among the different causes of sleep disturbance and to assess the severity of the disorder. A sleep apnea protocol is recommended. The study may show obstructive, central, and mixed sleep apneas, hypoventilation with oxygen saturations under 89%, or profound REM sleep-related desaturation of oxygen events that indicate diaphragm failure. The sleep architecture may reveal fragmentation of sleep with many arousals and awakenings, many of them associated with episodes of respiratory interruption.

Sometimes nocturnal disruption occurs as an independent abnormality translating nocturnal postural discomfort in a weak, incapacitated, sometimes deformed patient. If daytime excessive somnolence is prominent, a multiple sleep latency test should follow the nocturnal study. The daytime test may show excessive daytime somnolence proportionate to the nocturnal alteration or, as in the case of myotonic dystrophy, may show excessive daytime somnolence that is not explained by the nocturnal findings. This suggests an intrinsic form of hypersomnia, which, in some cases, is associated with REM sleep abnormalities.

Therapeutic goals should define whether or not therapy is directed at elimination of excessive daytime somnolence, improvement of nocturnal desaturation, reconstruction of sleep architecture with elimination of arousals, or correction of respiratory and heart failure. Noninvasive positive airway ventilation has revolutionized the treatment of most nocturnal respiratory abnormalities found in patients who have neuromuscular disorder. Positive pressure breathing corrects obstructive sleep apnea, improves hypoventilation, and assists diaphragm failure. Supplemental oxygen via a mask is recommended when positive air pressure therapy is insufficient to overcome mean levels of hypoventilation of 89% or less. Bilevel positive airway ventilation is tolerated better by patients who have weak chest walls and diaphragm and who cannot overcome expiratory forces. Supplemental oxygen via nasal cannula may be sufficient in some cases to correct REM sleep-related desaturations.

Patients who have advanced restrictive lung disease, severe chest-wall muscle weakness, loss of sleep-related respiratory drive, and diaphragm paralysis pose special problems that may need to be resolved individually using a combination of therapeutic maneuvers. Tracheostomy may be indicated in a few cases, but the dependence that it causes and the complications that it conjures have to be weighed against the benefits. Ethical considerations of prolongation of undignified life versus improvement of quality of life may have to be addressed in patients who have terminal neuromuscular disease. Children under age 6 tolerate nasal ventilation poorly [59], so other therapeutic measures may have to be considered [57,58], including temporal use of tracheostomy.

Protriptyline at bedtime improves muscle tone and is of some value in patients who have obstructive sleep apnea with weak pharyngeal walls. There is some evidence that methylphenidate and modafinil control excessive daytime somnolence in patients who have myotonic dystrophy and do not respond to the application of noninvasive positive airway ventilation.

References

[1] Guilleminault C, Stoohs R, Quera-Salva MA. Sleep-related obstructive and nonobstructive apneas and neurologic disorders. Neurology 1992;42(Suppl 6):53.

[2] Vargervik K. Experiments on the interaction between orofacial function and morphology. Ear Nose Throat J 1987;66:201.

[3] Smith PEM, Edwards RHT, Calverley PMA. Mechanisms of sleep-disordered breathing in chronic neuromuscular disease: implications for management. Q J Med 1991;296:961.

[4] Heckmatt JZ, Loh L, Dubowitz V. Nocturnal hypoventilation in children with nonprogressive neuromuscular disease. Pediatrics 1989;83:250.

[5] Carroll JE, Zwillich C, Weil JV, et al. Depressed ventilatory response to oculocraniosomatic neuromuscular disease. Neurology 1976;26:140.

[6] Wilson DO, Sanders MH, Dauber JH. Abnormal ventilatory chemosensitivity and congenital myopathy. Arch Intern Med 1987;147:1773.

[7] Plum F, Swanson AG. Abnormalities in central regulation of respiration in acute and convalescent poliomyelitis. J Arch Neurol Psychiatry 1958;80:267.

[8] Cosgrove JL, Alexander MA, Kitts EL, et al. Late effects of poliomyelitis. Arch Phys Med Rehabil 1987;68:4.

[9] Guilleminault C, Motta J. Sleep apnea syndrome as long term sequela of poliomyelitis. In: Guilleminault C, Dement WC, editors. Sleep apnea syndromes. New York: Alan R. Liss; 1978. p. 309–15.

[10] Steljes DG, Kryger MH, Kirk BW, et al. Sleep in post-polio syndrome. Chest 1990;98:133.

[11] Gay PC, Westbrook PR, Daube JR, et al. Effects of alterations in pulmonary function and sleep variables on survival in patients with amyotrophic lateral sclerosis. Mayo Clin Proc 1991;66:686.

[12] Arnulf I, Similowski T, Salachas F, et al. Sleep disorder and diaphragmatic function in patients with amyotrophic lateral sclerosis. Am J Respir Crit Care Med 2000;161:849–56.

[13] Meyrignac C, Poirier J, Degos JD. Amyotrophic lateral sclerosis with respiratory insufficiency as the primary complaint. Eur Neurol 1985;24:115.

[14] Lechtzin N, Gowda N, Anderson F, et al. Non-invasive positive airway pressure ventilation prolongs survival in patients with amyotrophic lateral sclerosis. Presented at the 57th Annual Meeting of the American Academy of Neurology. Miami Beach, April 2005.

[15] Bourke SC, Bullock RE, Williams TL, et al. Non-invasive ventilation in ALS: indications and effect on quality of life. Neurology 2003;61:171–7.

[16] Barthlen GM, Lange DJ. Unexpectedly severe sleep and respiratory pathology in patients with amyotrophic lateral sclerosis. Eur J Neurol 2000;7:299–302.

[17] Quera-Salva MA, Guilleminault C, Chevret S, et al. Breathing disorders during sleep in myasthenia gravis. Ann Neurol 1992;31:86.

[18] Gajdos P, Quera-Salva MA. Respiratory disorders during sleep and myasthenia. Rev Neurol 2001;157:S145–7.

[19] Mier-Jedrejowicz A, Brophy C, Green M. Respiratory muscle function in myasthenia gravis. Am Rev Respir Dis 1988;138:867.

[20] Keesey JC. Does myasthenia gravis affect the brain? J Neurol Sci 1999;30:77–89.

[21] Barthlen GM. Nocturnal respiratory failure as an indication of noninvasive ventilation in the patient with neuromuscular disease. Respiration (Herrlisheim) 1997;64(Suppl 1): 35–8.

[22] Amino A, Shiozawa Z, Nagasaka T, et al. Sleep apnea in well-controlled myasthenia gravis and the effect of thymectomy. J Neurol 1998;245:77–80.

[23] Phemister JC, Small JM. Hypersomnia in dystrophia myotonica. J Neurol Neurosurg Psychiatry 1961;24:173.

[24] Coccagna G, Marinelli P, Lugaresi E. Sleep and alveolar hypoventilation in myotonic dystrophy. Acta Neurol Belg 1982;82:185.

[25] Park YD, Radtke RA. Hypersomnolence in myotonic dystrophy. Neurology 1992; 42(Suppl 3):352.

[26] Broughton R, Stuss D, Kates M, et al. Neuropsychological deficits and sleep in myotonic dystrophy. Can J Neurol Sci 1990;17:410.

[27] Laberge L, Begin P, Montplaisir J, et al. Sleep complaints in patients with myotonic dystrophy. J Sleep Res 2004;13:95–100.

[28] Meché FGA, Bogaard JM, Sluys JCM, et al. Daytime sleep in myotonic dystrophy is not caused by sleep apnea. J Neurol Neurosurg Psychiatry 1994;57:626.

[29] Hansotia P, Frens D. Hypersomnia associated with alveolar hypoventilation in myotonic dystrophy. Neurology 1981;31:1336.

[30] Martínez-Rodríguez JE, Lin L, Iranzo A, et al. Decreased hypocretin-I (Orexin -A) levels in the cerebrospinal fluid of patients with myotonic dystrophy and excessive daytime sleepiness. Sleep 2003;26:287–90.

[31] Meché FGA, Boogard JM, Berg B. Treatment of hypersomnolence in myotonic dystrophy with a CNS stimulant. Muscle Nerve 1986;9:341.

[32] Mac Donald JR, Hill JD, Tarnopolsky MA. Modafinil reduces excessive somnolence and enhances mood in patients with myotonic dystrophy. Neurology 2002;59:1876–80.

[33] Culebras A, Feldman RG, Merk FB. Cytoplasmic inclusion bodies within neurons of the thalamus in myotonic dystrophy: a light and electron microscopy study. J Neurol Sci 1973;19:319.

[34] Culebras A, Segarra JM, Feldman RG. Eosinophilic bodies within neurons in the human thalamus: An age-related histological feature. J Neurol Sci 1972;16:177.

[35] Glantz RH, Wright RB, Huckman MS, et al. Central nervous system magnetic resonance imaging findings in myotonic dystrophy. Arch Neurol 1988;45:36.

[36] Martin JJ. Thalamic syndromes. In: Vinken RJ, Bruyn GW, editors. Handbook of clinical neurology, vol. 2. Amsterdam: North Holland Publishing; 1969. p. 469.

[37] Friedlander WJ, Bittenbender JB. EEG findings in myotonia dystrophica. Electroencephalogr Clin Neurophysiol 1964;17:564.

[38] Broughton R, Stuss D, Kates M, et al. Neuropsychological deficits and sleep in myotonic dystrophy. Can J Neurol Sci 1990;17:410.

[39] Finnimore AJ, Jackson RV, Morton A, et al. Sleep hypoxia in myotonic dystrophy and its correlation with awake respiratory function. Thorax 1994;49:66.

[40] Gilmartin JJ, Cooper BG, Griffiths CJ, et al. Breathing during sleep in patients with myotonic dystrophy and non-myotonic respiratory muscle weakness. Q J Med 1991;78:21.

[41] Takahashi Y, Kipnis DM, Daughaday WH. Growth secretion during sleep. J Clin Invest 1969;47:2079.

[42] Culebras A, Podolsky S, Leopold NA. Absence of sleep-related growth hormone elevations in myotonic dystrophy. Neurology 1977;27:165.

[43] Sassin JF, Parker DC, Mace JW, et al. Human growth hormone release: relation to slow-wave sleep and sleep-waking cycles. Science 1969;165:513.

[44] Rancurel G, Garma L, Hauw JJ, et al. Familial thalamic degeneration with fatal insomnia: clinico-pathological and polygraphic data in a French member of Lugaresi's Italian family. In: Guilleminault C, Lugaresi E, Montagna P, et al, editors. Fatal familial insomnia: inherited prion diseases, sleep and the thalamus. New York: Raven Press; 1994. p. 15–26.

[45] Maayan Ch, Springer C, Armon Y, et al. Nemaline myopathy as a cause of sleep hypoventilation. Pediatrics 1986;77:390.

[46] Smith PEM, Edwards RHT, Calverly PMA. Ventilation and breathing pattern during sleep in Duchenne muscular dystrophy. Chest 1989;96:1346.

[47] Redding GJ, Okamoto GA, Guthrie RD, et al. Sleep patterns in non-ambulatory boys with Duchenne muscular dystrophy. Arch Phys Med Rehabil 1985;66:818.

[48] Hukins CA, Hillman DR. Daytime predictors of sleep hypoventilation in Duchenne muscular dystrophy. Am J Respir Crit Care Med 2000;161:166–70.

[49] Wilson DO, Sanders MH, Dauber JH. Abnormal ventilatory chemosensitivity and congenital myopathy. Arch Intern Med 1987;147:1773.

[50] Kotagal S, Archer CR, Walsh JK, et al. Hypersomnia, bithalamic lesions, and altered sleep architecture in Kearns-Sayre syndrome. Neurology 1985;35:574.

[51] Martin RJ, Sufit RL, Ringel SP, et al. Respiratory improvement by muscle training in adult-onset acid maltase deficiency. Muscle Nerve 1983;6:201.

[52] Dedrick DL, Brown LK. Obstructive sleep apnea syndrome complicationg oculopharyngeal muscular dystrophy. Chest 2004;125:334–6.

[53] Mellies U, Ragette R, Dolma Schwake C, et al. Long-term noninvasive ventilation in children and adolescents with neuromuscular disorders. Eur Respir J 2003;22:631–6.

[54] Parhad IM, Clark AW, Barron KD, et al. Diaphragmatic paralysis in motor neuron disease. Neurology 1978;28:18.

[55] Bennett JR, Dunroy HM, Corfield DR, et al. Respiratory muscle activity during REM sleep in patients with diaphragm paralysis. Neurology 2004;62:134–7.

[56] Chan CK, Mohsenin V, Loke J, et al. Diaphragmatic dysfunction in siblings with hereditary motor and sensory neuropathy (Charcot-Marie-Tooth disease). Chest 1987; 91:567.

[57] Garrido-García H, Mazaira Alvarez J, Martín Escribano P, et al. Treatment of chronic ventilatory failure using a diaphragmatic pacemaker. Spinal Cord 1998;36:310–4.

[58] Stolk J, Versteegh MI. Long term effect of bilateral plication of the diaphragm. Chest 2000;117:786–9.

[59] Heckmatt JZ, Loh L, Dubowitz V. Night-time nasal ventilation in neuromuscular disease. Lancet 1990;335:579.

ELSEVIER
SAUNDERS

Neurol Clin 23 (2005) 1225–1253

NEUROLOGIC
CLINICS

Cumulative Index 2005

Note: Page numbers of article titles are in **boldface** type.

A

ABC. See *Activities-Specific Balance Confidence (ABC).*

Absence epilepsy, during sleep, 1134

Abuse
  alcohol
    neuropathy due to, 377–379
    parkinsonism due to, 438
  drug, neuropathy due to, 377–379

Acceleration, in aviation environment, 543–544

Acetylcholine, effects on sleep, 972–975

Acid secretion, during sleep, 1012–1013

Acoustic neuroma, surgical treatment of, 887–889

Acrylamide, neuropathy due to, 384

Activities-Specific Balance Confidence (ABC), 793–794

Acute disseminated encephalomyelitis, 92–93
  MS and, 93–96

Acute hemorrhagic leukoencephalitis, 93

Acute lymphoblastic leukemia (ALL), therapeutic irradiation for, impact of, 581–582

Acute nonrecurring spontaneous vertigo, in children, 810

Acute quadriplegic myopathy, 414–416

Acute radiation syndrome, 573

Addict(s), frozen, 345–348

Adhesion molecules
  in circulation, OSA and, 1067–1068
  in MS, selective expression of, 158

Agent Orange, neuropathy due to, 385–386

Aging
  change-in-support reactions due to, 759–762
    mechanisms of, 763–764
  CNS effects of, 791–792
  effects on vestibular system, 791

Agrypnia excitata, 1119

Alcohol abuse
  neuropathy due to, 377–379
  parkinsonism due to, 438

Alcoholic myopathy, 419–420

ALL. See *Acute lymphoblastic leukemia (ALL).*

ALS. See *Amyotrophic lateral sclerosis (ALS).*

Alternative agents, for insomnia, 1159

Aluminum
  ALS due to, 465
  Alzheimer's disease due to, 490–492
  myoclonus due to, 442–443
  Parkinson's disease and, 503
  toxicity of, 359

Alzheimer's disease
  aluminum and, 490–492
  copper and, 492–494
  environmental exposure effects on, 488–497
  heavy metals and, 490
  iron and, 492–494
  magnetic fields and, 494–496
  manganese and, 492–494
  pesticides and, 494
  smoking and, 496–497
  solvents and, 488–490
  zinc and, 492–494

Amiodarone, amphiphilic drug myopathy due to, 405–406

Amphetamine(s), neuropathy due to, 379–380

Changing Your Address?

Make sure your subscription changes too! When you notify us of your new address, you can help make our job easier by including an exact copy of your Clinics label number with your old address (see illustration below.) This number identifies you to our computer system and will speed the processing of your address change. Please be sure this label number accompanies your old address and your corrected address—you can send an old Clinics label with your number on it or just copy it exactly and send it to the address listed below.

We appreciate your help in our attempt to give you continuous coverage. Thank you.

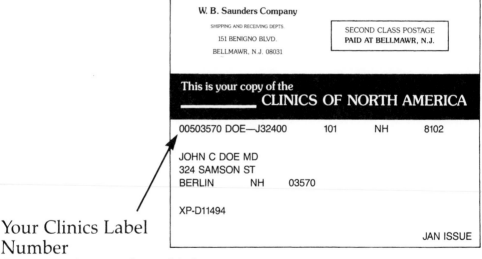

Your Clinics Label Number
Copy it exactly or send your label along with your address to:
W.B. Saunders Company, Customer Service
Orlando, FL 32887-4800
Call Toll Free 1-800-654-2452

Please allow four to six weeks for delivery of new subscriptions and for processing address changes.